AF842723

The Psychotherapy of Personality Disorders

Psychodynamic Psychotherapy and Assessment in the Twenty-First Century

Series Editors: Steven Tuber, City University of New York at City College

Mission Statement

Psychodynamic Psychotherapy and Assessment establishes a milieu for the presentation of scholarly clinical work through a developmental lens. The emphasis throughout the series is on the integration of scholarship and practice through writings that are informed by both sources of learning. This domain includes works that document both evidence-based and traditional approaches within the field and applies these approaches to work with infants, children, adolescents, and adults. Efforts that link assessment to treatment are especially welcome, as are integrations between neuropsychological (brain-based) and psychological (mind or self-based) formulations about personality development and its aberrations. The impact of trauma, both chronic and acute, on the psychological lives of its victims is also an important area of study within this domain. New voices within the field are encouraged to write about the interface between the content and process of their emergent thinking and practice. In addition to the areas mentioned above, more experienced clinical scholars are encouraged to write about the supervisory process and its impact on both theory and practice. Works that focus on specific developmental processes and paradigms at points throughout the lifespan are another welcome area for contributions.

Titles in the Series

The Psychotherapy of Personality Disorders: Emergent Systems Theory as an Integrative Framework, by Lisa J. Cohen

Obsessive-Compulsive Disorder and Uncertainty: Struggling with a Shadow of a Doubt, by Moshe Marcus and Steven Tuber

Psychodynamics Commencing in Early Childhood: The Case for an Additional Tripartite Complex, by Joseph Newirth

From Sign to Symbol: Transformational Processes in Psychoanalysis, Psychotherapy, and Psychology, by Marvin P. Osman

The Psychotherapy of Personality Disorders

Emergent Systems Theory as an Integrative Framework

Lisa J. Cohen

LEXINGTON BOOKS
Lanham • Boulder • New York • London

Published by Lexington Books
An imprint of The Rowman & Littlefield Publishing Group, Inc.
4501 Forbes Boulevard, Suite 200, Lanham, Maryland 20706
www.rowman.com

86-90 Paul Street, London EC2A 4NE

Copyright © 2022 by The Rowman & Littlefield Publishing Group, Inc.

All rights reserved. No part of this book may be reproduced in any form or by any electronic or mechanical means, including information storage and retrieval systems, without written permission from the publisher, except by a reviewer who may quote passages in a review.

British Library Cataloguing in Publication Information Available

Library of Congress Cataloging-in-Publication Data

Names: Cohen, Lisa J., author.
Title: The psychotherapy of personality disorders : emergent systems theory as an integrative framework / Lisa J. Cohen.
Description: Lanham : Lexington Books, [2022] | Series: Psychodynamic psychotherapy and assessment in the twenty-first century | Includes bibliographical references and index. | Summary: "Lisa J. Cohen introduces an integrative model of divergent treatments for personality pathology. Implications for assessment, diagnosis and treatment are discussed and illustrated with case examples"—Provided by publisher.
Identifiers: LCCN 2022004535 | ISBN 9781793610102 (cloth) | ISBN 9781793610119 (ebook)
Subjects: LCSH: Personality disorders—Treatment. | Psychotherapy. | System theory
Classification: LCC RC554 .C64 2022 | DDC 616.85/8—dc23/eng/20220323
LC record available at https://lccn.loc.gov/2022004535

Contents

Figures

Tables

Acknowledgments

I would like to thank the many people who reviewed parts of the manuscript and gave me valuable feedback, without which I daresay, this manuscript would be virtually unreadable. Thank you to Morrel Cohen for correcting my mathematics in Chapter 1; to Julie Evans for her enthusiasm; to Sarah Bloch Elkouby for the information on psychotherapy integration research; to Igor Galynker, Megan Rogers, Jenelle Richards, Lauren Loveras and the Tuesday research meeting for their invaluable feedback on what did and did not make sense; to Liza Rimsky for her feedback, editing, and very helpful PDF's; to Temma Ehrenfeld for the reporter's viewpoint; to Kate Levin for the lay point of view, to Colin Pugh for the information on psychedelics; to Naomi Zack for her sage advice and to Kasey Beduhn, a patient and supportive editor. Thanks also to Steve Tuber for giving me this opportunity. I must also thank my students, who, to paraphrase D. W. Winnicott, paid to teach me (though they didn't pay me exactly). Finally, to my patients, who also paid to teach me and without whom this book would not exist. Thank you for trusting me with your stories.

Lastly, to Edward. Wherever you may be now, I know you are always with me. And if it's not you who is sending me weird texts, then my phone is getting hacked.

Introduction

There is an old Hindu parable about the blind men and the elephant. It goes something like this. Four blind men approach the elephant. The first grabs the elephant by the tail and says, "Oh, the elephant is very much like a rope." The second grabs the elephant by the trunk and says, "No, the elephant is very much like a snake." The third grabs the elephant by the leg and says, "You're both wrong. The elephant is very much like a tree." Finally, the fourth man puts his hand against the side of the elephant and says, "No, I'm afraid the elephant is very much like a wall." In the Hindu tradition, this parable illustrates our limited understanding of the ultimate unity of reality. We are all blind men grasping at different parts of the elephant.

Perhaps this is an apt metaphor for the current state of psychotherapy, and particularly so for our students. Student clinicians today are confronted with a plethora of different models of psychotherapy. There are the acronyms, such as CBT, DBT, ACT, ERP, and IPT. Older schools of thought, including psychoanalysis, Gestalt therapy, and family systems, coexist with newer developments such as mindfulness and mentalization-based therapies. Within psychoanalysis alone, there are many branches, including classical psychoanalysis, object relations, self-psychology, and relational psychoanalysis.

While we can argue the more the merrier and that more options can only be good for our patients, the sheer breadth of possibilities can be overwhelming for beginning therapists and even for more seasoned ones as well. How do we know which ones are best? And for which patients? Moreover, each of these modalities has an implicit, or even explicit, model of the human mind which can starkly contradict the models of other modalities. Again, the beginning therapist can be stymied. Who's right? Who's wrong? If they're all right, how do we explain the contradictions between them?

In the face of these challenges, many people simply pick a camp and stick to it, sometimes with religious fervor. (The elephant is very much like a tree.) Other people, perhaps the largest portion of the field, pick aspects of different models then throw them into their grab bag to be used in an ad hoc manner without any unifying framework (See Stricker, 2010).

Purpose

The purpose of this book, therefore, is to propose a unifying framework for the diverse approaches to psychotherapy. I propose that the mind/brain is one entity, one elephant so to speak, and that the different models of the mind are simply addressing different parts of it. My focus will be specifically on personality pathology, though setting it within a biopsychosocial context. In the first section of the book, I will present the theoretical framework, entitled *Emergent Systems Theory*. The second part of the book will address the clinical implications of this framework with regard to both assessment and treatment.

Extant Integrative Frameworks

This is far from the first attempt at an integrative framework for psychotherapy. Indeed, there is a long and illustrative history of this (Gold, 2013; Stricker, 2010), and the Society for the Exploration of Psychotherapy Integration (SEPI) has been in operation since 1983 (Stricker, 2010). As early as the 1970s, Paul Wachtel sought to integrate behavioral therapy with psychoanalysis (Wachtel, 1977). Christopher Muran and Jeremy Safran have continued that approach, particularly by synthesizing the psychodynamic focus on the therapeutic relationship with techniques from the cognitive tradition (Muran, Safran, Eubanks & Gorman, 2018). Further, many of the developments within cognitive behavioral therapy incorporate components of alternative modalities. In fact, the so-called third wave of cognitive behavioral therapy, including dialectical behavioral therapy (Linehan, 1993, 2015), schema focused therapy (Young, Klosko & Weishaar, 2003), and acceptance and commitment therapy (ACT; Hayes, 2015), explicitly incorporate Eastern meditational traditions, Gestalt therapy, object relations theory, and/or attachment theory. Other researchers have attempted to find common factors linking the different therapeutic modalities (Gold, 2013), such as the therapeutic alliance (Safran & Muran, 2003); therapists' empathy, warmth, communication skills, and cooperativeness (Wampold, Baldwin, Holtforth, & Imel, 2017); as well as client focus, positive expectancy, and the provision of hope (Stricker, 2010). In general, psychotherapy integration encompasses three major domains, integration of techniques, integration of theory and elucidation of common factors (Bloch-El Kouby, Knopf, Gold, & Muran, 2016; Stricker, 2010). In this book, I aim to provide an integrative theoretical framework to guide selection of therapeutic techniques. Although I am certainly not the first to do this, to my knowledge, few integrative models utilize a general systems approach within a broad neuro-evolutionary framework. And that is my intention here.

EMERGENT SYSTEMS THEORY

Emergent Systems Theory is drawn from models of general biology, neuropsychology, computer science, and family systems theory. This model holds that human psychology is a dynamic *system*. A system is an integrated whole created by the interactions of its component parts. Each system serves as the component subsystem of higher-level systems. Different system levels affect one another from both top-down and bottom-up directions. Higher-level systems have greater power to efficiently regulate the functioning of lower-level systems, much as an executive can coordinate and manage a large organization. Lower-level systems are fundamental to the overall structure, however, and serious dysfunction at lower levels prevents the functioning of higher levels.

Nonetheless, while a system is comprised of its component subsystems, it is not *reducible* to them; the whole is greater than the sum of its parts. Likewise, systems develop from simplicity to complexity through the process of *emergence*. This is a rather mysterious process in which something complex emerges from a simpler level of organization. It is a process of creativity, one that is never entirely predictable. As such, Emergent Systems Theory is essentially a *developmental* theory. This theory posits that the structure of the human mind reflects development across the lifespan, particularly in childhood, but also across the evolution of the species.

In fact, the process of evolution is central to Emergent Systems Theory. To a certain extent, the brain is layered like an archaeological dig. The deepest parts of the brain are the oldest and most conserved across evolution while the highest and outermost are the newest and most elaborated. Moreover, to some degree, each layer of the brain mediates its own set of psychological functions with its corresponding types of psychopathology. This has tremendous implications for both differential diagnosis and treatment selection. In this book, I argue that appropriate diagnosis requires us to locate the pathology in question at the correct level of the mind/brain. Likewise effective treatments must also engage with the appropriate level.

How does this relate to psychotherapy? Well, first, we can understand human psychology as a system nested within a larger arrangement of hierarchically-organized systems, ranging from the cellular to the societal level of organization. Likewise, we can understand *personality* as a system nested within the larger system of human psychology. This is to say that personality represents only a part of the totality of human psychology. Not all psychology is personality. More specifically, not all psychological systems function at the level of personality. For example, classical conditioning is a primitive (and evolutionarily ancient) cognitive system that operates at a lower level of psychological organization. Many anxiety disorders are attributed to faulty fear conditioning and thus can be anchored at this same system level. Likewise, systematic desensitization utilizes classical conditioning and is the treatment of choice for most anxiety disorders.

This notion is extremely important when differentiating between what is and is not personality pathology. Just as we treat cancer (pathology at a cellular level) differently than we treat a broken arm (pathology at the level of a large body part), we treat bipolar disorder (pathology at a fundamental affective level) differently from borderline personality disorder (pathology at the level of interpersonal representations). Note that many people equate bipolar disorder and borderline personality disorder, but the research literature shows that they are very different disorders.

Definition of Personality

So let us return to the question of personality. First, we need to define it. What *is* it, exactly? I will define personality as a combination of both character and temperament, consistent with the work of Cloninger (Cloninger, Svrakic & Przybeck, 1993). Temperament refers to inborn, genetically-determined styles of responding to the environment, including traits such as extraversion and introversion. It is an evolutionarily older psychological system, mediated in large part by deeper and older regions of the brain. Character, on the other hand, likely makes up the predominant part of personality. It is a function of learning and involves newer, cortical regions of the brain and more complex psychological functions. Consistent with many other schools of thought, such as object relations, attachment theory, and schema therapy, I will suggest that character is at base a system of *interpersonal representations*.

Similarly called early childhood schemas, object representations, or internal working models of attachment, these are templates, maps, or schemas of emotionally salient relationships between the self and significant other people. They are a kind of script of how people interact, which serves to guide the person's affective, cognitive and behavioral responses in relevant situations. They are, in effect, a short cut to negotiating our way through the world. Interpersonal representations develop in early childhood based on lived experience with emotionally important people in our lives. They operate largely outside of consciousness but can become conscious with effort (and often psychotherapy). When these representations are dysfunctional, personality pathology is the result.

Psychotherapy Informed by the Emergent Systems Model

So now we return to the question of how Emergent Systems Theory can inform psychotherapy of personality pathology. As discussed above, we have to select our treatment based on the level of the system where the pathology is located. If we see significant pathology at lower levels of affect, cognition or behavior, say with substance abuse, poor anger management, or panic disorder, then we have to address those problems directly, using (or referring for) substance abuse treatment, dialectical behavior therapy, behavior therapy, or other appropriate therapies. But these treatments, while extraordinarily helpful for the specific symptoms, will not treat the underlying interpersonal representations. The root of the personality pathology will still remain. Additionally, our verbal and intellectual abilities operate outside of our core interpersonal representations. They are grounded in a higher and evolutionarily newer level of our brain. This explains why intelligence and personality pathology are clearly separate phenomena. It also explains why intellectualized insight does not always lead to change, although verbal concepts can be valuable tools for regulating behavior.

Sometimes pathology at one level of organization can spread either upwards or downwards to another level. Then we have comorbid conditions, which may or may not require interventions at both levels. Typically, we focus on the primary locus of pathology before addressing the secondary effects. In this book, I will go into greater detail about how different forms of psychopathology can be mapped onto different levels of human psychology and the associated implications for diagnosis and treatment.

Once the dysfunction in lower levels of the mind/brain are stabilized—for example, when emotional lability and impulsivity are under control—we can foster the development of greater levels of organization in our patients' interpersonal representations. We can facilitate the *emergence* of greater complexity at that system level. More specifically, we want our patients to develop increased nuance, consistency, and accuracy in their understanding of themselves and the people in their world. Why is this important? Because there will be beneficial effects in both a top-down and bottom-up direction. Both (top-down) regulation of affect, cognition, and behavior and (bottom-up) regulation of interpersonal and social relations will be strengthened. Ultimately, we want our patients to develop a more mature understanding of self and other so that they can engage in the world more effectively. In this book, we will discuss the different methods of facilitating such personal growth and when and how to select treatment modalities to address the many different types of pathology attributable to different levels of the mind/brain.

SUMMARY

To summarize, this book will propose a unifying framework for the diverse therapeutic approaches to the treatment of personality pathology. This framework, termed Emergent Systems Theory, has the following core tenets:

- Human psychology is a dynamic system, defined by the interaction patterns of its component parts.
- This system is nested within a larger arrangement of hierarchically-organized systems, ranging from the neurobiological to the societal level of organization.
- Systems develop from simplicity to complexity through the process of *emergence*.
- Effective treatment and assessment must locate the pathology in question at the appropriate level(s) of the mind/brain.
- Personality pathology reflects disturbance at the level of *interpersonal representations*.
- Once control of lower level behavioral systems is achieved, the goal of psychotherapy is to facilitate the development of interpersonal representations towards greater levels of organization.
- Better organized interpersonal representations allow for more effective top-down regulation of cognition, affect and behavior—in essence, for better functioning within the world.

In the first chapter, we will explore the principles of Emergent Systems Theory and place it in the context of prior literature. In the second chapter, we will take a walk back through human evolution, going all the way to the beginning of life. Why go back so far? Because for one, it will illustrate how the earliest stages in evolution are integrated into the fabric of our brains now. Secondly, by reviewing each successive stage of our brain evolution, we can best understand how the human mind/brain is structured today. Drawing from the seminal work of Jaak Panksepp and Paul MacLean, I will present a 5-level model of the human mind/brain, with each level reflecting a successive stage in human evolution. After a more detailed discussion of personality and personality pathology (Chapters 3 and 4), Chapters 5 through 8 will explore assessment and treatment in the context of these proposed five levels as well as the neighboring levels, lying directly above or below the mind/brain proper. Finally, Chapter 9 will address the socio-cultural level of the human system and the myriad ways that it influences all lower levels in a top-down manner.

It is my hope that this model can provide a road map for clinicians, to help them navigate the complexities of assessment and treatment selection.

Chapter One

Emergent Systems Theory

The aim of this book is to present an integrative model of the many different approaches to psychotherapy, specifically with regard to personality disorders. In this chapter we will explore the primary tenets of this framework, which I have termed *Emergent Systems Theory*. First, we will discuss the 6 basic principles of this theory and then review prior literature on complex systems, drawn from the diverse fields of psychology, psychiatry, cognitive science, and biology. When you read this chapter, you may find it quite abstract and even wonder how it is relevant to the psychotherapy of personality disorders. But I hope to show how these basic principles can deeply enrich our understanding of our mind/brain, both in health and pathology. In later chapters we will explore how Emergent Systems Theory can help guide actual assessment and treatment with regard to personality pathology.

Principle 1: Definition of Systems

We will start by defining the term system. What exactly is meant by this term? We can define a system as *a whole comprised of the patterns of interactions between its component parts*. A system is a coherent entity. It is a thing in itself. But it is comprised of its member parts and the characteristics of the whole derive from the patterns of interactions of its members. For example, a family is composed of the members within it and the characteristics of the family, whether the family is close or distant, fractious or companionable, are defined by the interactions among them. Our solar system is defined by the orbits of planets circling the sun. Likewise, an atom is defined by the movement of electrons interacting with one another and the atom's nucleus. As you can see, the structure of a system is not limited by size or domain. Systems are found throughout all of nature. (See Figure 1.1.)

Principle 2: Emergent Properties

Emergent properties refer to those features of the whole that are only found at the level of the whole. These same characteristics are not found at the level of the component parts. For example, the structure of the atom is not found

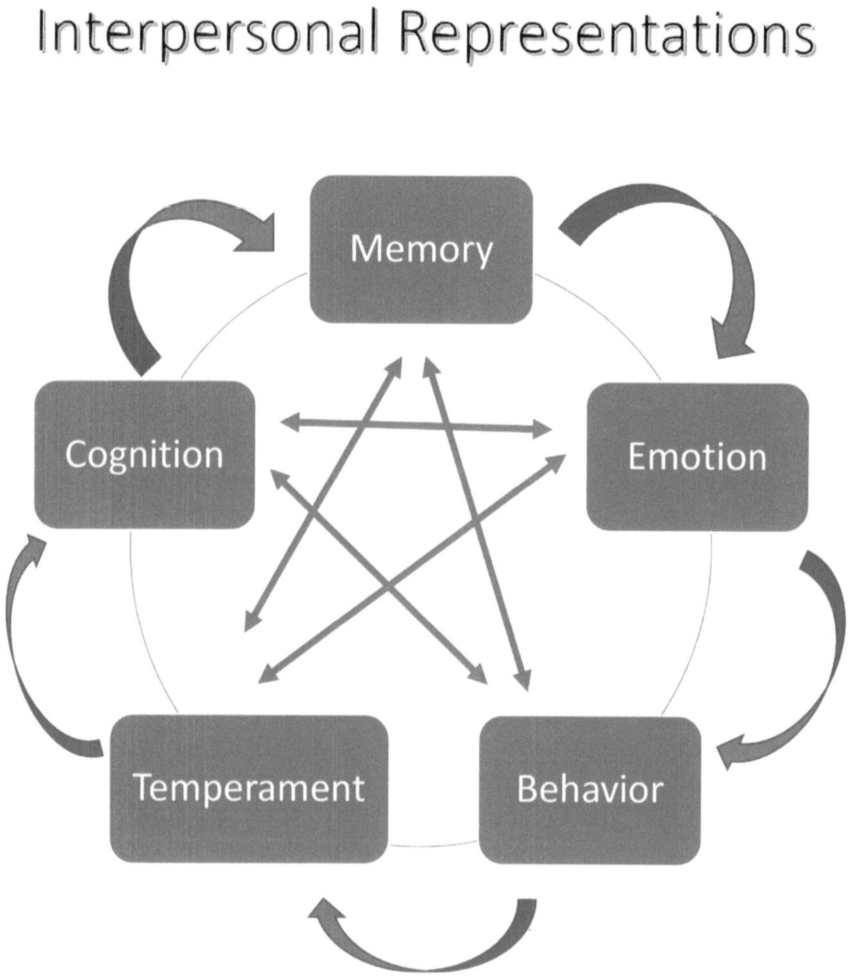

Figure 1.1. System diagram. A system is an integrated whole created by the interactions of its component parts. For example, the system of interpersonal representations contains the interacting subsystems diagramed above. Image created by Lisa J. Cohen.

in the electrons or in the nucleus; it is only in the atom itself. The same can be said for the structure of the solar system. The planets alone do not account for the shape of the solar system. It is the interaction *between* the planets and the sun that makes the solar system what it is. Thus, when a whole is created by the interaction of its component parts, it brings something *new* into the picture. These new qualities are known as emergent properties. They *emerge* out of the interaction of the system's parts. As the Gestalt psychologists said over 100 years ago, the whole is more than the sum of its parts. Indeed, many students of the mind have considered the notion of emergence with regard to the relationship between mind and body. More specifically, the philosophical concept of *emergent materialism* proposes the mind to be an emergent property of the brain (Dennet, 1991; Harnad, 1995; Searle, 1992; Stein, 2021).

The question of emergence has tremendous philosophical implications. To what extent are our personalities, our hopes, dreams, loves and hates, reducible to the electrical impulses of neurons? To reduce the whole to the behavior of its parts in a way is to kill it. It robs the whole of its identity. Feinberg and Mallatt touch on this question when they distinguish between weak emergence and strong emergence (Feinberg & Mallatt, 2016). Both positions hold that the system's emergent features can be described without reference to its component parts. In other words, we can describe the behavior of the system as a whole without *reducing* it to the behavior of its parts. We don't have to account for molecules when describing the behavior of biological organisms; we don't have to account for atoms when describing the behavior of chemicals. And most relevant to our purposes, we don't have to account for neurobiology when describing personality pathology. It is undoubtedly illuminating to reference neurobiological processes when discussing personality pathology, and we will certainly do so in this book. But we do not *need* to do so in order to describe personality-disordered behavior.

Nevertheless, in weak emergence, each system is ultimately explainable by its component parts provided there is sufficient information to do so. Systems can be very complex, and we may not have the computational power to break down system behavior adequately. In weak emergence, therefore, all emergent systems are *potentially* reducible to the behavior of their component parts. That would mean that ultimately, when (and if) the science advances far enough, we will be able to explain all of psychology (including personality pathology) by analyzing the behavior of neurons.

In contrast, with strong emergence the emergent features are in principle *irreducible* to the behavior of its component parts. No matter how much information we have and how powerful our computational capacity, we will never be able to fully reduce the behavior of systems to those of its parts. This means that psychology will never be fully reducible to biology and biology will never be fully reducible to chemistry. We will never be able to predict all of psychological phenomena by analyzing neuronal behavior.

As to which position is true, we simply do not know. It's kind of a $64,000 question. We can account for some complex systems with highly sophisticated analyses of their component parts. This is how computer modeling of weather systems predicts the behavior of hurricanes with startling precision. However, no one yet has succeeded in reducing all the rules of chemistry to physics, all those of biology to chemistry, or all those of psychology to biology. The question of reducibility may not be something we can answer. As long as there are examples of successful reductive solutions, we cannot rule out weak emergence but as long as there are systems that have not yet been proven reducible, we cannot rule out strong emergence. Given the present state of knowledge, it seems wise to maintain an open mind but also to recognize that there are characteristic features of the whole that are not found within the component parts. On a practical level, it is generally most efficient to deal with the whole on its own terms. For example, doctors typically fix a broken arm with a splint rather than trying to re-engineer bone cell development by altering gene expression. In terms of psychology, we tend to treat family pathology in family therapy rather than in 5 different individual therapies.

From another perspective, there is an aesthetic aspect of emergence. There is something profoundly awe-inducing when we see something wholly new emerge out of what was there before. We feel this when we observe children develop. One day babies may be crawling and then the next day pulling themselves up by the furniture. We see this with our patients as well, when they achieve a new level of personal growth. Life itself is an emergent property. Somehow, out of a mass of chemicals, life begins. Regardless of the ultimate reducibility of emergent properties, it is important for us to keep in mind the sheer *beauty* of emergence. When we lose track of that, we lose an important part of life experience. I would suggest that we also lose an important part of our humanity.

Principle 3: System Hierarchy

Just as systems are comprised of their constituent parts, systems can join together with other systems to form a higher-order system. Each system can serve as a subsystem for a larger system. Likewise, each subsystem can be composed of its own subsystems. In this way, emergent systems tend towards hierarchy. For example, atoms are subsystems of molecules, which form subsystems of cells, which form subsystems of tissues which form subsystems of organs, which form subsystems of organisms, which can group together into colonies. Each level of the system is emergent from the one below and as such has unique properties not found at lower levels. The different fields and subfields of science reflect this hierarchical structure, for example with the distinct fields of physics, chemistry, biology, psychology and sociology. Subfields show finer divisions into hierarchical levels. Chemistry has inorganic, organic and biochemistry. Biology has micro- and evolutionary biology and psychology has neuro-, cognitive, personality and social psychology. (See Figure 1.2 for an illustration of system hierarchy.)

As has long been assumed in neuroscience, Emergent Systems Theory posits that the human mind/brain is organized in just such a hierarchical structure. It is a building with many floors. Moreover, as will be detailed in Chapters 4–6, this hierarchy has profound implications for diagnosis and assessment. This is because psychopathology can emerge at any level and as such will have features that cannot be explained by the behavior of lower levels. *Effective treatment therefore requires accurate identification of the level*

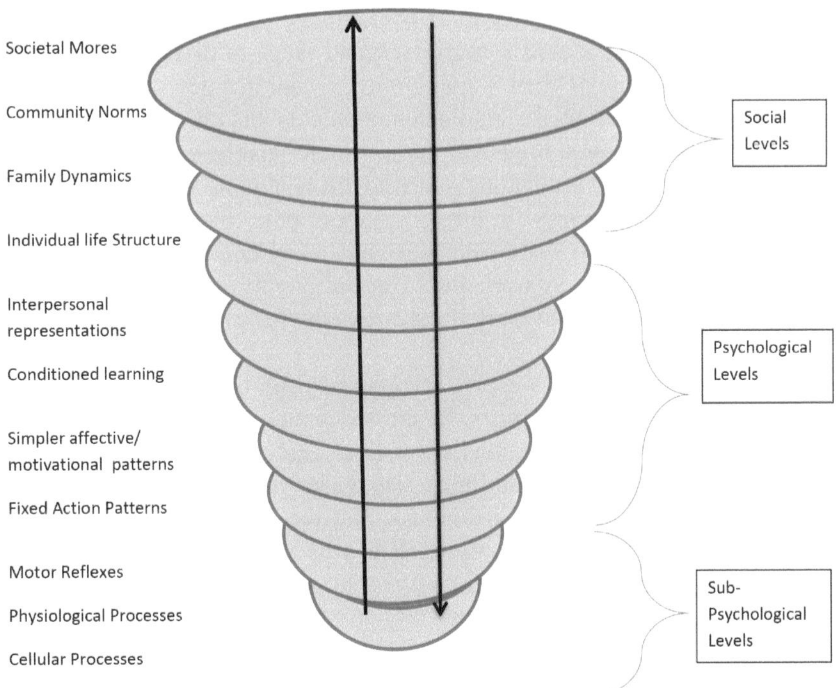

Figure 1.2. Human system hierarchy. Human psychology is a system nested within a larger arrangement of hierarchically-organized systems, ranging from the neurobiological to the societal level of organization. System influence can occur in both top-down and bottom-up directions. Image created by Lisa J. Cohen.

at which the system dysfunction occurs as well as selection of interventions designed for that specific level.

Principle 4: Top-down and Bottom-up Influence

It is important to keep in mind, however, that the different levels of a system do not exist in isolation from one another. System levels interact continuously. In this regard, such systems are *vertically integrated.* When higher-level systems exert influence on lower-level systems, we call that top-down causation or top-down influence. Bottom-up causation (or influence) occurs when lower-level systems affect the functioning of higher-level systems. As detailed by Sabelli and Carlson-Sabelli (1989), there are different qualities to the two directions of influence. Top-down influence has "supremacy," in that the greater reach over the entire range of subsystems allows for efficient and powerful centralized control. It also provides for greater flexibility and a broader range of possible responses. Think of a CEO in a well-organized corporation who has to confront a major challenge facing the firm. Let's call our CEO Janet. Janet is able to recruit a broad range of diverse resources to get a thorough picture of what is going on. She can then devise a wide range of plans, select the best fit, and implement it quickly and efficiently. Janet will be in a far better situation to respond to any major challenge to the firm than will Joe, who works in accounting and who has neither access to information nor decision making ability for any department other than his own. This is the benefit of complexity and explains why so many organisms have evolved towards greater complexity over time. But complexity is expensive in terms of time and energy (and CEOs are literally expensive) so there are advantages to simplicity.

In our own mind/brains, we have retained both simple and complex levels for use in different circumstances. When facing a challenging new situation, our frontal lobes come on line and allow us to analyze the situation with the full force of our cognitive capabilities, while also recruiting all other parts of the brain needed to accomplish this task. But the frontal lobes take a great deal of energy to work effectively. That is why we feel so tired after concentrating on a demanding task for several hours. Therefore, once a task is well known and becomes routine, we rely on older and less complex parts of the brain to get the work done. Our work becomes automatized and far less energy intense.

Of course, bottom-up influence is also important. Top-down is not the only game in town. Sabelli and Carlson-Sabelli refer to the "priority" of lower-level systems as they are essential for the functioning of the system as a whole.

Because they form the foundation of all systems built on top of them, disturbance at lower levels can have far reaching effects across the system as a whole. Think of a pyramid of cheerleaders. Now imagine what would happen if the bottom row suddenly stood up. Everyone above them would fall down. Another example is cancer, which is a disorder at the level of DNA, the lowest level of organization of life forms. Mutations in DNA lead to runaway reproduction of mutant cells, eventually destroying the entire animal if not stopped.

Principle 5: Development of Emergent Systems through Integration, Differentiation, and Articulation

In order to understand the structure of a complex system, it is critical to understand how it developed. Indeed, we will rely on such a developmental framework to understand personality pathology and how to treat it. In general, emergent systems tend to develop from relative simplicity to relative complexity. While systems do not always move in this direction, and there are many examples of systems simplifying, there is a widespread tendency, particularly among biological systems, to develop towards greater complexity. As postulated in Werner and Kaplan's orthogenetic principle (1963), organisms develop towards relative complexity through the coordinated process of integration and differentiation (and here we add the process of articulation).

In the human mind/brain, we see tremendous development of complexity both across evolution and across the lifespan. In fact, there are dramatic parallels between evolutionary and lifespan development, also known as phylogeny and ontogeny, respectively. We will explore this concept in depth in Chapter 2, where we will consider how the human mind/brain grew in complexity through the specific processes of integration, differentiation and articulation. Moreover, throughout this book we will pay considerable attention to these three processes as they will prove central to the treatment goals of psychotherapy with personality disordered patients. This will be explained in Chapter 5. But for now, we will simply define these processes and show how they relate to complexity.

Integration refers to coordination between the parts. The different parts interact with one another and start to influence each other. When the different parts act in a coordinated way, we can say that they are integrated. When bees in a hive coordinate to feed the queen and fill the hive with honey, they form an integrated system. If your cardiologist and your primary care doctor integrate their medical records system, then they can read each other's reports on your health, making sure to coordinate your care. Likewise, if you link your credit card accounts to your checking account, you can move money between the different accounts more easily than if they were not integrated. As you can see, the process of integration is ubiquitous across nature and across our daily life. It is a key component of complexity.

It is also important to distinguish between integration and aggregation. In aggregation, there is no interaction between the parts. Think of an array of rocks in a field. They all just sit there and will not move unless acted upon by some external force. They do not interact with one another. However, imagine now that a flock of Canada geese land on these rocks. They will interact with one another, squawking, fighting, and following each other's lead when they spot food. Moreover, when they take off, they will fly in a V formation, exhibiting a property of the whole flock that is not evident in any individual goose.

Differentiation refers to separation between the parts. It describes part to part relationships within a system. An important tradition within psychodynamic theory addresses the issue of self-other differentiation. This concept is similar to that of theory of mind, which originated in developmental psychology. Prior to the age of 4, children have little understanding that they have a mind that other people do not share, that what is in their mind is not in other people's minds. If you ask a 3-year-old child who his or her mother is, the child might answer "Mommy." If you ask young children where they live, they will tell you "my home." They are not trying to be difficult. They simply do not realize that their perspective is different from yours. Of note, differentiation may be defined otherwise in different fields, for example in developmental biology. But for our purposes here, we are defining it as above.

The process of *articulation* is similar to differentiation, but it describes part to whole relationships within the system instead of part-to-part relationships. Articulation refers to the process by which a global unity comes to have many different components. The crude becomes nuanced. For example, at the earliest stages of embryonic development, the brain is a long tube with three simple bulges. As the embryo develops, those three bulges divide into many different parts, eventually producing the vast array of distinct and specialized brain regions that make up the human brain. In this way, the uniform becomes multifaceted and variegated.

Thus, by the coordinated processes of integration, differentiation and articulation, simple systems move from crude, simplistic, and isolated units to multi-faceted and coordinated structures, with enhanced efficiency and a wider array of possible behaviors. In living organisms, complexity allows for greater flexibility, a broader behavioral repertoire and improved adaptability to changing conditions.

Principle 6: Nonlinear Rate of Change

As psychotherapists, our goal is to help our patients change. We wish to ameliorate suffering, heal psychopathology and promote healthy psychological growth. Therefore, the question of rate of change, of how quickly and even how predictably our patients change, is highly relevant to us.

Emergent systems are nonlinear, which means that they do not have a constant rate of change. Linear change reflects a constant relation between input and output. For every hour that you work you are paid a specified amount. Mathematically, a linear relationship can be expressed as $y=ax$. If your salary is $30.00 per hour and you work 40 hours, you will be paid $1,200.00 (1,200 = 30 × 40). If you graph the relationship between hours worked and money earned, you will have a straight line, which is why these relationships are called linear. (See Figure 1.3.) With linear rates of change, outcome is very easily predictable. If you know how many hours you work, you can easily predict how much money you will make.

Emergent systems, however, are not always linear. For the most part, complex systems like the mind/brain do not behave in linear ways. In these conditions, there is no constant relationship between input and output. For example, we cannot predict how well and how quickly a person will change depending on the number of psychotherapy sessions we provide. We can hope that more psychotherapy produces more positive change, but we know that different patients change at different rates. We also know that change is not always incremental, occurring at a steady pace. Sometimes people slog away for a while without any appreciable change but then suddenly turn a corner with a burst of growth. We cannot predict the response to therapy in a linear way.

As noted above, emergent systems commonly behave in non-linear ways. This is because systems are made up of interacting parts. Every time one part of the system (Part A) changes, there are ripple effects throughout the system. The other parts (B, C, and D) are changed as well. And because all parts are interactive, the behavior of Parts B, C, and D affects Part A, the original part that was changed. In this way systems are *recursive*, their own activity feeds back on itself. If A is activated, then it bumps against B, which then bumps back against A. In this case, the rate of change is *exponential;* it is accelerating. Mathematically, this can be expressed as $y=e^{ax}$, which is known as an exponential equation.[1] The exponent is the number of times the initial number is multiplied by itself. But exponential processes can be inhibitory as well as escalating. A's activity may be slowed down when it bumps against B which then bumps back and further slows A down.[2] The more A occurs, the less likely it is to recur.

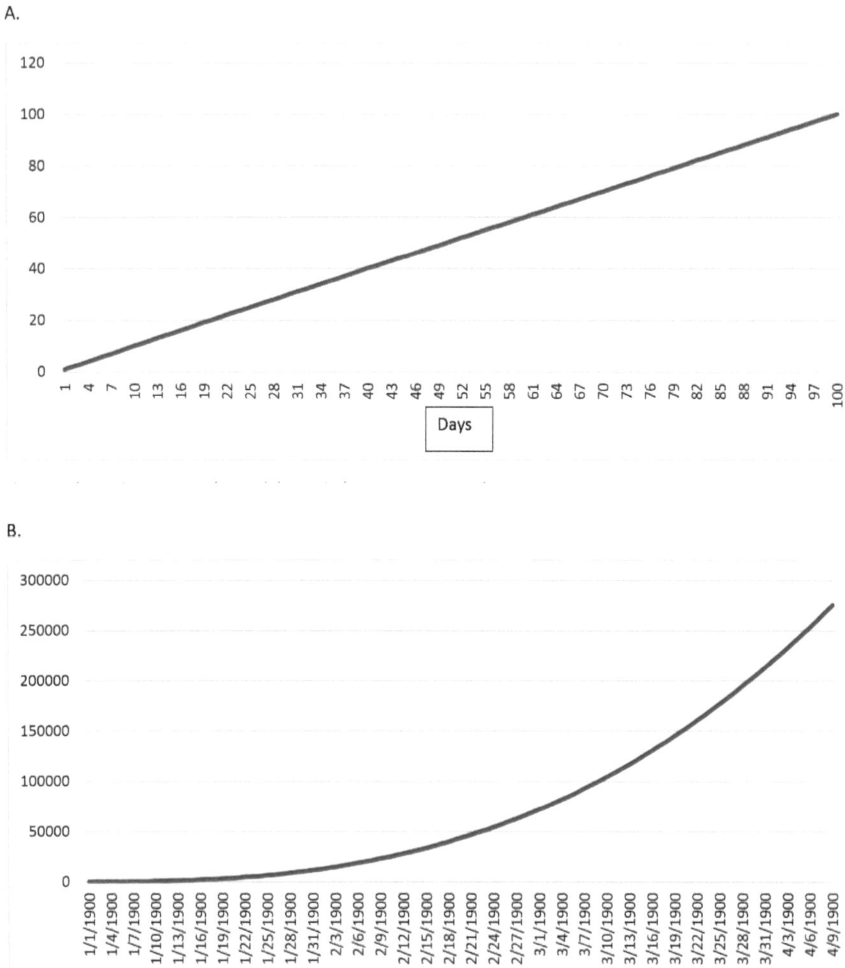

Figure 1.3. Linear and exponential curves. The top figure (A) represents a linear function; growth occurs at a constant rate. The bottom figure (B) represents non-linear or exponential growth. Notice the explosive rate of growth over a 3-month period. Image created by Lisa J. Cohen.

A perfect example of a nonlinear process involves David Barlow's theory of panic attacks (Barlow, Craske, Cerney, & Kiosko, 1989). In this model, there is a three-part system incorporating physical symptom, catastrophizing cognition and the emotion of anxiety. The person experiences some minor physical symptom, such as shortness of breath, then interprets the physical symptom in a catastrophic way (There's something wrong with me. I think I'm sick). This elicits anxiety, which activates the autonomic nervous system resulting in additional physical symptoms, such as rapid heartbeat and perspiration. This in turn intensifies the catastrophizing cognitions (I'm having a heart attack! I think I'm going to die!), which only further intensifies the anxiety. This cycle can feed on itself until it escalates into a full-fledged panic attack. Importantly, the panic attack does not build gradually, at a steady pace. It can escalate very quickly, leading the person to believe it came out of nowhere with no known cause.

If we graph exponential equations, they do not create a straight line (See Figure 1.3). In fact, they create a curved line and the shape of the curve varies tremendously depending on the magnitude and sign of the exponent "a." The higher its magnitude, the steeper the curve. When "a" is positive the curve points upward, when "a" is negative the curve points downwards. As emergent systems involve many, many interacting parts, there may be many variables in the equation, all with their own exponential equations. In this way it is very difficult to predict the behavior of emergent systems with precision.

But all is not lost. Nonlinear systems have specific properties that we can harness effectively in psychotherapy. As above, when the coefficient "a" is positive, there is an abruptly escalating rate of change. This is known in biological systems as a *positive feedback loop*. Examples include any addictive behavior. The more you engage in an addictive behavior, the more you want to do it. Barlow's theory of panic attacks also describes a positive feedback loop. The physical symptoms lead to catastrophizing cognitions which lead to anxiety which in turn increase physical symptoms. Another term for this would be a *vicious cycle*. These are also common in marital relationships; the more one partner wants to be close, the more the other partner pulls away, which leads the first partner to demand more attention, which in turn elicits more escape behavior from the second partner. This has been described as a "dodge and chase" pattern in the marital therapy literature. Identification of these vicious cycles offers many opportunities for intervention, as small steps in interrupting the feedback loop can have a large effect cumulatively. Simply stopping a single action from recurring can move patients onto a corrective path, in time turning a vicious cycle into a "virtuous" one. Likewise, intervention at an early stage can often stop the escalation before it becomes unmanageable.

In a negative feedback loop, the more the behavior occurs, the less it is likely to repeat.[3] The behavior inhibits itself. This can be a positive step, preventing behaviors from escalating out of control, as feelings of satiation inhibit overeating. Our body has many negative feedback loops. For example, the hypothalamic-adrenal-pituitary (HPA) axis activates under stress, releasing corticotropin-releasing hormone (CRH) into the blood stream, which essentially steps on the gas, preparing our body for the fight/flight response. However, CRH also stimulates the release of cortisol, which then steps on the brakes, preventing our engine from overheating, so to speak. Negative feedback loops can also be problematic, however, if they reinforce avoidance of constructive activity. The more someone avoids airplanes, for example, the less likely they are to take a trip that requires air flight. In fact, avoidance creates powerful negative feedback loops with regard to motivation to engage with the environment.

HISTORY OF COMPLEX SYSTEMS THEORIES

Now that we've covered the basic principles of Emergent Systems Theory, we can place them in the context of prior literature. These 6 principles were drawn from a range of fields grappling with the concept of complexity and emergent processes. Although interest in complexity has popped up from time to time for at least a century, for example with the Gestalt psychologists' focus on holistic perception, the topic did not flourish until the 1980s and 1990s, greatly aided by the computer revolution. In order to appreciate the full significance of contemporary systems theories, however, it is necessary to consider the general scientific paradigm which preceded it. This is very important as the same paradigm permeated our understanding of the human mind, of our psyche.

Throughout the history of science, a spirit of *reductionism* has held enormous sway. This might go back as far as the ancient Greeks. For example, the pre-Socratic philosopher Democritus (c.460–370 B.C.E.) proposed that the world was made up of tiny, invisible and irreducible particles called atoms. But historically, a key turning point occurred when Isaac Newton presented his treatise *Philosophae Naturalis Principia Mathematica* to the Royal Society of London in April of 1686. Certainly, since that point a bias towards reductive thinking has pervaded the natural sciences. Although Isaac Newton famously credited his predecessors (e.g., Kepler, Copernicus, and Gallileo), claiming to be "standing on the shoulders of giants," his contribution was seen by many as the basis of modern science. Newton's work was based on the assumption that the universe is composed of particles, or bodies in motion, and that there are universal laws prescribing the movement of bodies in space. In the *Principia*, Newton presented his three universal laws of motion, expressed in mathematical language. From these three laws and the law of universal gravitation (a central concept of gravity), the behavior of any body in space could be predicted. The movement of ocean tides, planets, and grains of sand as well as the trajectories of cannon balls could all be predicted, allowing for profound advances in human control over the natural world. Newtonian physics obtained its predictive power through reducing the universe to fundamental laws about elemental parts. Consequently, it was through the predictive power of Newtonian physics that reductive reasoning gained its dominant influence on scientific epistemology.

In general, science proceeds through both *analysis* and *synthesis*. In reductive reasoning, the complex whole is broken down into its constituent parts. Knowledge is analytic. In synthesis, the simple parts are put together to build up a complex whole. Knowledge is integrative. Newtonian physics is a triumph of reductive science. Although it is neither fair nor accurate to state that synthetic thinking has played no role in science over the last 300 plus years, many people believe that there has been a bias within science to overvalue an analytic or reductive approach and overlook, if not devalue, a synthetic approach. This bias is known as reductionism.

Freeman Dyson, a preeminent physicist, described just this viewpoint in a paraphrasing of his debate with Brian Green, another prominent physicist.

> Theoretical science may be divided roughly into two parts, analytic and synthetic. . . . Green was saying that only analytic science is worthy of the name of science. For him, synthetic science is nothing but practical problem solving . . . He said . . . when we know the fundamental equations of physics, everything else, chemistry, biology, neurology, psychology, and so on, can be reduced to physics and explained by using the equations. (The New York Review of Books, May 13, 2004, p. 19)

Similarly, Leon Lederman, a particle physicist, explains that there is a hierarchy in science (Lederman, 1993).

> A discernible hierarchy exists, though it is not a hierarchy of social value or even of intellectual prowess. Frederick Turner, a University of Texas humanist, put it more eloquently. The exists, he said, a science pyramid. The base of the pyramid is mathematics . . . because mathematics does not rest upon or need any of the other disciplines, whereas physics, the next layer of the pyramid, relies on mathematics. Above physics sits chemistry, which requires the discipline of physics; in this admittedly simplistic separation, physics is not concerned with the laws of chemistry . . . Then comes biology, which rests on an understanding of both chemistry and physics. The upper tiers of the pyramid become increasingly blurred and less definable: as we reach physiology, medicine, psychology, the pristine hierarchy becomes confused . . .
>
> The pyramid may be disrespectfully summed up by an old saying: the physicists defer only to the mathematicians, and the mathematicians defer only to God (though you may be hard pressed to find a mathematician that modest). (p. 12–13)

Thus, even though Lederman takes pain to deny that the pyramid reflects differences in social value or intellectual rigor, the last statement reveals quite a different cultural attitude within the hard sciences.

Moreover, this paradigm was not limited to the hard sciences but permeated the social sciences just as deeply. In psychology, it is most evident in the earliest forms of behaviorism, in which all of learning was reduced to the simple relationship between stimulus and response. The mind was referred to as the black box. Because it was assumed that intangible mental processes could not be measured objectively, they were dismissed rather contemptuously as irrelevant to science. The theories of Sigmund Freud, whose seminal work influenced much of 20th century thought, were also reductionist in important ways. The reductionism of Freudian theory is most evident in his attempt to reduce all complex psychological behavior to the vicissitudes of an ultimate and fundamental motivational force. Libido, a generalized sex drive, served as the essential drive, although Thanatos or the death drive was added following the carnage of WWI. Both were explained in terms of energy discharge.

Thus, an implicit epistemology of reductionism has pervaded many branches of the human sciences.[4] In fact, I would argue that reductionism still holds considerable influence within psychology. For example, within the science of dreaming, many investigators reduced dream imagery to the random firing of neurons in the brain stem, dismissing the richly personal meaning of dreams as coincidental byproducts. Although newer dream researchers reject that simplistic reductionism, embracing the complex meaning of dreams, they still must grapple with the earlier paradigms (See Jarvis, 2021).

In sum, while the benefits of the analytic method underlying reductionism are incontrovertible, having produced enormous advances in science and technology over the last several centuries, the limitations are also significant. Most importantly, this paradigm provided an inadequate understanding of complexity. In effect, we continuously missed the forest for the trees. Reductionism also fails to address the transformation from states of simplicity to states of complexity. And without such models in psychology, we can have little understanding of change and development. We cannot know our history.

Gestalt Psychology

Throughout the period of peak reductionism, say in the late 19th and early 20th century, there were some islands of holistic thinking. Gestalt psychologists, based in Germany in the early 20th century, were interested in the tricks of perception. In studying perceptual illusions, scientists such as Max Wertheimer, Wolfgang Kohler, and Kurt Koffka discovered how perception depends on *pattern making*, illustrating how the mind actively creates an integrated whole out of discrete parts, sometimes making mistakes in the process. The term "gestalt," in fact, refers to a holistic pattern. Moreover, it was the Gestalt psychologists who gave us the phrase, "The whole is bigger than the sum of its parts."

The Role of Computer Science

The real turn towards systems theory, however, comes out of developments in computer science in the middle of the 20th century. In their 1995 book *Frontiers of Complexity*, Peter Coveney and Roger Highfield review this history.

Cellular Automata

In the 1950s, Stanislaw Ulam conceptualized a computer program later termed the cellular automaton, a simple program that created complex visual patterns. The automaton consisted of a grid of cells, in which each cell would behave according to local rules that took into account not only its own state but the states of its neighbors. Neighboring cells would *interact*; changes in one cell would precipitate changes in its neighbor which would then demand changes in the original cell. Thus, through the mechanism of feedback loops, this simple computer program showed how complexity could emerge out of the behavior of parts. Using very simple principles, local rules could generate enormously complex and variegated patterns. In this way, extraordinary complexity arose out of simplicity. John von Neumann, another founding father of computer science, hypothesized that similar bottom-up processes may underlie the evolution of life.

In the early 1980s, Stephen Wolfram was interested in the variety of macroscopic patterns generated by simple local rules. He found that out of an infinite set of local rules, four distinct classes of patterns emerged, reflecting different degrees of regularity and change. He proposed that a combination of regularity and irregularity may be most suggestive of living systems, as without regularity there is no consistent form but without irregularity there is no change or development.

Out of these and similar constructs evolved the fields of chaos theory, self-organizing systems, and complexity theory. The power of such theories was in their ability to model extraordinarily complex systems. For the first time the patterning of zebra stripes, weather patterns, stock market growth and contraction, chemical reactions, cell growth and neural networks could all be simulated. Nonetheless, despite the elaborate nature of the patterns generated by algorithms utilizing feedback loops, these programs did not really introduce anything *new* that could not be predicted from the initial rules. In this way, there were exemplars of *weak* emergence.

Neural Networking

Building on the idea that models of complexity could tell us something profound about the workings of the brain, computer scientists developed the notion of the neural network, a type of computer algorithm that modeled the interactions of the brain's neurons. Neural networks advanced the work of cellular automata to incorporate input from the environment and in so doing introduced the notion of complex *adaptive* systems. Like cellular automata, neural networks use local rules and feedback loops to generate highly complex patterns from the interaction of simple parts. Additionally, however, neural networks can simulate the emergent property of *learning*, the system's self-modification in the face of new information. The brain, like a cellular automaton, is comprised of a fabric of interacting cells, or neurons. Both neurons and automaton cells are characterized by intercellular communication and a largely binary (off/on) activation system.

Based on this model, Warren McCulloch & Walter Pitts developed a computer program as early as 1949, in which a set of input "neurons" fire until a critical threshold is reached in an output "neuron," causing it to fire in response. In the early 1960s Frank Rosenblatt addressed the fundamental property of self-modification (i.e., learning) by incorporating feedback mechanisms into his computer program which he called the Perceptron. In response to a given external stimulus, input neurons fire into output neurons, stimulating a new pattern of firing. Externally derived information on the accuracy of the resulting firing pattern is then fed back into the input neurons, such that correct connections are strengthened and incorrect ones weakened. Repeated cycles of firings and corrective feedback lead to closer and closer approximations of the intended pattern. The imprint of this early computer program is found in all types of artificial intelligence today, including voice recognition programs.

Ludwig von Bertalanffy and the Study of Biology

The biologist Ludwig von Bertalanffy brought the concepts of complexity and self-organizing systems out of the realm of computer algorithms and into the study of actual living organisms. In 1969, he published a book entitled *General Systems Theory*, which summarized his writings of the previous three decades. Von Bertalanffy was interested in an approach to biology that addressed properties such as wholeness, organization, growth and development, and self-regulation. In his view, such phenomena had been long disregarded in the mechanistic and reductionist framework of "classic science." Von Bertalanffy linked his own theoretical contributions to a wider holistic trend spreading across scientific disciplines and ranging from math and physics to psychology and sociology. Importantly, von Bertalanffy applied principles of general systems theory to the study of actual living organisms.

Von Bertalanffy defines a system as a coherent entity comprised of interacting parts. Systems have characteristic properties which are irreducible to those of its component parts. Moreover, systems can be either open or closed. Open systems are characterized by interaction with the environment, specifically the exchange of material and energy across system boundaries. All living systems are open systems, dependent upon a constant input of energy. Closed systems, on the other hand, are entirely self-contained. Closed systems follow the second law of thermodynamics, in which all systems tend towards negative entropy. This refers to the loss of energy and the degradation of order and structure over time. An example of this would be a spinning top. The top is set in motion by a human movement, but without additional force the top will spin until it runs out of energy and then fall down flat. In contrast, open systems continue to function and to maintain their internal organization as long as they sustain a constant input of energy. The human body is a perfect example of this. Dependent on food and oxygen to survive, we literally die and decompose if deprived of external sources of energy. Von Bertalanffy asserts that only open systems grow toward greater complexity, as such development depends on a surplus of energy only possible with continuous external input.

Von Bertalanffy was also interested in the conservative nature of systems, in the remarkable degree to which systems preserve their structure across time and across different conditions. He was particularly concerned with *homeostasis*, the capacity of organisms to self-regulate in the face of perturbations to the system. Homeostasis depends on feedback of information about the state of the system back into the system. In response to this, the component parts then readjust to bring the larger system back into a steady state. In other words, homeostasis depends on negative feedback loops, in which the output, as it feeds back into the input, reduces the rate of activity. Examples include the body's temperature control as well as individual cells' regulation of sodium and potassium levels. We can see parallels with this concept in psychological systems as well, in terms of people's reluctance to change their fundamental ways of functioning in the world.

Von Bertalanffy also proposed two underlying principles of system development. *Progressive segregation* refers to the tendency of organisms to develop from simple homogeneous systems into segmented structures with increasingly independent components. In the embryo, for example, a mass of identical cells develops into highly specialized organs and tissues. This is essentially analogous to the process of articulation described earlier. *Progressive centralization* refers to the tendency for a "leading part" to emerge and centralize control of the rest of the organism, much like the central nervous system in embryonic development. This is similar to the process of integration discussed earlier. Relatedly, complex systems tend towards hierarchical order. Although von Bertalanffy is rather vague about the underlying mechanisms, he observes that all complex organisms incorporate many hierarchical levels, such that each system level forms the component subsystem of the next highest level.

Family Therapy

Within psychology, it was in the relatively new field of family therapy that the principles of complex systems first flourished. The practice of family therapy arose independently in several areas across the United States, uniting into an organized movement in the late 1950s. In the 1960s the movement took off, rapidly becoming a pivotal force in psychology, psychiatry and other mental health disciplines. The child of many parents, family therapy has no single progenitor. The overall body of work is attributed to a group of clinician/researchers known as the "pioneers," which includes Gregory Bateson, Donald Jackson, Murray Bowen, Nathan Ackerman, Salvador Minuchin, Jay Haley, Virginia Satir, and several others. The pioneers' perceptions of theoretical developments in other fields shaped the paradigm in which they conceptualized their work. They were particularly influenced by von Bertalanffy's General Systems Theory.

A number of basic ideas unite the several branches of family systems theory. The first tenet is that individuals function as members of a larger system, specifically the family, and thus an individual's psychopathology cannot be understood in isolation from its immediate interpersonal context. In fact, the symptoms of "the identified patient" frequently serve a function for the larger family system, as a child playing truant at school may bring parents in a strained, distant marriage back into interaction. Secondly, the family system has its own characteristics which are irreducible to the level of the individual. Such features include boundaries and a hierarchical structure, which regulate the flow of information and power. Boundaries exist between the family and the outside world, between the individuals within the family, and between subsystems within the family, such as the parents and the children. In Minuchin's structural family therapy, family pathology is often attributed to disruptions in appropriate boundaries and hierarchies, as when a child is elevated into the parental subsystem. Thirdly, family systems act to preserve homeostasis, such that individual members will reorganize to bring the family system back into equilibrium when the system is disrupted. In this way, families often resist change. For example, a wife may suddenly refuse to return to treatment after her husband and son relinquish their long-standing conflict.

Murray Bowen, another pioneer, was interested in the concept of differentiation, how individual family members may disentangle themselves from enmeshment with the family into more mature relationships based on a better articulated and more distinct sense of self. This notion of differentiation of separate parts out of a global whole is similar to von Bertalanffy's ideas of progressive segregation.

Santa Fe Institute: Complex Adaptive Systems

In 1984, a multidisciplinary group of scientists established the Santa Fe Institute to study complex adaptive systems, which refer to complex systems that change in response to their environment. Their research covered physical, computational, biological, and social systems but they had a particular focus on artificial intelligence (AI). This involves using computer programs to model the workings of the human brain. The Santa Fe Institute brought the computer science approach closer to the domain of psychotherapy, particularly via their interest in mental representations.

In the published proceedings of a 1993 Conference, institute members laid out their approach (See Morowitz & Singer, 1994). In the Introduction, Jerome Singer stipulated that the study of complex adaptive systems reflected a scientific paradigm shift in the 1980s and 1990s away from the simple, reductionist and linear view of cause and effect that had pervaded many fields. He described this work as a cross-discipline endeavor, extending to astrophysics, quantum mechanics, cellular biology, evolutionary biology, archaeology and economics. Despite some variation in terminology, there was general agreement about how to define complex adaptive systems, largely in keeping with principles set forth by John Holland.

Holland, a formative influence in this movement, listed several basic principles of complex adaptive systems. These systems are defined by the collective behavior of numerous interacting constituent parts (or agents) whose activity cannot be described linearly. Therefore, the behavior of the whole system cannot be predicted by summation of the behavior of the parts (again echoes of the Gestalt psychologists). There is also considerable variation in shape, form and function of these agents, as found in the different regions and cell types in the brain. However, the system is entirely interconnected so that removal of one agent will cause the system to reorganize in order to compensate for the loss of the missing part (consistent with von Bertalanffy's focus on homeostasis). Moreover, systems are constantly evolving, resulting in the continuous appearance of newly emergent features and structures.

Importantly, a defining feature of complex adaptive systems is their creation of internal models of their environment, which provide a series of rules governing their behavior within the environment.

Murray Gell-Mann, a physicist who won the Nobel prize for physics in 1969, addressed these internal models in greater depth. Gell-Mann purported that all complex adaptive systems gather data from their environments and then search for regularities, or repeated patterns. In fact, he refers to adaptive systems as pattern-recognition machines. The identified regularities are compressed into *schemata*, another word for internal models of the environment. Schemata provide a set of rules about how the environment works which then guides the system's behavior within it. In this way, schemata serve descriptive, predictive and prescriptive functions. When schemata are applied, the results of the ensuing interaction with the environment are then fed back to update and modify the relevant schemata. In this way, there is continuous feedback and modification. However, schemata necessarily simplify the information about the environment. In order to be useful, they need to be streamlined. As a consequence, they can make errors. Systems can detect regularities where none exist, for example with superstitious behavior, where people insist on connections between random events. Alternatively, they can miss regularities and overlook patterns that do exist. Critically, Gell-Mann's notion of schemata powerfully parallels the concept of interpersonal representations, which is central to many models of personality pathology, as will be discussed throughout the book.

Gell-Mann also suggested that schemata compete with one another as if in a Darwinian race for survival of the fittest. Schemata that are reinforced by the environment are strengthened but those that are not are weakened. Interestingly, he suggests that some subordinate schemata remain latent and can re-emerge if circumstances change and they become newly relevant. In terms of personality, we might see this when childhood views of relationships that were buried suddenly re-emerge when the environment produces relevant cues. Surely, we've all had the experience of being brought back to an earlier time and to a long-forgotten way of seeing oneself when suddenly faced with reminders of that previous time. High school reunions, for example, often have this effect.

Cognitive-Affective Science

In his 2021 book, Dan Stein explores the current state of cognitive-affective science, which aims to advance computer-based models of the mind/brain relationship beyond reductionistic paradigms and towards a more holistic approach (Stein, 2021). He criticizes the earlier computer models, in which the mind was seen as a self-enclosed computational machine, with no attention to emotion or context. He notes that the current such computer models, encompassed under the umbrella term of cognitive-affective science, present the mind as emergent from the brain, embodied (in the brain and the rest of the body) and embedded (in the interpersonal and other context). Such an approach is highly consistent with the basic tenets of Emergent Systems Theory.

Psychodynamic Theories

Returning to the domain of psychotherapy, we can see how similar concepts play out within the realm of psychodynamic theory. While not focused on systems theory per se, psychoanalytic theorists were certainly focused on mental representation, and accordingly on the development of the human mind within its interpersonal context. By the second generation of psychoanalysts after Freud, there was a convergence of ideas about the role of internal representations of early childhood relationships, both in health and psychopathology. Through decades of case studies and in-depth psychotherapeutic treatments, analysts realized that much of their adult patients' struggles came from the picture of the world they had internalized from their primary relationships during childhood. Indeed, this insight has remained the bedrock of contemporary psychodynamic thought and has even spread to other schools of psychotherapy, such as Beckian cognitive therapy and Jeff Young's schema therapy. This book also endorses this view and holds further that dysfunction at the level of interpersonal representations is the primary source of personality pathology and therefore the ultimate target of psychotherapy for patients with this pathology.

A number of psychoanalytic theorists, such as Irene Fast and Sid Blatt, addressed the process of *development* of these representations, such that they attributed adult psychopathology, or what we would now call personality pathology, to inadequate development within these representations. Specifically, they explored how failures of integration and differentiation of self and other representations underlay their patients' difficulties, concepts we will explore in greater detail in Chapters 3 and 4.

Since the heyday of complexity theories in the 1980s and 1990s, the issue has slipped from discourse within the larger popular culture. In some fields it has become thoroughly integrated into the general worldview, almost taken for granted. This is particularly the case within neuroscience where the assumption that the brain is organized in a hierarchical structure and demonstrates emergent properties is widely accepted. Within clinical psychology and psychiatry, however, the principles of complex systems have faded from view to a much greater extent. To my mind, this is highly unfortunate, and this book therefore is intended to address this gap.

To summarize, this chapter introduced the 6 basic principles of Emergent Systems Theory and placed them in the context of prior literature. These 6 principles reference: 1) Systems definition, 2) Emergent properties, 3) Hierarchical structure, 4) Top-down and bottom-up influences, 5) System development through integration, differentiation, and articulation, and 6) Nonlinear rate of change. In the following chapters we will show how these principals can illuminate the psychotherapy of personality pathology, both in terms of diagnosis and treatment. In short, Emergent Systems Theory purports that the mind/brain is a hierarchically-organized, emergent system and that different forms of psychopathology are located on different levels of organization, each with their own emergent and non-reducible characteristics. As such, each form of psychopathology requires uniquely suited interventions for effective treatment. Personality pathology can be located at the level of *interpersonal representations*, a higher-order level of the human mind/brain. This is a relative latecomer in the evolution of our species, and as such exerts top-down influence (supremacy) over earlier and lower-level functions of thought, emotion and behavior. However, interpersonal representations emerge fairly early in the individual lifespan and therefore carry the traces of our earliest childhood. Change in these representations can be accomplished in psychotherapy, using both top-down and bottom-up processes, as will be described in detail later.

In the next chapter we will explore how our current mind/brain came to be the way it is. Because each level of organization emerges from earlier and lower levels, the very structure of our mind/brain contains our entire history, dating back billions of years. To understand how our mind/brain is constructed and how the different levels relate to each other, it therefore is critical to understand its full history. In this way, Emergent Systems Theory offers a profoundly *developmental* model of our psychology. We will look at our development both across phylogeny, the evolution of the species, and across ontogeny, the individual lifespan. And we will see how developments billions of years ago at the level of single cell organisms still play critical roles in our mental health.

NOTES

1. The mathematical term "e" refers to a constant that appears throughout mathematics and rounds up to 2.71828. The coefficient "a" measures the number of times the changes feedback on themselves; it measures the strength of the feedback.

2. Mathematically this is expressed as $y=e^{-ax}$.
3. Negative feedback loops occur when the coefficient "a" is negative.
4. Indeed, the problem of reductionism in psychology has been addressed by numerous theorists and philosophers of mind (Rees & Rose, 2004; Satel & Lilienfeld, 2013; Stein, 2021; Tallis, 2014).

Chapter Two

Beginnings

In this chapter, we're going to take a journey. We're going to go all the way back to the beginning of life to see how the extraordinary complexity of our mind/brain evolved from remarkably simple origins. Moreover, we'll see how at every step of the way, new structures emerged via the processes of integration, differentiation, and articulation. We will also see how our earliest origins continue to live on in the very structure of our psyches. Why do we have to go back so far, 3.8 billion years to be precise? Because this gives us the long view, and it is my contention that only through taking the long view can we best see the entirety of our mind/brain as a unified and hierarchically-organized, emergent system.

MIND VS. BRAIN

Before we get started, I want to address a few points. The first pertains to terminology. I have been using the term "mind/brain" to refer to human psychology. Other authors have used this or similar terminology (See Panksepp, 1998; Panksepp & Biven, 2012; Stein, 2021). Why use this term here? In psychotherapy we are interested in the individual's subjective world so it is reasonable to use the term mind. But the mind does not exist without the brain. There simply is no mind without brain. However, in contrast to a group of philosophers known as the neurophilosophers (See Churchland, 2002), I am not suggesting that the mind is equal to the brain. Mind and brain are not interchangeable. Although there may be no mind without brain, there is definitely brain without mind. Much of what the brain does is not mental. Most of our brain processes do not reach consciousness, particularly those involved with physiological functions, such as temperature regulation and hormone release. Moreover, the mind is more than the brain. The content of the mind includes the world around us. Therefore, the mind is an *emergent property* of the interaction between brain and world. However, because of the inextricable relationship of mind to brain and because study of the brain can reveal so much about the mind, I have elected to use the term mind/brain to encompass the broader system, the whole kit and kaboodle.

The relationship of the brain to the mind is only the latest version of the mind/body problem, a question that has vexed philosophers since time immemorial. And frankly we are no closer to solving it now than when we explained it by referencing animal spirits. While we have made tremendous progress in understanding the *neural correlates* of psychological processes, that is, what happens in the brain when various psychological processes take place (e.g., perception, cognition, etc.), we are still stymied by the question of *qualia*. Qualia refer to the subjective experience of psychological processes, such as the yellow of yellow. We know that we perceive the color yellow when light waves of a certain frequency hit our retina, activating certain neural responses. But that tells us nothing about why anything looks *yellow* to us. Ultimately, we have no idea how objective neural behavior translates into subjective experience. As above, subjective perception is an emergent property of neural activity, one which has never been and may never be reduced to its component parts. Nonetheless, understanding more about the behavior and history of neural structures can still illuminate an enormous amount about complex mental processes, such as personality pathology. Therefore, we will put the issue of qualia aside and march on.

Methods of Examining Evolutionary History

How do we determine the sequence of evolution? How can we possibly figure out what happened billions of years before our species even existed? There are multiple means of extracting an evolutionary timeline. The first is by examining the fossil record. By studying fossilized remains of extinct species and noting the geological layers in which they are found, we can gain some sense of the time course of the ancestors of today's species. Comparative anatomy is also a critical resource. Examination of similarities and differences between living species allows us to deduce common origins. Interestingly, the notion of comparative anatomy is rather recent. As explained by Stephen Jay Gould, in the 18th century, Carl Linnaeus created a taxonomy of all living species based on comparative anatomy rather than anthropocentric views of their relevance to mankind. He thus provided a necessary foundation for later evolutionary investigations. Linnaeus's taxonomic system is still in use today although with significant modifications. A third source of evolutionary data comes from embryonic development. As noticed by 19th century biologists, widely divergent species share remarkably similar patterns of embryonic development. The timing of divergences in early development (for example when fish embryos start to look different from chicken embryos) sheds light on the time course in which different species branched off from common ancestors. Very recently, in fact only since the early 2000s, we also have been able to study the entire genomes of different species and calculate the percentage of shared genes between them. We have even been able to extract viable genetic material from remains of extinct species, such as Neanderthals. Thus, our understanding of the evolutionary history of living animals, our own species included, is based on multiple methods, some dating back several hundred years. When the findings from different methods converge, we can be extra confident in our conclusions. The review that I am about to present is based on multiple sources, some recent and some less so. Given the rapid pace of technological development, it is possible that some of the details may be out of date. Moreover, the dating of events millions to billions of years in the past is far from precise and often lacks consensus. I believe that this is less important, however, than the general storyline, for which we can feel quite confident, as it based on almost three centuries of scientific research.

Human Brain Anatomy

Just one more detour before we begin our journey proper. Here, we will briefly review the basic anatomy of the human brain. This should make it easier to follow as we discuss brain evolution. While we will explore brain anatomy in more detail at the end of the chapter, for now a brief overview will set the stage for our journey. The brain is an extremely complicated network of interacting neurons (brain cells) that science is only beginning to understand. The human brain weighs about 3 pounds (2 to 3 percent of the average person's body weight) but it uses a disproportionate amount of our daily energy consumption. For example, our brain requires about 15 percent of the blood pumped out by our heart and 20–25 percent of the oxygen and glucose used by our bodies.

All vertebrate brains develop from a three-part brain structure, comprised of the forebrain, midbrain, and hindbrain. The forebrain has developed the most in humans and is the largest region of our brain. It is also most central to our conscious mental life. The forebrain is made up of two general regions: the telencephalon (cortex, limbic system, and many subcortical areas) and the diencephalon (thalamus and hypothalamus). The telencephalon is the largest part of the forebrain and the *neocortex* the largest part of the telencephalon.

The neocortex makes up the outer layers of the brain and looks kind of like a wrinkled boxing glove (See Figure 2.1 for a diagram). This 6-layer tissue is the most recently evolved part of our brain and the most complex. It is critically important for all high-level psychological functions.

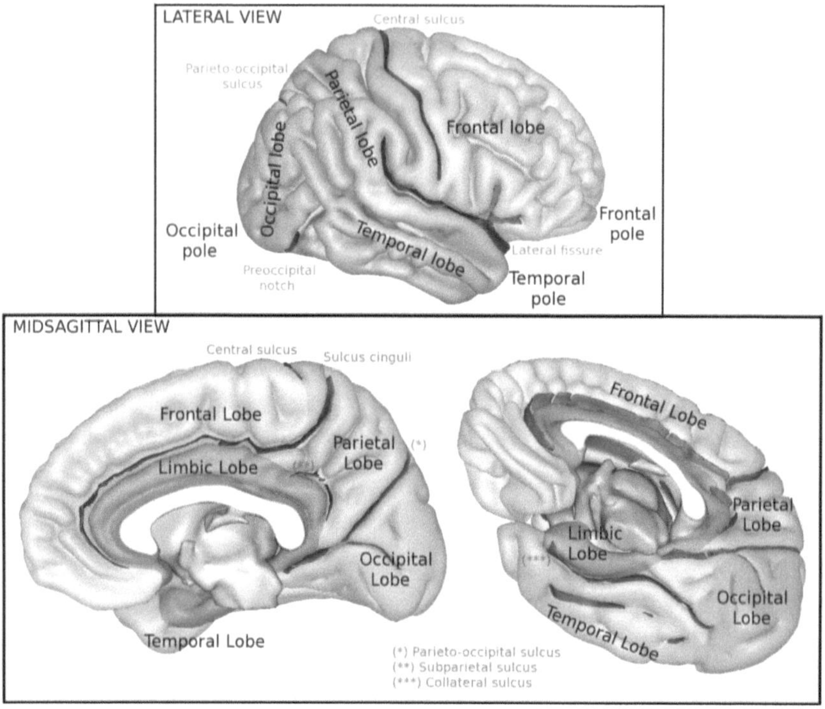

Figure 2.1. Neocortex. Outer (lateral) and inner (medial) view of the human cortex. Sourced from Sebastian203, Creative Commons. 2011. commons.wikimedia.org/wiki /File:LobesCapts.png

The neocortex is divided into 4 lobes. The occipital lobe is in the back of the brain. The parietal lobe lies in front of the occipital lobes, on the sides of the brain. The temporal lobes extend across the bottom and outer sides of the brain, like the thumbs of a clenched fist. These three lobes are critically involved with perception. The frontal lobe takes up the front half of the neocortex. It is the seat of complex thought as well as intentional and planned action. The neocortex is only a segment of the larger cortex, however. There are also inner regions of the cortex, known as the mesocortex and allocortex. They include such structures as the cingulate gyrus and the hippocampal regions. These are evolutionarily older areas of the cortex and serve to link memory, emotion and cognition. For our purposes, we will refer to these regions as the limbic lobe.

All areas beneath the cortex are known as *subcortical regions.* The distinction between cortical and subcortical processes is an important one in neuroscience. See Figure 2.2 for a diagram of subcortical regions. Beneath the neocortex and limbic lobe are a host of brain regions involved with memory, emotion, and motivated behavior, including the amygdala, basal ganglia, and nucleus accumbens. The diencephalon, a smaller and older section of the forebrain than the telencephalon, lies in the middle of the brain. It includes the thalamus, which controls what sensory information gets to the cortex, and the hypothalamus, which connects our emotional/motivational states with physiological arousal.

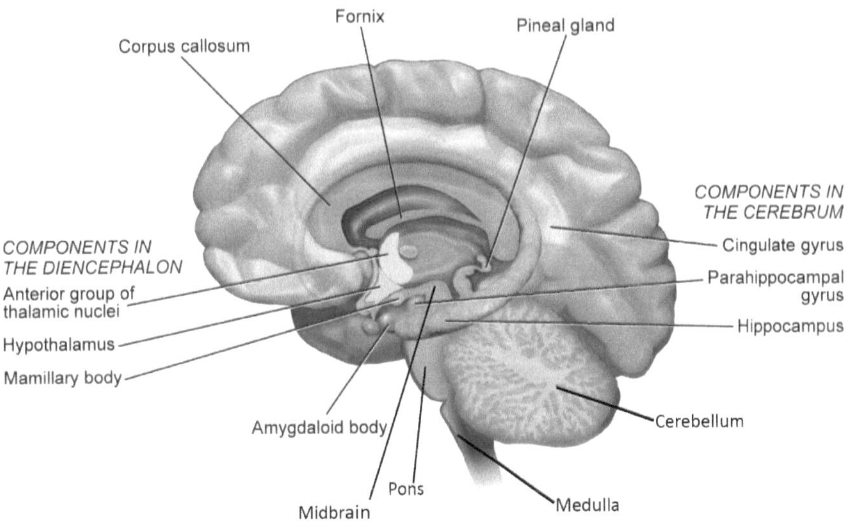

Figure 2.2. Subcortical areas. The subcortical regions of the brain. Note that the medulla and pons are parts of the brain stem. Blausen.com staff (2014). "Medical gallery of Blausen Medical 2014." *WikiJournal of Medicine* 1 (2). DOI:10.15347/wjm/2014.010. ISSN 2002-4436.

The midbrain lies below and behind the forebrain, closer to the spinal cord. It is a small region in the human brain but contains some structures important for emotional functioning. The hindbrain lies at the bottom of the brain, closest to the spinal cord, and includes several fairly large structures. The brain stem, comprised of the pons and the medulla oblongata, controls basic physiological processes, such as respiration and body temperature. The cerebellum is the large, wrinkled bulb projecting out from underneath the back of the neocortex. It is involved with motor control as well as some cognitive functions.

As we will shortly explore, the brain evolved from back to front, from inner to outer, and from bottom to top, so that the deepest, innermost, and lowest regions of the brains are the most conserved across evolution. Likewise, the furthest forward, highest, and outermost regions have changed most across evolution and contain the most complex structures.

HOW IT ALL STARTED

At this point, we will begin our journey, proper. We will start by going all the way back to the origins of life, about 3.8 billion years ago (bya). The beginning of life on earth is typically attributed to the emergence of self-replicating molecules, which are thought to have been ribonucleic acid (RNA). DNA (dioxyribonucleic acid) is believed to have evolved out of RNA. Let's stop and consider this for a moment. DNA, which forms the basic building blocks of all life on earth and which controls so much of our biological functions, was first formed almost 4 billion years ago. Astoundingly, it has made remarkably few changes across this huge span of time. DNA works the same for human beings as it does for green algae. DNA is shaped like a double helix, a kind of twisting ladder. The rungs of the ladder are made up of different pairs of four smaller molecules: adenine, thymine, guanine, and cystosine. A triplet of pairs codes for an amino acid. A gene is made up of the sequence of triplets that code for a protein. From this simple beginning, the rest of life unfolds. In fact, the size of the genome (an organism's total number of genes in a cell) has changed very little from the fruit fly to our own species, 14,000 vs. about 20,000 genes (Willyard, 2018). This is a tiny difference, when we consider that there are perhaps 100 billion neurons in the human brain and 100 trillion neuronal synapses (junctures where different neurons connect). In other words, the earliest and most basic level of organization of the human body has been remarkably conserved across billions of years of evolution.

Single-Celled Organisms

The first single-celled organisms evolved about 3.5 bya. This required the development of a membrane to encase the DNA (along with RNA and related proteins) and thereby to form a boundary between the inside and the outside of the cell. By the time multicellular organisms arrived on the scene about 780 million years ago (mya), much of the structural components of the modern neuron were already present. In this way the rudimentary architecture of our own brain cells was in place at the level of single-celled organisms, hundreds of millions of years before brains themselves even existed.

Prokaryotes are single-celled organisms without a nucleus and include such primitive organisms as bacteria and archaea. Eukaryotes evolved about 1.8 bya. The earliest eukaryotes were single-celled organisms with a nucleus. Eukaryotes later evolved into an enormous range of organisms. In fact, all complex forms of life are classified as eukaryotes, including plants, animals, fungi and protists (a group of primarily single-celled organisms). Moreover, the basic cell structure of the first eukaryotes is maintained in every cell in our body, including our neurons.

Astoundingly, the prokaryote bacteria, among the most primitive of organisms, utilize a basic behavioral toolkit. They process chemical information from the environment to determine the presence of either food or toxins and then approach or avoid accordingly. And note, they do this without brains. In fact, when they sense either resources or hazards in the immediate environment, they do a little dance-like movement and shift their flagella (tail-like appendages), which sends them zipping off in another direction.

This also merits some reflection. Bacteria's behavioral toolkit reveals two fundamental dimensions that organize brain function in all higher animals. The first is the sensory-motor dimension. Organisms seek out and process information about their environment (sensory) and then they act upon it (motor). In humans this is largely handled by our cortex. The posterior or back regions process sensory information, and the anterior or frontal regions process planned motor behavior. The second dimension has to do with *value*, what is beneficial vs. harmful to the organism. As explained by Antonio Damasio, it is value that directs the organism's interactions with the environment (1999). In humans this is handled by our emotions, largely mediated by subcortical regions, which signal what is good and what is bad for us. Human personality (and personality pathology) reflects the interaction between these two dimensions, as manifested in our patterns of information processing, emotion, and behavior.

But let us return to single-celled organisms and what they reveal about the most fundamental level of organization of the human mind/brain. Bacteria process chemical information about their milieu through molecular receptor sites on their cell membranes. Does this sound familiar? It is the basic structure of our neuronal synapses. Our brain cells take in information about their environment and also communicate with one another via molecules landing on receptor sites on their cell membranes.

Very early on cells developed the ability to exchange genetic material, the basis of sexual reproduction. Exchange of genetic material proved highly advantageous, as it provided alternative traits that could come in handy when the environment changed. Therefore, according to Bownds (1999), cells evolved ways to communicate with each other in order to promote genetic exchange. Specifically, cells released pheromones into the environment (which was the ocean) to communicate their availability to other cells for sexual reproduction, sort of like posting an ad on a dating website.

This parallels another basic property of modern brain function. Just as primitive single-celled organisms released chemicals into the sea to communicate with one another, our brain cells release hormones into the blood stream to communicate with other cells in our body. For example, our stress response is mediated by the hypothalamic-pituitary-adrenal (HPA) axis. By releasing hormones into the blood stream, the HPA axis activates a chain reaction from the brain down to the adrenal glands next to the kidneys.

Yet neurons communicate with each other not only through chemical messengers but also through electrical impulses called action potentials. A neuron receives chemical messengers on multiple receptor sites. This eventually triggers an action potential. The action potential travels down the length of neuron's axon, an arm-like extension (See Figure 2.3). This then stimulates the release of more chemical messengers at the end of the axon (the axon terminals). Though the neuron per se did not evolve until later, the precursors for neurons were definitely present in single-celled organisms. All of these features, chemical messengers, receptor sites, action potentials and axon-like projections, have been found in single-celled organisms.

Thus, we see that the most fundamental level of organization of the human mind/brain, namely the neuron, corresponds with developments at the earliest stage of evolution.

Multicellular Organisms

Around 780 mya, multicellular organisms evolved (date from Kristan, 2016). This may have come about through several mechanisms. We know that single-celled organisms formed colonies. For example, tightly integrated colonies of bacteria and yeast are evident today. It is possible that the individual members of the colonies became so interconnected that they ultimately functioned as a single unit and were able to reproduce as such. Alternatively, larger organisms may have swallowed up smaller ones. For example, mitochondria in our own cells have their own DNA, suggesting that they may have once been separate organisms. In fact, recent theories hold that most multicellular organisms descended from archaea, rather than bacteria, and that the mitochondria in our cells descend from bacteria that were ingested by the larger archaea (Youle, 2019). These developments illustrate the process of *integration*. The processes of *differentiation* and *articulation* also came into play, however, as previously identical cells diverged into different forms and functions.

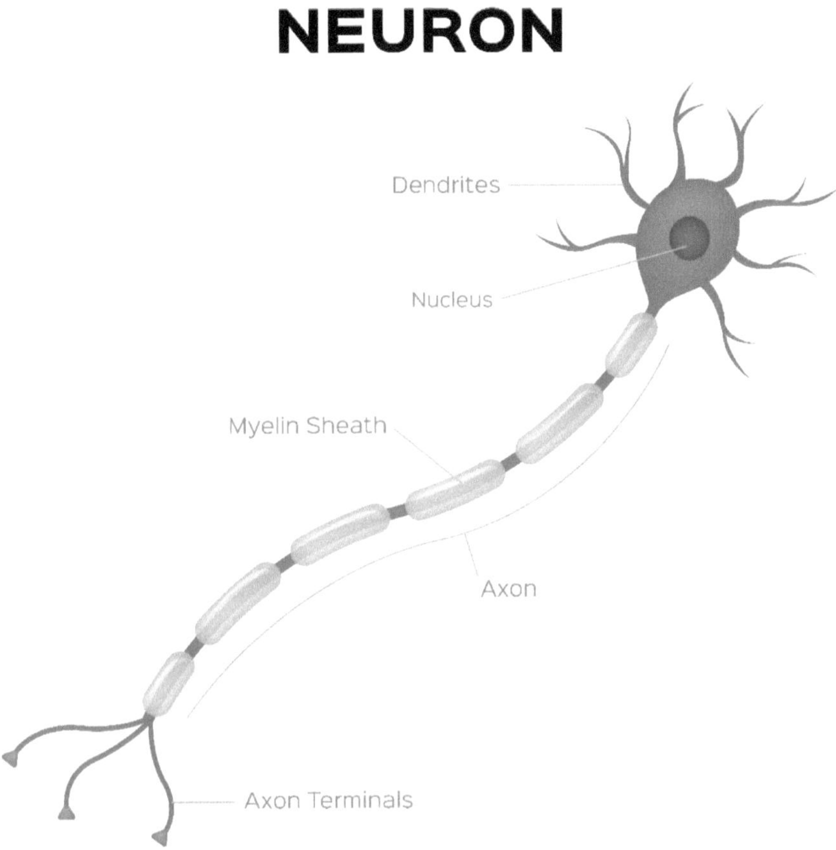

Figure 2.3. Neuron and synapse. The structure of the neuron. gritsalak karalak. Shutterstock.

Sponges may have been one of the earliest multicellular organisms, dating back about 635 (Feinberg & Mallatt, 2016) to 780 (Kristan, 2016) mya. These basically functioned as water filters, extracting nutrients from the water flushing past their cells, with little differentiation of component cells. They had neither nervous systems nor neurons.

According to Kristan (2016), neurons likely evolved between 640–720 mya. Neurons offer tremendous advantages in terms of negotiating the environment. A neuron coordinates input from multiple sources into a single binary reaction, combining breadth of information with efficiency of response. Moreover, its action potentials allow for fast reactions and the long axon permits communication between neurons at a distance from one another.

The first system of neurons was likely the reflex arc, in which a receptor cell acts directly on an effector cell. Sensory input directly leads to motor response and only two neurons are involved. Humans have maintained simple reflex arcs as part of our own motor systems. When your doctor hits your knee with a hammer and your knee jerks, that is a reflex arc. Interneurons, inserted between two other neurons, later created a longer chain of neuronal communication. As more interneurons were inserted into the chain, this allowed for exponential increases in the complexity of information processing and behavioral responses. Interneurons make up a significant portion of the human brain.

The first neurons were likely organized into loose nerve nets, kind of like how the internet forms a network of individual computers. This is how we find neurons in jellyfish, the simplest form of animal with a nervous system. The next step was for individual neurons to group together into ganglia (ganglion in the singular), which would control specific functions or body parts.

Bilaterians and Chordates

The clade of bilateria evolved about 600 mya. (A clade is a group that descends from a common ancestor.) This includes all symmetrically organized organisms and encompasses all vertebrates. One of the first bilaterians was likely a worm, shaped like a hollow tube. At the front end of the tube was the mouth and at the end, the anus. The rest of the tube was gut. Importantly, a nerve cord, that is a line of ganglia, stretched along the inside of the tube. A particularly large ganglion at the mouth end of the tube served as a rudimentary brain. According to Bownds (1999), brains tend to evolve close to the mouth of an organism. Certainly, our own brains are close to our mouths. To give a sense of how primitive these early nervous systems were, the nematode, a small worm that has been studied extensively, has only about 300 neurons.

The phylum chordata, to which humans belong, evolved out of the bilaterian clade about 560 mya. Chordates are characterized by the presence of a notochord, a long rod-like structure that, in vertebrates, later evolved into the spine. At the level of chordates, therefore, we see the beginnings of a central nervous system. A long line of ganglia topped by a master ganglion is attached to a supporting rod. In vertebrates, the nervous system threads through the notochord to form the spinal cord. Once again, to show how our earliest history retains its traces in our bodies today, notochords are still present in early embryonic development and only later develop into parts of the spine.

Cambrian Explosion

About 560 to 520 mya, there was an explosion in the diversity of life. Most of the animals alive today evolved from phyla[1] that emerged during this period. Although there are other explanations, Feinberg and Mallatt attribute the Cambrian explosion to a kind of arms race between predator and prey, in which both evolved enhanced sensory capabilities to be able to track, hunt and/or evade one another. Similarly, Kristan notes that around 525 mya, the fossil record shows animals with hard shells and spiky protrusions, suggestive of adaptations to predator-prey relations. Kristan also notes that the first nervous tissue was evident in the fossil record at this time, with indications of well-formed eyes and the faint outline of a nervous system.

Vertebrates

The Cambrian explosion gave us the first vertebrates, dating back about 525 mya. These were jawless fish, tiny animals with a spinal cord, back bone, head, tail, and simple three-part brains, who were probably filter feeders and became adept at rapidly swimming toward food and away from predators. The three-part brain deserves some consideration as this remains the fundamental brain structure of all vertebrates, including our own species. The earliest brains were simple tubes topped by a series of three bulges, the hindbrain, midbrain, and forebrain. (See Figure 2.4.) Although many fish species have pretty much conserved this original form, in higher animals, particularly mammals, this simple structure has become elaborated to the point that it is almost unrecognizable. Nonetheless, embryos of all vertebrates begin with this structure, again illustrating how our ancient history retains its traces in our present form.

The advent of vertebrates brought a big leap in sensory processing. There was a proliferation of sense receptors, generally placed on the surface of the body. Primitive receptors for light, sound, odor and pressure on the body then evolved into complex sense organs for vision, hearing, smell and touch. As the capacity to receive sensory information increased, areas of the brain to process all this new information evolved in concert.

This is when the dorsal or upper parts of the brain made their first appearance, particularly in the midbrain and forebrain. In the midbrain, the optic tectum evolved, which likely served in visual processing. The telencephalon evolved out of the forebrain. This area of the brain has had the most elaboration in birds and mammals. In mammals, the neocortex, limbic system, and basal ganglia develop out of the telencephalon, all regions that are highly significant for human psychology. In the jawless fish, a rudimentary cortex made its first appearance.

It is likely that the telencephalon originally evolved to process smell. In most mammals (except primates), the sense of smell still takes up a large part of the forebrain. For the early jawless fish, smell offered many advantages.

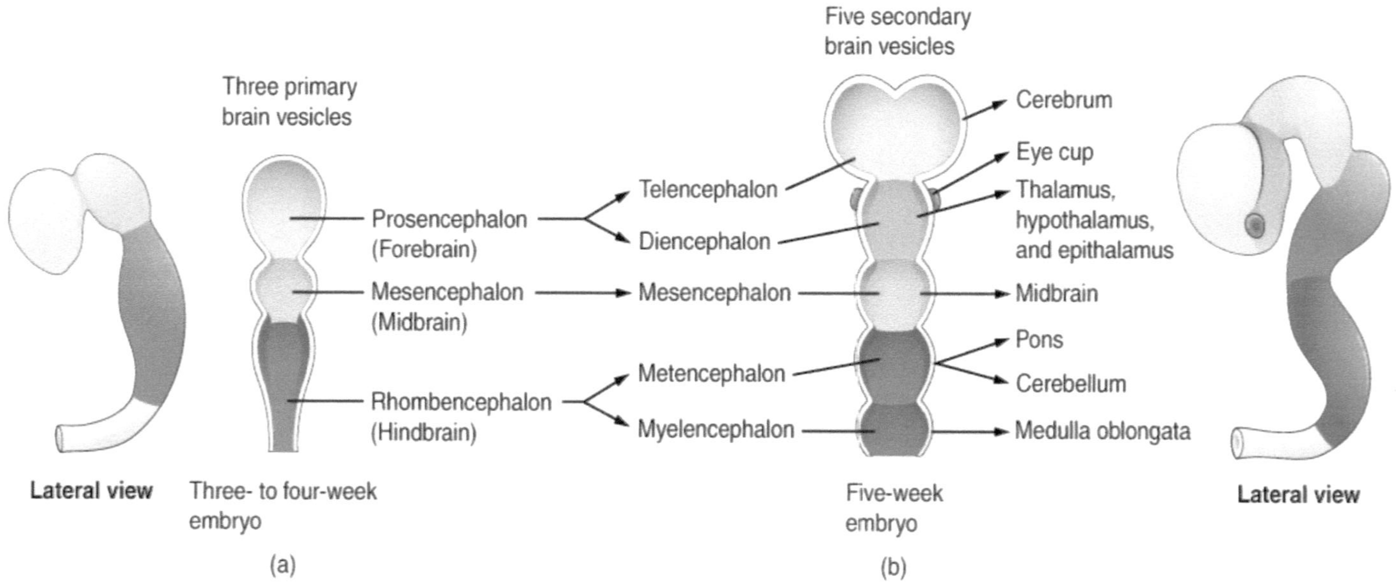

Figure 2.4. The three-part structure of the brain. This earliest brain structure in vertebrate evolution is seen in the initial period of human embryonic development. Here we see that ontogeny truly does recapitulate phylogeny. Sourced from OpenStax. Creative Commons. 2016. cnx.org/contents/FPtK1zmh@8.25:fEI3C8Ot@10/Preface.

Sightlines are limited under water and sound is often muffled. Smell, which processes chemicals that waft through the water, is well suited to a watery environment. It is also a natural outgrowth of the chemical receptors that had been in operation for billions of years. Because of its ancient role in brain processes, even in humans, smell retains close ties to older brain regions processing emotion and memory.

Another critically important innovation in vertebrates was myelin, although this probably did not appear until the advent of fish with jaws. This is a fatty sheath that coats the neuron's axon and serves to greatly increase the speed of action potentials. It is more energy efficient and also prevents different axons' electrical impulses from interfering with one another. Because the speed of action potentials depends on the diameter of the axon, myelinated neurons could be as fast as larger neurons that were not myelinated, thus allowing more neurons to be packed into a small space. In another instance where development mirrors evolution, myelination takes place quite slowly in human maturation. In fact, the frontal lobes are not fully myelinated until about the age of 25 (which explains a good deal about adolescent behavior).

Of critical relevance to our focus on interpersonal representations in personality, it was in the early vertebrates that the brain started to create *maps* or *representations* of the environment. The sensory organs recorded the spatial and temporal patterning of light waves, sound waves, odor or physical pressure on the body and then transmitted that information up to the brain. The brain then *repeated* this patterning across space and time in its own configuration of neuronal firing. Multiple neurons in the brain coordinated their firing to recreate the same pattern in which the original sensory stimulation hit the sense organs. Feinberg and Mallatt date the emergence of sensory consciousness to this time as they propose that these brain maps were sufficiently complex to create subjectively experienced vision, hearing, smell, or touch. In other words, they believe that the first (very rudimentary) form of consciousness dates back over 500 million years. Certainly, our own consciousness emerges out of this same basic structure. Our sense organs record the spatial and temporal patterning of sensory information and the brain maps and then repeatedly remaps these same patterns into increasingly complex patterns. Of course, at the level of human beings, the brain maps are many orders of magnitude more complex than those of the earliest jawless fish. In humans, our brain mapping reaches the extraordinary complexity of *cognition*, so that we not only create representations of the world around us but we can manipulate those representations in our mind. Nonetheless, the basic process of brain mapping or of representing the environment has remained the same across half a billion years.

Evolution of Consciousness

Let us now take a moment to reflect on the evolution of consciousness, as it is at this point in evolution where we see the initial flickers of a subjective life. Feinberg and Mallat list three categories of consciousness, exteroceptive, interoceptive and affective. Exteroceptive pertains to sensory representations of the external world. Through sensory/perceptual circuitry, the animal creates a map of the external world which is subjectively experienced as "out there." The interoceptive system processes sensations about the body's internal states, including feelings of muscle tension, rapid heartbeat, intestinal distress, etc. This system also processes feelings of physical pain. These feelings are experienced as "in here," within the animal's own body. In higher animals, interoceptive consciousness is elaborated in the cortex.

Affective consciousness is not located in space like the other two systems. It involves subjective experiences of core motivational states related to survival, such as fight/flight and appetitive drives, including hunger, thirst, and sex. Affective consciousness reflects the subjective experience of *value,* of pleasure vs. pain, desirable vs. undesirable. While a rudimentary system of value can be identified as far back as bacteria, there is no reason to think that the chemically induced approach/avoidance behavior of bacteria required consciousness. Bacteria do not have brains.

Feinberg and Mallatt date core affective consciousness to the emergence of vertebrates, about 525 mya. They state that the core brain regions involved are present in all vertebrates, even in ones as primitive as fish. These include specific regions in the hindbrain, midbrain and the lower (ventral) portions of the forebrain. In mammals and birds, expansion of the telencephalon in the upper (dorsal) forebrain led to far greater complexity in affective consciousness. In these cortical regions our more complex social and self-related emotions are processed. Nonetheless, even our most sophisticated emotional responses are built on top of more primordial emotional systems and it is in the interplay between the ancient and newer emotional systems where we find our patients. But there is still a world of difference between the mental life of fish and human beings so we now resume our journey across evolution.

From Jaws to Legs

Around 460 mya, jawed fish evolved. Jaws provided a significant advantage for fish as it allowed them to grasp food. As evolution progressed and fish gained more complexity and a broader range of adaptations, they spread out to a greater variety of environments, including shallow water.

Some fish developed air bladders, which helped in buoyancy in water and eventually evolved to help breathe on land. Around 420 mya, fish with lobed fins appeared. These are fleshy fins, covered in skin, in which bone and muscle are attached. They look like stumpy legs and indeed formed the precursors of legs. The clade of tetrapods, including all animals with four legs, evolved about 395 mya. Tetrapods include amphibians, reptiles, birds, and mammals. Some tetrapods later returned to the water and lost their legs (whales, dolphins) or simply reverted back to legless form (snakes). Nonetheless, these species are still classified as tetrapods as they evolved from species with four legs.

The four legs of tetrapods allowed for one of the most momentous changes in evolutionary history, the move out of the ocean onto land. This occurred about 390–360 mya. Amphibians, the oldest of the tetrapods, were the ones who made this transition. Once tetrapods came on land, there were numerous changes to adapt to the new environment, including the loss of gills and reduction of the tail. The shape and form of the vertebrae also changed, for example to aid locomotion on land and to create a neck, which allowed animals to turn their head. Environmental conditions on land were more variable than under water, which led to enormous variety in evolutionary adaptations, as demonstrated in the branching lines that led to reptiles, birds and mammals. But it is the evolution of mammals that interests us the most.

Mammals

Mammals first appeared about 170 million years after amphibians crawled onto land, 200–225 mya. About 70 mya after amphibians came ashore, say 290–320 mya, the first reptiles appeared. Three separate lines of descent evolved from the early reptiles: the synapsids, anapsids, and diapsids. Mammals evolved from the synapsids, turtles from the anapsids, and birds, dinosaurs and living reptiles from the diapsids. These initial lines of descent were distinguished from each other by the shape of the skull and jaw. About 248 mya, an enormous mass extinction wiped out about 95 percent of the species on Earth. It was probably caused by massive volcanic explosions precipitating an abrupt change in the Earth's temperature. One group of survivors was called the cynodonts, based on their doglike teeth. These fairly small predators were common in their time and have left a rich fossil record. While they are not classified as true mammals, they are the close ancestors of mammals and likely exhibited a number of mammalian features.

For one, there is good evidence that they were warm blooded. John Allman (1999) argues that much of mammalian evolution was jumpstarted by both the benefits and requirements of internal temperature regulation. In contrast to the sea environment, life on land involved significant shifts in temperature. This is highly problematic for the body's biochemistry as all the chemical reactions upon which the body depends (e.g., metabolism, respiration) require a constant temperature. And because these processes are inter-dependent and rely on various positive and negative feedback loops, a small perturbation can have very large effects. Hence some animals became warm blooded, allowing the body to maintain control over its own temperature via a process of negative feedback loops. But as with all else in life, being warm blooded entails trade-offs. Temperature homeostasis requires an enormous amount of energy. Allman states that birds and mammals, who are both warm blooded, expend 5–10 times as much energy as cold-blooded reptiles. Hence a range of adaptations followed to enable warm blooded animals to thrive. These included improved sensory abilities (particularly sense of smell or olfaction), differentiated types of teeth to bite, grind and chew better, anatomical changes supporting simultaneous breathing and chewing, a curled-up sleeping position to preserve heat, and of most interest to our purposes, parental care.[2] The energy requirements of temperature self-regulation, growth and development were too much for juvenile cynodonts to satisfy on their own. Hence maternal care provided warmth as well as food. A range of evidence points to parental care in cynodonts, including the fossilized remains of a small cynodont nestled next to a larger one. Additionally, the shape of the cynodont skull suggests well developed muscles around the snout and lips, which could be used for suckling mothers' milk.

Parental Care

Parental care became central to mammals' survival, a critical adaptation to their environment. In fact, mammals are named for their mammary glands, the body parts through which mothers feed their infants. Mammary glands evolved out of sweat glands, which serve to cool the body, another link between parental care and temperature regulation. Because parental care was so important to mammalian survival, numerous additional adaptations arose to support and facilitate it, including specific motivational/emotional systems in both the mother and infant.

As maternal care is extremely costly for the mother in terms of energy and time expended, she needs to be powerfully motivated to take the time and effort to care for her infant. She needs overriding motivation to make sure to do it. Hence, we see strong maternal attachment to infants across mammalian species. Likewise, infants' very survival depends on their mother's care, so they also need powerful motivation to seek out their mother, maintain close contact and elicit her care. As separation from the mother could easily mean death, infants developed strong aversive emotional responses to separation, expressed in vigorous distress calls. Moreover, parental care appears to be the foundation out of which many other types of social bonds later evolved, including pair bonding and family groupings.

Jaak Panksepp studied the neurobiology of emotion for many decades. Specifically, he detailed how the primary emotional/motivational systems of CARE and PANIC serve to promote maternal and infant attachment, respectively. These systems, found in all mammals, operate largely in the older and more ventral (lower) parts of the forebrain with involvement of the midbrain. In humans they are elaborated at the level of the cortex.

Relatedly, the work of John Bowlby and the subsequent field of attachment research have documented the powerful role of infant attachment and separation distress in humans. More recent work has shown the formative impact of early mother-child attachment well into adulthood. In fact, multiple research domains in psychology converge to support the central role of early attachment experiences in overall personality development. Thus, we now arrive at a point in our journey where evolutionary developments are directly related to human personality structure.

Now a note about birds. Birds also provide parental care to their young. Further, some species exhibit long-term pair bonding and paternal involvement in tending the young. However, as the common ancestor of birds and mammals probably did not exhibit parental care, it is likely that these behaviors evolved separately in birds and mammals.

What parts of the brain are involved with parental care? The female hormones estrogen, prolactin, and progesterone are related to maternal behavior in mammals, particularly right before and after giving birth. In this way, hormones related to the female reproductive system are also involved with maternal care. In fact, Panksepp suggests that the CARE system in mammals evolved from sexual motivational systems present in ancestral reptiles. The neuropeptide oxytocin plays a particularly important role in maternal care as well as other types of social bonds. Consequently, the brain regions that manufacture oxytocin, including parts of the hypothalamus and the extended amygdala, are central to maternal care. Both of these regions fall within lower (ventral) and older regions of the forebrain. Additionally, oxytocin links up to the dopaminergic reward and endogenous opioid systems, which mediate desire and pleasure (or pain relief), respectively. Thus, oxytocin connects desire and pleasure to interpersonal bonds.

In terms of the infant's bonds with the mother, many of the same regions are involved. However, infants' distress at separation is also an important part of the system. This seems to be linked to older pain and distress regions in the midbrain, specifically the periaqueductal grey. In this case, the emotional pain of loss and separation seems to have evolved out of older systems that process physical pain from bodily injury.

In sum, the attachment system in mammals evolved out of older emotional/motivational systems for fight/flight and appetitive drives (food, sex) that were present even in fish. Subsequently, the entire complex of social emotions in humans evolved out of mammalian parental care. It is the position of this book that these social emotions form the basis of human personality structure, with early attachment experiences playing a pivotal role. As this position is not universally held, it will be explored in depth in the next chapter.

But when mammals first came on the scene about 200 mya, they were not the dominant group of animals. It was only after the extinction of the dinosaurs about 65 mya that the mammalian class came into its own. This success led to a great diversification into a plethora of new subclasses, genera,[3] and species. Today's mammals range in size from the tiny mouse to the gigantic blue whale. They live on the ground, in the trees, in water and in caves at the edge of cliffs. They walk, swim and fly. Their social organization also diversified, with some mammals retaining simple mother-infant bonds and little additional social interactions except during breeding times (platypuses, moles, leopards) while others live in large, complex social groups with dominance hierarchies, alliances, and cooperative behavior (baboons, wolves, elephants, and humans). Pair bonds are also found in some mammalian species, in which males and females cooperate in the raising of the young. Some may mate for life, like gibbons and humans.

As these social structures evolved into greater complexity, the brain evolved in concert, providing greater ability to process social cues and a broader repertoire of social behaviors. Emotional/motivational systems also evolved to facilitate new social interactions, including dominance hierarchies, cooperative endeavors, emotional communication, and social play.

Fixed Action Patterns

Early emotional/motivational systems were fairly fixed reactions to stimuli, what animal behaviorists call fixed action patterns and what is colloquially referred to as instincts. There is a pre-set reaction to a specific type of stimulus. The animal does not have a goal in mind, just an urge to behave a particular way to a specific stimulus. Because of this stimulus-bound quality, there is not always goal correction when there is a mismatch between the behavior and the result. For example, cats are well known to cover their urine and feces. This likely serves to hide their tracks from predators. However, the cat is not *aware* that this is the purpose, it just feels an *urge* to perform a behavior in the context of a stimulus. When the behavior is completed, there is likely a reduction in tension, a sense of "OK, I'm done now." For example, I once owned a cat that used to jump into my bathtub after defecating in her kitty litter. She would energetically scrape at the bathtub walls until satisfied and then happily run out of the room, leaving her feces in the kitty litter entirely exposed. She made no connection between the goal of her behavior and its actual outcome. In humans, however, most of our behavior is goal-oriented. We have a goal in mind when we embark upon an action. Nonetheless, we do see re-emergence of fixed action patterns in human psychiatric disorders, such as obsessive-compulsive disorder and trichotillomania, a disorder of hair-pulling. The re-emergence of even more primitive reflex behaviors is shown in frontal release signs, a symptom of brain deterioration that occurs in severe dementia.

Learning and Memory

Nonetheless, mammals do learn and remember. They are not automatons without any mental processes at all. In fact, some forms of memory have been present for hundreds of millions of years. In 2000, Eric Kandel won the Nobel prize for his work on memory in the humble sea slug. He showed that a learned change in behavior was mediated by structural changes at the neuron's synapse. This process reflects habituation, the ceasing of a reflex response after a certain amount of repetition, and is perhaps the most primitive form of learning. Motor skill learning is another important form of learning, and is processed to a large degree in the striatum or basal ganglia, a region of the forebrain. This involves the learning of behavioral routines or motor programs. In humans this is subsumed under the category of procedural memory (how to do something) and is mediated by the striatum, thalamus, and cortex. Episodic memory is a more advanced form of memory and likely arose later in evolution. This includes explicit, conscious memory of lived events.

In mammals, one of the most common forms of learning is called *classical conditioning*, which was first studied by Ivan Pavlov in his research on dogs and salivation responses in the late 19th and early 20th century. Classical conditioning involves the pairing of a neutral cue with an emotionally salient stimulus. In this way the previously neutral cue now elicits the same emotional or behavioral reaction that the salient stimulus originally did. For example, dogs can learn that leashes spell going for a walk; cats can learn that the sight of the vacuum cleaner signals a loud and terrifying noise. In response to these conditioned stimuli, dogs will jump up and down and run in circles, while cats will run away and hide under the bed.

In classical conditioning the cue and the salient stimulus must be presented simultaneously. There is little to no delay between neutral or *conditioned* cue and the salient or *unconditioned* stimulus. In this way, the animal does not need to recall the conditioned stimulus, it only has to recognize it. It doesn't need to think about the leash or the vacuum cleaner, it only has to react when faced with it. Therefore, the animal does not need to maintain a mental representation of the stimulus outside of the immediate experience of it.

Classical conditioning is mediated by a range of subcortical regions in the lower and older parts of the forebrain. Fear conditioning is mediated by the amygdala as has been shown in the work of Joseph LeDoux. Reward conditioning, that is recognition of cues that signal desired rewards, is mediated by the dopaminergic reward system. This is a tract of dopamine neurons that course from the ventral tegmental area in the midbrain to the nucleus accumbens in the basal forebrain (a specific area in the lower, frontal forebrain). The dopaminergic reward system underlies the desire to pursue any rewarding stimuli, such as food, sex, or even crossword puzzles if you happen to like them. This system is also involved with addictions. During addiction, the dopamine reward system is co-opted by the object of addiction, which becomes the only thing the person desires, an extreme and pathological form of classical conditioning.

Operant conditioning is another type of learning and is associated with the work of B. F. Skinner. This occurs when the *consequence* of an animal's behavior, that is whether the behavior is rewarded or punished, determines the likelihood of the animal repeating the behavior. Reward increases the likelihood of the animal repeating the behavior while punishment decreases it. Operant conditioning is generally considered more advanced than classical conditioning because it affects volitional, intentional behavior rather than reflexive responses. It is not found in as many phyla as is classical conditioning. Feinberg and Mallat state that operant conditioning involves a range of ancient subcortical regions but that it also seems to be dependent on cortical regions. Rats who have been decorticated, that is their cortex has been disconnected from lower brain regions, are still able to learn by classical conditioning but not by operant conditioning.

Of note, in operant conditioning, the behavior and its consequences are frequently separated in time. In fact, operant conditioning loses its potency as the time between the behavior and the consequence increases. Therefore, if the consequence does not immediately follow the behavior, the animal has to maintain a mental representation of the behavior in order to connect it to the consequence. It has to keep the behavior in mind. Such mental representations of behaviors and behavioral goals are largely mediated by the frontal lobe. Indeed, the orbital frontal cortex, a region on the underside of the cortex, above the eyeballs, has been implicated in the ability to control or correct behavior in response to rewards and punishment, particularly when the nature of rewards and punishments changes (Rolls, 2004).

Even in higher animals, operant conditioning is not equally prevalent across species. Cats respond fairly well to training by classical conditioning but less so to operant conditioning. Dogs, however, respond very well to operant conditioning which is why they are trained with dog treats. Desired behavior receives a dog treat, which encourages more of that behavior. Likewise, operant conditioning is the dominant form of conditioning used in training human children.

Both classical and operant conditioning are utilized in psychotherapy for a range of conditions, such as anxiety disorders and impulse control problems. However, as will be discussed in later chapters, these forms of learning fall at a lower level of mind/brain organization than do interpersonal representations. They fall below personality per se. When using these techniques with personality disordered patients, therefore, therapists are not treating personality pathology itself, but rather its top-down effects.

Primates

With the emergence of primates, significant changes take place that move us much closer towards the human mind/brain. Primates, who evolved about 55 mya, started out as tiny arboreal mammals, climbing across tree branches and feeding on fruits, insects, and likely small vertebrates, such as lizards. The first group of primates are known as prosimians, and include the living species of tarsiers, lemurs, galagos, and lorises. "Prosimian" means before the monkeys. Monkeys evolved in Africa about 37 to 30 mya, followed by apes, who arrived on the scene about 17 mya.

Primates diverged from other mammals in two important ways, likely as an adaptation to their niche as arboreal predators. They developed large, forward-facing eyes with concomitant expansion of the visual processing regions in their cortex. This allowed primates to see further and to detect motion more sensitively. Overlapping visual fields for each eye permitted enhanced depth perception. Primates also developed color vision, which would have come in handy when distinguishing fruit from leaves. In this way, the primary sensory modality shifted from olfaction (smell) to vision. Indeed, the olfactory bulb is far smaller in primates' brains than in those of many other mammalian species.

Another key development was long and physically separate fingers, nails rather than claws, and opposable thumbs.[4] This allowed primates to traverse the branches with ease and to scamper across the tops of trees in search of fruit and prey. The integration of manual dexterity and visual acuity led to better visual-motor coordination. This expanded primates' options for interacting with the environment, including the capacity for reaching, grasping, and defensive maneuvers. Ultimately this led to tool use.

These anatomical changes required modifications in the brain to support new abilities. With primates, we see a series of very important developments that take us a long way on our journey towards the human mind/brain. In general, we see significantly larger brain to body ratios. Specifically, there was rapid growth of the telencephalon. Mainly this was reflected in expansion and elaboration of the neocortex, the 6-layer tissue that is only found in mammals. Visual areas as well as sensory and motor areas, particularly of the hand, also expanded and became more complex. Additionally, and of great relevance to our purposes, the prefrontal cortex expanded. This is the region that processes complex social information. It is also the site of cognition per se, which involves the capacity to create representations of the environment that can be held in mind and acted upon mentally. This capacity allows for much more complex and variegated behaviors.

To a lesser extent, primates also expanded the inner regions of their cortex, known as the limbic lobe (Elston, 2007). These include the cortical areas that circle the thalamus, an egg-shaped structure that sits atop the midbrain. The whole notion of the limbic system is controversial in neuroscience and there are as many definitions of it as there are neuroscientists. However, a ring of structures around the thalamus, including the cingulate gyrus and the hippocampal regions, appear to have expanded and elaborated in primates and thereby enhance primates' processing of emotion and memory.

Thus, we see complex elaboration of the brain systems underlying emotional/motivational systems. These systems became better integrated with learning and memory, which is critical for ongoing social relationships. Importantly, these developments *build upon* the earlier emotional systems of the midbrain and ventral forebrain but do not replace them. Both older and newer systems work together as an integrated whole.

Advances in Cognition

As noted above, we see a leap in cognitive abilities in primates. This is typically attributed to expansion of the frontal cortex but I will also suggest that it is linked to changes in the nature of memory. Specifically, we see elaboration of the capacity for *episodic memory*. At some point in primate evolution, episodic memory grew towards the form we see in humans. Now let's take a moment to focus on memory as this has profound implications for the development of human personality structure. In humans, cognitive psychologists distinguish between declarative and non-declarative memory. Declarative memory is accessible to consciousness. It includes both episodic and semantic memory. Episodic memory refers to memory of personally experienced events, while semantic memory refers to knowledge about facts, words, concepts and information. Episodic memory also includes autobiographical memory—knowledge about what happened to the self. Non-declarative memory stores information about how to do things. It is not dependent on consciousness. Examples include procedural, conditioning, and priming memory. The forms of memory discussed earlier in the chapter, classical conditioning, operant conditioning, and muscle memory, are included in this category (c.f. Fujii & Suzuki, 2009).

Non-declarative memory likely evolved earlier than declarative memory and is observable in phylogenetically older and simpler animals. This type of memory is mediated by subcortical structures, such as the nucleus accumbens, amygdala, and basal ganglia. Declarative memory (and episodic memory in particular) is more complex and likely a more recent evolutionary phenomenon, although more rudimentary forms of episodic memory are evident in many species (Allen & Fortin, 2013). Episodic memory is mediated by the hippocampus, a part of the limbic lobe. In many species, the hippocampus plays a role in place memory, allowing animals to remember where they encountered either rewarding or aversive stimuli. For example, it helps rats remember how to navigate mazes.

More recently, the hippocampus evolved towards more elaborated forms of episodic memory, including detailed memories of lived events and autobiographical information. Damage to the hippocampus in humans prevents creation of episodic memory but does not prevent other kinds of memory, such as fear conditioning. The phylogenetic recency of episodic memory is further supported by its relatively late arrival in childhood. Babies are not born with intact episodic memory; it typically matures during the 3rd to 5th year of life. Think about your earliest memory. Can you remember anything before the age of 2? Or even 3?

Many theorists believe that concepts, that is abstract ideas about our self and the world, derive from episodic memory. Before you can form ideas about an event, you need to remember what happened. The capacity for concepts underlies the enormous intellectual achievements of homo sapiens. I maintain that it also underlies the structure of human personality, in that personality is based on concepts of interpersonal relationships. Thus, at some point in primate evolution, we see movement towards the cognitive complexity necessary for human personality, both healthy and pathological.

But let us return to the evolution of primates. How do these changes in cognitive capacities affect primate behavior?

Advances in Social Behavior

For one, there are significant developments in primates' social abilities. Primates have larger and more complex social groups. There are multiple generations within a troop; juveniles do not automatically leave the social group upon maturity as in many other mammals. As such, infants have relationships with a range of family members and not just with their mother and littermates. Juvenile primates have relationships with older siblings, cousins, aunts, and grandparents as well as their own fathers. Keeping track of these relationships requires increased socio-emotional processing capability as well as enhanced memory for faces and emotionally significant interactions. For example, primates need to keep track of which animal was friendly or hostile in what circumstance.

Within their larger, more complex social groups, primates also have to negotiate dominance or status hierarchies. These are found in both males and females and have transgenerational implications. In various monkey species, the offspring of high-status females are at an advantage compared to offspring of lower status females. The troops also have a network of sometimes shifting alliances. Grooming behaviors serve as bonding rituals to cement alliances or gain favor with higher status troop members. The forward-facing eyes also make it easier to read subtle changes in facial expression. Indeed, primates have evolved a greater number of facial muscles to produce a broader palette of facial expressions than is found in other mammals. Again, increased memory and cognitive capacities help primates track these events and respond accordingly.

Most primate females give birth to singletons rather than litters. Moreover, primate young tend to have a longer time to maturity. This way infants spend more time in close proximity with their mother and benefit from her exclusive attention. This allows infants to learn from their mother as well as from the other members of the troop. Likewise, postnatal brain development occurs more slowly in primates and is more dependent on environmental input. In this way, primates are more dependent on *learning* than are most other mammals. This reliance on learning (which is dependent on sophisticated memory capacities) is a defining feature in humans.

Because of the complex social organization, individual animals need to understand their own place in a network of social roles. They need some kind of representation, or concept, of the self in the social world. We can speculate that this task marks the beginning of emotionally colored self- and other-representations, a central element of human personality.

Tool Use

The combination of cognitive development, visual-motor coordination and fine motor coordination produced significant changes in primates' capacity to manipulate the *non-social* world as well. In a remarkable move forward, primates show the beginning of instrumental tool use and cultural learning. A range of primate species are known to use simple tools. Capuchin monkeys use rocks to open nuts and chimpanzees strip branches to poke into termite mounds, a task called "termite fishing." Primates also learn new skills from observing others. For example, a troop of Japanese macaques taught each other to wash sweet potatoes. This is a critically important advance because it shows the beginnings of cultural evolution. Behavior can change through culture and not just genetic mutations.

As noted above, primates are more intelligent than many other mammal species, a product of the expansion of their cerebral cortex as well as their limbic lobe. Many primates show the basic capacity for thought, that is the ability to maintain and manipulate mental representations (or concepts) of objects and events that are not immediately present. This is the beginning of a conscious sense of *time*, of the future and the past. This capacity is illustrated in a charming video, easily searchable on Youtube, in which a baboon in a zoo shows amazement when a magic trick confounds its expectations. In another video, an orangutan bursts into what can only be called laughter when surprised by a magic trick. These animals have an expectation of what will happen next based on what has led up to the present moment. When the magic trick contradicts their expectations, they have an emotional reaction of surprise coupled with anger or even delight.

Great Apes

The superfamily of hominoids, otherwise known as apes, evolved around 17 mya. Apes are divided into two families, the lesser apes, which encompass the various gibbon species, and the great apes, which include orangutans, gorillas, chimpanzees, bonobos, and humans. In other words, not only are great apes our closest living relatives, but we ourselves are great apes. Of these species, we are most closely related to chimpanzees, with whom we share approximately 98.8 percent of our genes. We share 98.4 percent of our genes with gorillas, and 96.9 percent with orangutans. In comparison, we share about 99.9 percent with other humans, 93 percent with rhesus monkeys, and 75 percent with chickens (Potts & Sloan, 2010). The family of great apes (Hominidae in Latin and hominids in English) evolved about 14 mya (Ayala & Cela-Conde, 2017).

In apes we see ongoing progression towards larger brains, increased social and emotional sophistication, enhanced manual dexterity and greater intelligence. Besides humans and gorillas, all apes are at least partly arboreal although many apes are also at home on the ground. Anatomically, apes are generally larger than other primates and have lost their tails. Apes also have longer arms and greatly enhanced shoulder rotation, such that they can lift their arms above their shoulder. This allows them to swing from branches with grace and ease. Thus in apes, manual dexterity seems to have overshadowed the reliance on prehensile feet and tails for negotiating the forest. While neither humans nor gorillas swing from branches, it is likely their shoulder structure evolved from the same arboreal adaptation. Thus most apes have long arms, highly sensitive and dexterous hands, and shorter legs. When walking on the ground, this pushes their torso upright, so that their spine is almost vertical. In contrast, most other mammals walk with their backs horizontally aligned, parallel to the ground. This foreshadows a momentous change in later human evolution, the shift to bipedalism or to walking on two feet. While all great apes can walk on two feet, non-human apes typically prefer to use their arms in a kind of knuckle walk.

The move towards bipedalism offered a number of advantages. Primarily, it freed the hands for gestures as well as for carrying, catching and manipulating objects and ultimately for greater tool use. With the enhanced shoulder rotation, apes can also throw objects effectively. We see this in aggressive displays among orangutans, chimpanzees, and gorillas. This strengthened ability to manually affect the environment has been credited as a prime factor shaping brain evolution in humans.

Brain evolution in apes followed the trajectory first shown in other primates. There was an increase in brain size and complexity. We also see a notable increase in crenellations (wrinkles) in the neocortex, which provides an efficient way to increase surface area in a small cranium. In this way, the brain can expand dramatically without requiring a much larger skull.

The time to maturity in the great apes is longer than in other primates. Chimpanzees, orangutans, and gorillas reach full maturity in their mid-teens whereas macaques (a monkey species) do so in about half that time. This means that brain growth continues for a decade and a half after birth during which time the brain is significantly shaped by environmental input. Thus, all great apes are heavily dependent upon learning.

Relatedly, in ape species we see progressive complexity of social organization and capabilities. Communication becomes more complex. While monkeys show a range of facial expressions, the facial expressions of (non-human) great apes are more subtle and nuanced. In fact, they are remarkably human-like.

We also see tremendous growth in cognitive capacities. As noted above, the prefrontal cortex mediates the creation of concepts, representations of an object or event that can held in mind even when the stimulus is not present. To a much larger degree than with other primates, apes' understanding of their environment is removed from the constraints of space and time. Remarkably, the (non-human) great apes have demonstrated the capacity for language. They do not appear to create language on their own but they have shown the ability to learn when taught from a young age by humans. Koko the gorilla and Washoe the chimpanzee provide two well-known examples. Non-human apes cannot speak as they do not have the vocal apparatus, but they can learn to recognize symbols and to arrange them to express original thoughts.

Language is modular and combinatory. This means that it is composed of small parts that can be combined in virtually infinite ways to express unlimited ideas. While many animal species have a variety of vocalizations and behaviors that communicate important information, these modes of communication are largely fixed. They cannot be combined and rearranged to create novel ideas. The gorilla Koko, who learned manual sign language, was even reported to lie. In a particularly amusing example, she blamed another trainer for damage she caused to her own sink, signing, "Kate there bad." This means that she was able to separate the expressed idea from the known event to the extent that she could deliberately falsify her communication. Additionally, her ability to distinguish what *she* knows about a specific event from what *someone else* might know speaks to some capacity for theory of mind, a critical achievement in human development and one that is highly relevant for personality development. It must be noted, however, that these observations have been questioned and it is possible that non-human ape behavior is not as sophisticated as these reports suggest. Nonetheless, it seems safe to conclude that within these close cousins of ours, we see the precursors to our own extraordinarily complex linguistic capabilities.[5]

Likewise, non-human great apes demonstrate increased use of tools. For example, chimpanzees use different types of tools to fish for ants or termites, to pull water out of an enclosure, to crack open nuts and to access objects that are out of reach. In a 2010 study, Gruber and colleagues list 52 tool use behaviors in chimpanzees and/or bonobos. Tools were used in the context of feeding, play, grooming, aggressive encounters, and even sexual stimulation. Moreover, tool use is often performed in multigenerational family groups, providing opportunities for juveniles to learn critical skills.

We also see sophisticated problem solving in non-human great apes. The gestalt psychologist Wolfgang Kohler was interested in insight learning. He wanted to show that learning can take place holistically and not solely step by step via classical or operant conditioning. Kohler successfully demonstrated this in chimpanzees, such that they would figure out how to stack boxes on top of each other in order to reach bananas hanging from the ceiling. In chapter 8, we will consider this same kind of insight learning in the practice of psychotherapy.

Finally, some non-human great apes show a clear concept of self. This is demonstrated by the mirror test, in which a mark is made on the animal's face. Animals who understand that the mirror reflects their own body will touch their face when shown their reflection. Animals who do not understand this touch the image in the mirror, ignore it altogether, or even growl at it as if at another animal. Animals from all great ape species have passed this test though the pass rate varies across species. Most other animals do not pass the test. Even human children do not typically pass it until around 18 months. As mentioned before, the development of a self-concept is a critical milestone in the journey towards a human personality structure.

Now let's consider for a moment what we mean by a concept of self. There are many aspects to self-representation. We can assume that all sentient animals have a bodily sense of self; they know where their body starts and stops in space and that their sensory/motor experiences are located within their bodies. In all vertebrates, the brain creates a seamless experience of body moving through space by mapping and remapping sensory information. But that is very different from a *concept* of self, which refers to an idea that can be thought about separate from the immediate sensory/motor experience. This is why the mirror test is so powerful, because it beautifully separates those animals with a concept of self from those without. It also shows us how this aspect of interpersonal representation is a veritable newcomer in evolutionary terms, unlike the core affective systems which are far, far older. It is also important to note that our capacity to *feel* emotions long predated our capacity to *label* them with language. As we shall see, the varying phylogenetic ages of these different psychological capacities are highly pertinent to the psychotherapy of personality disorders.

Hominins to Humans

There is surprisingly little consensus as to how to classify recent human ancestors in the evolutionary tree. I will use the solution suggested by Ayala and Cela-Conde (2017). The family of Hominidae includes great apes and humans. The subfamily of Homininae includes chimpanzees and the human lineage. About 6 mya, the ancestral lines of humans and chimpanzees diverged. The resulting human lineage is classified under the tribe of *Hominini* and that of chimpanzees under the tribe of Panini. There have been multiple genera in the Hominini tribe, most of which have led to dead ends. The two genera most relevant to us are Australopithecus and Homo.

At the current moment in evolution, we are the only hominins (members of Hominini tribe) left. All other hominin species are extinct.[6] Because we are the only remaining species or even genus of this tribe, we cannot compare our brains or behavior with sister species. Instead, we examine the fairly sparse record of skeletal remains and material found nearby. Further, although we cannot measure the brains of our hominin ancestors directly, we can create what is called endocasts from their skulls. In the past 20 years, we have also been able to analyze genetic material from earlier hominin bones.

What do we know about our hominin ancestors? Several genera preceded Australopithecus. These included Sahelanthropus, Ororrin, and Ardipithicus, who lived between 7 and 4.4 mya in East Africa. About 4 mya, Australopithicus emerged in East Africa and ultimately spread to a wider region. The genus Homo likely evolved from Australopithicus about 2.6 mya. Homo species were avid travelers. Even prior to Homo sapiens, they dispersed out of Africa to cover much of Eurasia.

The major change from the great apes to hominins was the move towards bipedalism. Earlier hominins remained partly arboreal, with long ape-like arms and shorter legs. However, as they evolved towards more consistent bipedalism, they transferred from the trees to the ground, eventually able to walk long distances across the savannahs of East Africa. As the hominins became more fully bipedal, a number of anatomical changes occurred. They grew longer legs and proportionately shorter arms. Further, the shape of the pelvis changed to support their new posture, a development with far reaching impact.

The new pelvis was narrower than the ape pelvis, providing less room in the birth canal for the infant's head. This reinforced the earlier trajectory for infants to be born with incomplete brain development, requiring even more neural development to take place after birth. Consider that macaques achieve 65 percent final cranium capacity at birth, chimps 40.5 percent, and humans only 23 percent. With so much development occurring after birth, the brains of hominins were that much more shaped by the post-natal environment, particularly the mother-infant relationship. In this way, children became acculturated to the world they were born into. This process allowed for much more rapid adaptations to changing environments than can happen through genetic evolution alone. As above, hominins traveled across wide distances. We can speculate that their enhanced dependence on learning facilitated this process.

One fascinating method by which hominins evolved bigger brains was through the process of *pedomorphy*. In his 1977 book, Stephen Jay Gould suggested that evolutionary changes typically occur through alterations in the *timing* of embryonic development, either by speeding it up or slowing it down. In hominins, the rate of skull development was greatly slowed, so that adults preserved infantile cranial proportions. In other words, adult human heads are shaped like babies' heads. If we compare the adult and juvenile skulls of humans and chimpanzees, we see that the heads of human adults resemble those of the juveniles of both species more than it resembles adult chimpanzees. Likewise, the infant chimpanzee is morphologically more similar to the adult human than to the adult of its own species. Infants of both species have small, flat, vertically aligned faces with small jaws, high foreheads and large brain cases. So do adult humans. In contrast, adult chimpanzees have horizontally-aligned faces with large, protuberant jaws, low foreheads and proportionately smaller brain cases. Across the 6 to 7 million years of hominin evolution, hominin heads progressively transformed from an ape-like skull towards the more infantile skull of modern humans. Concomitantly, their brain size more than tripled.

Brain size did not increase that much in Australopithecines, only taking off after the Homo genus appeared on the scene. Australopithecus brains ranged from about 400 to 500 cubic centimeters (cc). Homo habilis (handy man) lived from about 2.3 to 1.6 mya and had a brain size of about 600–700 cc. Homo erectus (standing man) lived from about 1.8 mya to 300 thousand years ago (kya) with a brain size about 900–1100 cc. Homo erectus is associated with the use of fire, more elaborate hand axe technology, and seasonal base camps. They also had the first major migration out of Africa. Homo neanderthalensis (Neanderthals) lived from about 300 to 50 kya. Their brain size was actually larger than that of modern humans, about 1600 cc. They likely shared some advanced cognitive capacities with our own species, such as use of symbols, burial of the dead, and decoration of artifacts. Our species, Homo sapiens, emerged about 200 kya and has an average brain size of about 1300 cc. More specifically, across hominin evolution, both the frontal and temporal lobes expanded and became more crenellated.

In concert with this relatively rapid brain growth, intellectual capacities mushroomed. Despite lack of direct evidence of hominin cognition, we have a fairly extensive record of tool making practices. As far back as Australopithecines, we find large caches of stone tools. Hand axes were chipped off of flint cores. This differs from the tool use found in apes in important ways. For one, hominins used tools to make tools. In this way, we have the onset of *technology*. Also, central tool making sites suggest that tools were made in advance of their use, reflecting significant planning. Evidently, tools were carried to the kill site to cut, scrape, chop or hit. Further, the widespread use of these tools points to cultural transmission of this technology. The Olduwan technology dates back to about 2.6 mya. Acheulean technology, which produced larger and more carefully shaped hand axes, dates back to about 1.7 mya. Both technologies originated in East Africa.

The use of fire to cook food, provide heat and protect against predators also dates far back in hominin history. While there is strong evidence of fireplaces and hearths from about 700 thousand years ago (kya), the intentional and controlled use of fire may date back as far as 1.5 mya. Cooking expanded hominins' nutritional options considerably. It also supported more planned and socially organized eating practices.

About 500 kya, hominin technology took a fairly rapid jump in complexity, with evidence of wood spears, bone fishing hooks, and big game hunting. The use of pigments and bone needles to sew clothes followed. There was another leap in technology about 100 kya, well after the emergence of Homo sapiens. Within the last 100,000 years, unmistakably symbolic and artistic creations appeared, including stunningly beautiful and realistic paintings of large game in the caves of Europe from about 40 kya. Even Neanderthals, with whom we interbred to some extent, exhibited symbolic and ritualistic behavior, with burial of the dead and geometric markings on objects.

In our own time, humans have developed extraordinarily complex technology, based on entirely abstract concepts of things we cannot even see or touch (i.e., physics). This technological complexity relied upon the huge expansion of our neocortex across hominin evolution and its resultant intellectual development (See Figure 2.5). At the core of Homo sapiens' intelligence lies the capacity to create and manipulate concepts, mental representations of events and objects that can be separated in space and time from the events they depict. This allows us to anticipate the future and reflect upon the past. We can also imagine multiple alternative courses of action before acting, and consider the consequences of each one. Additionally, we can conceptualize recursively; we can have ideas about ideas and again about those ideas. In this way, our ideas grow increasingly abstract. Further we are capable of metacognition; we can think about thinking. We can also introspect; we can think about feeling. In this way, our conceptual abilities can regulate our cognitive, emotional, and behavioral responses in a top-down fashion. And it is in the interplay between these recently evolved conceptual abilities and our much older emotional and behavioral systems where we find personality.

We do not currently have the methods to establish when language first emerged in hominins but it was likely a gradual process that preceded Homo sapiens. It is hard to imagine the complex technology of Homo erectus and Neanderthals without the aid of language. Nevertheless, language clearly emerged after basic conceptual abilities were well established. In fact, language helps us elaborate, manipulate and communicate concepts. Thus, language can modify our core interpersonal representations in a top-down manner. Indeed, this is exactly what we do in the psychotherapy of personality pathology.

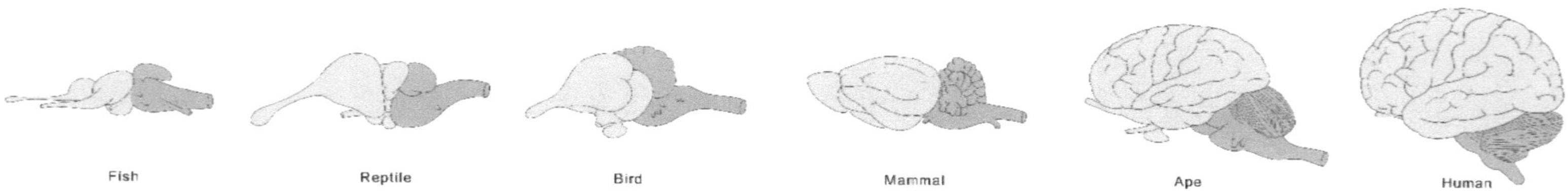

Figure 2.5. Evolution from fish to humans. Evolutionary changes in brain size and shape from fish to humans. Note how the forebrain enlarges and becomes more crenellated, eventually dominating the entire brain. Also note the proportional reduction of the olfactory bulb, the large protruding structure in the front of the brain. Aldona Griskeviciene. Shutterstock.

We have now reached the end of our journey through evolution. We have seen how over 3 billion years of evolution has produced the almost inconceivably complex, emergent system that is the human mind/brain. At different points across evolution, different brain structures emerged with their own associated behavioral systems. Later brain and behavioral structures arose on top of these earlier systems, as elaborations upon them. In general, developments progressed from the back of the brain to the front and from the bottom to the top. Our current mind/brain encompasses the totality of these systems and the interactions between them. The hierarchical structure of the human mind/brain therefore reflects the remarkable story of its entire phylogenetic history.

Ontogeny and Phylogeny

We can now ask how evolution is reflected in the development of the individual organism. In other words, how is *phylogeny* reflected in *ontogeny*? In the late 19th century, a German biologist named Ernst Haeckel popularized the idea that ontogeny recapitulates phylogeny. In other words, you can figure out the entire evolution of a species by looking at the earliest developmental stages of the modern animal. This is particularly evident in the embryonic stages. In fact, the earliest embryonic stages of the human, dog, chicken and even lizard look pretty much alike. It is only in the later stages of embryonic development that the species-specific traits become apparent.

Haeckel was a very good popularizer of science and the idea was intrinsically intriguing. The theory of evolution was still quite new and the thought that we could peer into our ancient history just by taking apart chicken eggs hit a nerve in the culture. Haeckel's theory spread widely and influenced many areas of the contemporary popular culture. Haeckel was right about the general principle; how animals develop does tell us something about how their species evolved, particularly in the earliest stages of development. However, he got a lot of the details wrong. It often happens that dominant theories later shown to be erroneous are treated very poorly after their fall from grace and Haeckel's theory was thrown into disrepute for most of the 20th century.

In 1977, another great popularizer of science, Stephen Jay Gould, brought attention back to the relationship between phylogeny and ontogeny. He reviewed Haeckel's work as well as that of his contemporaries and reconceptualized the relationship between phylogeny and ontogeny.

In particular, he noted how the earliest stages of ontogeny are most *conserved* across evolution, such that the earliest developmental stages of an animal are likely to reflect earlier stages in the evolution of its species. Why is this so? Because the earliest stages are the most fundamental; they create the foundation out of which all later stages develop. Mutations in these foundational structures have the most far-reaching effect and thus have most potential to destroy the entire organism. Think about a stack of blocks. It is much more dangerous to the integrity of the stack to remove a block on the bottom than on the top. Therefore, early stages in development tend to be conservative, and thus maintain their form across the evolution of a species. We will now consider how our phylogeny is reflected in the embryonic development of our brain.

DEVELOPMENT OF HUMAN BRAIN

Brain development in all vertebrates starts out the same way. In the earliest stages of embryonic development, a flat plate is formed. It is composed of three layers, the ectoderm, mesoderm, and endoderm. Some cells divide more rapidly than adjacent cells, which causes the layers of the plate to buckle and fold. The outer layer of the plate, the ectoderm, bends into a furrow until the outer edges of the furrow converge at the top. This forms the *neural tube* which then separates from the rest of the ectoderm. The neural tube is attached to the notochord, which develops into the spine. You may remember the notochord as the defining feature of our phylum, Chordata, dating back about 560 mya.

The neural tube is the initial starting point for the entire brain. At the top of the neural tube, there are three bulges called the hindbrain, midbrain, and forebrain (rhombencephalon, mesencephalon, and prosencephalon, respectively). This same three-part brain structure goes back over 500 mya (See Figure 2.4). The hindbrain is the most conserved across evolution. It develops into the pons, medulla oblongata, and the cerebellum. The pons and medulla are part of the brain stem, which regulates basic physiological processes and connects the brain's motor regions with the body's muscles. The brainstem also contains the reticular activating system, which underlies basic arousal, alertness, and consciousness. It is a narrow tract of neurons that runs through the center of the brainstem into the midbrain. Of relevance to our purposes, the brainstem also contains the cell bodies of key neurotransmitter tracts targeted by psychiatric medication, specifically serotonin and norepinephrine. Finally, the cerebellum is a bulbous structure that hangs off the back of the brainstem. It is involved with motor coordination, balance, and some elements of cognition. (See Figures 2.1 and 2.2 for an illustration of the adult human brain.)

The midbrain is divided into the tectum and the cerebral peduncle. It is less conserved than the hindbrain but more conserved than the forebrain. The tectum is an ancient visual processing region. In humans these areas are termed the inferior and superior colliculi and serve to stabilize eye movements. The cerebral peduncle contains the cell bodies of psychologically relevant neurotransmitters, specifically dopamine and acetylcholine. The periaqueductal grey is also in the midbrain. This plays a key role in our ancient emotional/motivational systems and is particularly involved with pain, fear, and rage responses as well as reproductive behaviors.

Importantly, the periaqueductal grey mediates the *subjective experiences* of these emotional systems as well as the relevant behaviors. For example, stimulation of the proper site in the periaqueductal grey can elicit pure, unadulterated feelings of terror. This is why neuroscientists no longer believe that our subjective experience of emotions, our qualia, so to speak, are a recent development restricted only to humans. Of course, any pet lover has long taken this for granted, but sometimes science takes a while to catch up with everyday knowledge.

Forebrain

The forebrain is where all the evolutionary action has taken place. This is the brain region that has most grown and elaborated across human phylogeny. The forebrain first divides into the *diencephalon* and the *telencephalon*, the former being more ventral (lower) and phylogenetically older. On the neural tube, the diencephalon lies behind the telencephalon. The two main structures of the diencephalon are the *thalamus* and the *hypothalamus*. The thalamus is a big egg-like structure that sits atop the midbrain. It is the gatekeeper for stimulation from the sense organs trying to reach the cortex. It protects our brains from being overwhelmed by sensory stimulation.

The hypothalamus sits just below the thalamus, hence the name *hypo*thalamus. The hypothalamus serves as the master gland and controls hormonal release into the rest of the body. It plays a central role in numerous physical drives, including hunger, thirst, and sexual arousal. It also activates the autonomic nervous system in response to emotional/motivational input. Likewise, it is a critical player in the body's stress response.

The telencephalon takes up the largest part of the brain. This region has changed the most over evolution and contains the most complex neurocircuitry. The telencephalon originally served to process olfaction (smell) and the lowest and oldest part of this region is devoted to processing smell. In humans this is a relatively small area labeled the rhinencephalon. The amygdala, a critically important region in emotional processing, originally evolved as part of the rhinencephalon. In mammals the amygdala became much more elaborated with rich connections to higher and evolutionarily newer regions.

Thus, it is typically grouped with higher level structures associated with emotion (Pabba, 2013).

The *basal ganglia* are a more dorsal and somewhat newer part of the telencephalon. These are a fairly large group of structures, some of which extend back into the brain stem. The basal ganglia are involved with motor behavior and coordination and play a key role in fixed action patterns in both mammals and birds.

The cortex is the largest part of the telencephalon and thereby comprises the largest section of the human brain. In the cortex, neurons are arranged in layers, which allows for an exponential increase in the complexity of neuronal interactions. The allocortex is the lowest and evolutionarily oldest region of the cortex. These regions have 3–4 layers and include olfactory and hippocampal regions. The mesocortex has 3–6 layers and includes the cingulate and the parahippocampal regions. The hippocampus and related regions are involved in memory and the cingulate gyrus is involved in decision making plus other cognitive and affective functions. For simplicity's sake, we will subsume both these regions under the term *limbic lobe*, a collection of cortical structures that serve central roles in processing memory and emotion. The limbic lobe is to be distinguished from the better-known and broader term, *limbic system,* which includes both cortical and subcortical regions involved in emotional processing (e.g., the hypothalamus, amygdala, and septal nuclei).

On top of the limbic lobe and taking up the largest portion of the brain lies the neocortex. This 6-layer neural tissue is found only in mammals and is the newest part of the telencephalon. The neocortex is divided into 4 lobes. The occipital lobe processes visual information, the parietal lobe processes touch and spatial information, and the temporal lobe processes auditory information and memory. The frontal lobe synthesizes input from all other lobes and also has extensive connections with subcortical regions. It processes volitional motor behavior and is the seat of executive functions, which include goal setting and shifting, planning, and response inhibition. The frontal lobe is also the seat of high-level cognition and abstract thought. Importantly, there is a difference between the dorsolateral (upper and outer) regions of the frontal lobe and the ventromedial (lower and inner) regions. The ventromedial regions are closer to the limbic system and play a larger role in emotional processes. The dorsolateral are more task-oriented and instrumental. This is where unemotional cognition (i.e., cold vs. hot cognition; Stein, 2021) is processed. It is likely the ventromedial regions of the frontal lobe that are most involved in interpersonal representations.

The neocortex is divided into two cerebral hemispheres, the right and the left. These hemispheres subserve different cognitive functions. In this way, our brain is *lateralized.* The right hemisphere processes spatial information and non-verbal emotional cues. It is far more involved than the left hemisphere in the processing of interpersonal and emotional information. The left hemisphere controls language. General cognitive processing styles also differ between the two hemispheres, as supported by numerous studies. The left hemisphere favors detail-oriented, sequential, and analytic information-processing, while the right favors holistic pattern recognition. In other words, the left hemisphere breaks the whole into parts and the right synthesizes the parts into an emergent whole. We will revisit this distinction in Chapter 8 when we discuss different modes of psychotherapy.

Systematizing Models

As you can see, the human brain is very complicated and it can be difficult to keep track of all the different structures. In the late 1960s, Paul MacLean proposed a model that consolidated the diverse brain regions into a simple 3-part scheme. His *triune model* posited that the levels of organization of the human brain reflect its evolutionary history. The *reptilian* brain is the oldest (and simplest) of the brain regions and contains the reticular system, midbrain, and basal ganglia. The *paleo-mammalian* region comes next. This contains what he termed the limbic system, a ring of subcortical structures involved in emotion. The limbic system is comprised of the limbic lobe plus the hypothalamus, amygdala, and septum. The *neo-mammalian* region contains the neocortex. While the specifics of MacLean's system have been challenged, the idea of grouping different brain regions according to their phylogenetic history was a seminal contribution.

Jaak Panksepp was heavily influenced by MacLean. As mentioned earlier in this chapter, Panksepp spent decades studying animal emotions. He proposed a three-tiered model of the emotional systems in the human brain, termed the Nested BrainMind Hierarchy. The *primary emotional systems* involve areas of the brain stem, mid-brain, and ventral forebrain. This system mediates genetically-based, largely fixed stimulus-response patterns that date back to the emergence of mammals, if not earlier. The *secondary emotional system* involves higher, subcortical regions, such as the amygdala, and pairs the primary emotional systems with conditioned learning. The *tertiary emotional system* includes the neocortex and superimposes conceptual capacities on top of the two lower emotional systems (Davis & Panksepp, 2018). We will revisit this model in later chapters.

Post-natal Growth

So, what happens to the brain after birth? While the creation and positioning of brain structures take place in utero and are largely genetically controlled, many synaptic connections between neurons take place after birth. These processes are experience-dependent. Myelination of axons is also incomplete at birth and continues for many years afterwards. Myelination of the frontal lobe is not complete until early adulthood.

In general, subcortical development completes before cortical development, which continues for years. Likewise, the cognitive capacities subserved by the neocortex take almost two decades to mature. Indeed, learning and emotional maturation continue throughout life.

The experience-dependent nature of human brain development and the slow maturation of the frontal lobe leave children very vulnerable to psychopathology in deleterious environments. In effect, the child is unable to put stressful events into proper perspective. This is because the emotional systems are going full bore while the cognitive systems are not in place to contain them. Consequently, the child's developing representations of self and others will be flooded by negative emotions that are poorly understood.

We are now ready to turn our attention to the role of interpersonal representations in personality structure. In the next chapter we will review the clinical and neurobiological evidence that supports this relationship and then consider the top-down influence that interpersonal representations exert on cognition, affect and behavior.

NOTES

1. Phylum (phyla in plural) is a classification of species derived from Linnaean taxonomy. It lies below kingdom and above class. Humans are in the chordata phylum.

2. Parental care per se is not unique to mammals. For example, some frogs and toads guard their eggs until they hatch and then transport them into the water. Crocodiles and alligators lay their eggs in nests which they cover with mud and protect from predators (Allport, 1997). Nonetheless, most non-mammalian species do not exhibit parental care much beyond incubation, such that the complexity of parental care in mammals and the length of time devoted to it clearly mark an advance from what came before.

3. Genera is the plural form of genus, which is the Linnaean classification just above species.

4. We see similar adaptations among rodents, who share a common ancestor with primates. The ancestral line of rodents and primates only diverged about 75 mya, more recently than the ancestral lines of cats and dogs diverged from that of primates.

5. After perusing YouTube, I can personally attest to the sophistication of ape communication. In one video, a man at a zoo tosses a banana to an orangutan sitting across a moat from him, perhaps a 15-foot distance. The orangutan catches the banana with one hand and deftly peels it. After finishing the banana, the orangutan holds its right

hand open and face up and looks directly at the man, clearly gesturing for another banana. As the hand is awkwardly placed for catching the banana but excellently placed for communicating a request, the gesture appears more symbolic and communicative than instrumental. When the next banana is not forthcoming, the orangutan pelts the man with a clump of sod. This exchange is repeated until the man runs out of bananas.

6. This is something we may want to keep in mind as we grapple with climate change.

Chapter Three

Interpersonal Representations

Now that we've covered Emergent Systems Theory in Chapter 1 and the evolution of our mind/brain in Chapter 2, it is time to take a closer look at what is meant by interpersonal representations. In this chapter we explore this concept in greater detail. Specifically, we will ask: How do we define the term? What is the history of the concept? What is the empirical evidence to support its role in personality pathology? And what are the possible neurobiological substrates?

DEFINITION OF PERSONALITY: CHARACTER VS. TEMPERAMENT

Let us first consider the definition of personality. In this we will borrow from the work of Robert Cloninger (Cloninger, Svrakic & Przybeck, 1993), who proposes that personality has two components, *temperament* and *character*. Cloninger defined temperament as unlearned response biases to risk, danger, reward and punishment. He saw it as a phylogenetically older system, based in procedural (or nondeclarative) memory, and mediated by cortico-striatal circuits. It is the part of the personality that is most genetically-based and most automatic. Character,[1] in contrast, is a conceptually-based system which filters responses to the environment through perceptions of the self. In other words, it is a system of interpersonal representations. This phylogenetically newer system is based in (potentially) conscious, declarative memory and is mediated by circuits connecting the limbic lobe, neocortex, and older subcortical regions. If you recall from Chapter 2, declarative memory incorporates both episodic memory of lived events and semantic memory of facts, ideas, and language. In Cloninger's view, character is more shaped by the environment than temperament but still has a substantial genetic component.

For our purposes, Cloninger's division of personality into two separate systems, one genetically-based and largely automatic, the other conceptually-based and highly influenced by the environment, marks an important conceptual advance. While we have so far stressed the role of *learned* interpersonal representations in personality pathology, it is important to acknowledge the genetic contributions as well. Indeed, there has been much research into the genetics of personality and the issue of how much is learned vs. inborn is an ongoing and sometimes contentious debate. Cloninger's system offers an elegant resolution to this controversy and one with some support from evolutionary neurobiology, as will be discussed later.

Alternative Models of Personality

In this vein it is worthwhile to consider other frameworks for conceptualizing personality before we delve into the literature on interpersonal representations. The primary alternative to the representational model of personality is one that focuses upon specific personality traits or dimensions. The Big 5 model is the best known of these approaches. The Big 5 refers to five personality dimensions extracted from factor analyses of normal personality traits. In other words, in samples of healthy, nonclinical research subjects, descriptors of personality traits consistently clustered into 5 larger categories of traits, labeled openness to experience, conscientiousness, extraversion, agreeableness, and neuroticism (i.e., OCEAN) (c.f. Matthews, Deary & Whiteman, 2003). Research suggests that the Big 5 model captures much of the individual variation in normal personality traits found in the population and that this system is valid across many different cultures. Moreover, these traits correlate in expectable ways with measures of psychopathology, with neuroticism the most closely associated.

Another trait-based approach to personality or at least to psychology involves the Research Domain Criteria (RDoC), proposed in 2009 as a collaborative scientific project sponsored by the National Institute for Mental Health (NIMH), the primary funding body for mental health research in the United States. The RDoCs were viewed as a way to streamline mental health research and to more easily integrate psychology and neurobiology (Cuthbert & Insel, 2013; NIMH, retrieved 11/22/2021). Indeed, they remain central to NIMH's research funding strategies and are seen as a corrective to the multiplicity, frequent redundancy, and arbitrary cut-offs of categorical diagnoses used in the DSM.[2] The RDoCs consist of 6 domains, negative valence, positive valence, cognitive systems, systems for social processes, arousal/

regulatory systems, and sensory motor systems. Each domain is further subdivided into constructs and subconstructs and can be studied at different levels of analysis: genes, molecules, cells, circuits, physiology, behavior, self-report, and paradigms.

Trait-based approaches are also inherent in much of brain imaging research. For example, Andrew Fox and Ned Kalin and colleagues have studied the neurobiology of anxious temperament (AT), using brain imaging as well as other techniques (Fox & Kalin, 2014; Fox et al., 2015). They have identified a circuit of neural structures that appear to underly this personality trait, specifically the peri-aqueductal gray, amygdala, hippocampus, and frontal lobe. This network cuts across all levels of the brain and ranges from the oldest regions, such as the brain stem and mid brain into the newest brain regions, such as the frontal lobe (Fox & Kalin, 2014; Fox et al., 2015).

Importantly, while all of these trait-based approaches have been fruitful for research, they have had little impact on psychotherapy (c.f., Stein, 2021) and thus are less relevant for our project here, to provide an integrated framework for the psychotherapy of personality disorders. Indeed, as will be discussed in Chapter 6, most psychotherapies for personality disorders focus specifically upon patients' maladaptive interpersonal representations. I will also suggest that many of the traits listed above may be better conceptualized as temperament rather than character, consistent with Fox and Kalin's terminology of anxious temperament.

Further, these trait-based approaches are inherently reductive in nature, reducing a vast array of psychobehavioral tendencies into a few umbrella categories. While this avoids the cacophony of different categories found in many diagnostic systems, I will argue that it does not consider the mind as a complex emergent system, although the RDoCs clearly imply a hierarchical structure within neurobiology (genes to molecules to cells). Finally, all of these approaches reflect what might be called *vertical integration* (a term commonly used in economics). Here, this refers to an emphasis on the whole brain system from the bottom levels of the hierarchical structure to the top. While this is an accurate depiction of how the mind and brain function, as the brain is a single integrated system, it may have less utility for differential diagnosis and thus for appropriate selection of therapeutic technique. It is the premise of this book that the mind/brain can be usefully differentiated into what might be called *horizontal levels*, reflecting different points in evolutionary history. The older, simpler regions of the brain mediate crude but fundamental psychological processes whereas the newer, more complex regions mediate more complex psychological processes that have top-down influence on the older and simpler functions (c.f. Sabelli and Carson-Sabelli, 1989). Proper therapy involves accurate identification of the primary mind/

brain levels involved in the presenting problem. This will be elaborated in greater depth in Chapters 5 through 7.

Genes vs. Environment in Personality

Importantly, the degree of genetic heritability may differ between the traits addressed in the trait-based approaches and the personality features derived from interpersonal representations. This is highly relevant to the study of psychotherapy as change through psychotherapy depends on the capacity to learn. Logically, inborn and unlearned behaviors should be less amenable to change through learning than are learned behaviors. There appears to be a strong genetic component to the Big 5. Twin studies, which compare the degree to which traits are shared between identical and fraternal twins, suggest that the Big 5 traits are about 50 percent genetic. Nonetheless, it has been difficult to identify specific genes associated with each trait. For example, a 2015 study by Power and Pluess looked for associations between each trait and over 500,000 polymorphisms (genes that vary across individuals). Only neuroticism and openness to experience showed significant genetic linkages. Moreover, these two traits were found to be only 15 percent and 21 percent heritable, respectively. The authors speculated that twin studies might overestimate heritability. Thus, the exact contribution of genes vs. environment to personality remains very much an open question.

Other personality traits have also been found to have relatively large genetic components, however, and some have even been linked to specific genes. These include impulsivity, antisocial behavior, anxiety, introversion, and shyness (c.f., Matthews et al., 2003).

Fox and Kalin (2014; Fox et al., 2015) suggest that anxious temperament is about 30–35 percent genetic, based on various measurement techniques. However, as explained later, there are likely both genetic and learned components to the actual measurable behavior, as how people respond to anxiety-provoking situations will be influenced both by learned experience and genetic tendencies. Specific genes have been linked to AT, however, supporting the importance of its genetic etiology (Fox & Kalin, 2014).

Although Cloninger stresses the shared genetic and environmental influence on both temperament and character (Zwir et al., 2020), I will maintain an etiological distinction between these two systems. Temperament will be seen as primarily *genetic* with some environmental influence and character as primarily *environmental* with some genetic influence (largely that of temperament). As will be explained in Chapter 5, character and temperament can be understood as distinct subsystems that lie on different levels of organization of the mind/brain. Moreover, I propose that it is character that provides the ultimate target for the psychotherapy of patients with personality pathology. Hence, our focus will primarily be on character, defined herein as *consistent patterns of thought, affect, and behavior derived from a system of interpersonal representations*. Likewise, we will attribute to temperament any personality traits that are substantially genetic and operate largely outside of the realm of character.

Interpersonal Representations

Now let us turn our attention back to the concept of interpersonal representations. We will consider this in some depth as it is so central to our model of personality pathology. This concept is certainly not new; rather, it is a widely shared idea. In fact, in 2013, the DSM-5 task force for personality disorders published a new diagnostic scheme in which disturbed self and/or interpersonal functioning served as the gateway criterion for any personality disorder. Ultimately, the earlier diagnostic system was retained in DSM-5 and the new one listed as provisional. Nevertheless, the task force's proposal of the new scheme demonstrates how broadly the viewpoint of personality pathology as grounded in interpersonal representations extends across the mental health field. While undoubtedly a transtheoretical construct now, the idea of interpersonal representations first developed in psychoanalytic theory. So, this is where we shall start our review.

Freudian Theory

Although the concept may have originated in psychoanalysis, Freud's own theories focused neither upon interpersonal representations nor personality per se. It was actually in the second generation of the psychoanalytic movement that the clinical focus shifted from narrowly defined symptoms to patients' overall personality structure. And with this shift, interpersonal representations became a central area of interest.

But first let us consider the primary points of Freud's theoretical framework (c.f. Gottlieb, 2012). As much of Freud's ideas do not fit smoothly into a modern world view, it is important to consider the context in which he was writing. First, Freud was a neurologist; as such, he was interested primarily in symptoms and syndromes rather than personality. Likewise, he was interested in the *biological* bases of behavior, leading him to search for biologically-based instincts underlying human motivation. Second, Freud made his major discoveries in the late 19th and early 20th centuries, an era far more sexually repressive and puritanical than our own. Hence the problem of repressed sexual feelings was quite salient, particularly for the middle-class women he tended to treat. Third, as a scientist from the turn of the 20th century, he fully identified with the reductionist ideals of his era. Hence, he aimed to explain complex human emotions and relationships by isolating a single biological cause, in this case the vicissitudes of the sexual instinct.

So, what did Freud have to say? Largely, Freud interpreted his patient's neurotic symptoms as *compromise formations* between instincts and societal inhibitions. He initially formulated libido, loosely defined as sexual pleasure, as the ultimate motivating force, but added Thanatos, the death drive, following the carnage of World War I. Thanatos was later interpreted as aggression. Hence, his clinical lens focused on patients' conflicts about socially proscribed sexual and aggressive feelings.

Additionally, Freud created a profoundly *developmental* model. Libido progresses through a predictable sequence of stages across childhood, moving through the oral, anal, phallic, and genital stages. Each of these psychosexual stages was also characterized by specific personality traits. Importantly, psychopathology was conceptualized in developmental terms, reflecting either developmental arrest or regression to an earlier stage.

How do these ideas relate to Emergent Systems Theory as I have presented it so far? For one, the developmental framework is consistent with the idea of the mind/brain as a hierarchical, emergent system. Developmental arrest and regression reflect movement between different levels of organization that evolved sequentially over time. Secondly, the emphasis on sexuality and aggression as core biological drives accords with both Paul MacLean's triune system and Jaak Panksepp's model of mammalian emotions. In MacLean's model, the instincts are mediated by the reptilian brain, the oldest part of the emotional system, while the uniquely human societal constraints are mediated by the neo-mammalian brain, specifically the neocortex.

In Panksepp's model, the sexual and aggressive instincts parallel the LUST and RAGE primary emotional systems.[3] The emotions of guilt and shame derive from the tertiary emotional systems of the neocortex, specifically the frontal lobe. Thus, in both MacLean's and Panksepp's models, the battles between id (instincts) and superego (morality) represent interaction between the phylogenetically ancient emotional systems of the lower brain regions and the newer, conceptually-based, inhibitory systems of the frontal lobes.

Nonetheless, this view of the mind is strikingly atomistic; it is not an *interpersonal* model. To the extent Freud does consider the role of the child's caretaker in development, it is as the *object* of the libidinal drives (hence the rather reprehensible term "object" for mother or other key attachment figure). It was the drives that shaped the child's growing psyche, far more than the child's *relationship* with the actual mother. It is not that Freud was oblivious to the child's relationships with family members—he did have 6 children himself—but that interpersonal relationships per se were not seen as central to the core motivational systems.

Object Relations Theory

This changed with the advent of object relations theory. Early object relations analysts maintained much of Freud's theoretical infrastructure but showed greater interest in the infant's feelings about the actual mother. While these early theorists retained a rather atomistic approach, focusing more on the child's internal mental processes than on the relationship with real people, they did depart from Freud in two important ways. 1) They insisted that infants' drives are object-oriented from the start. The object is not simply the convenient goal of the libidinal drive but intrinsic to the child's psyche. 2) Psychological development was less about a sequence of erogenous zones than about the child's representations of the interpersonal world. *Specifically, they looked at how the organization of interpersonal representations matures across childhood.* How does the way the child understand self and other grow and develop? Implicit in all theories is the belief that the child's representations develop from a relatively crude, simplistic state to a much greater level of complexity and sophistication. (See Williams (2012) and Britton (2012) for reviews of object relations theory.)

Melanie Klein (1882–1960) was a pioneering object relations theorist. Building on the work of Karl Abraham, a first-generation analyst, she focused on the infant's conflicting feelings of love and hate towards the mother, or more specifically, the mother's breast. Klein believed that infants create *introjects*, or internalized images, of their mothers and that these introjects are strongly colored by the infants' emotions. Early introjects are of "part-objects," that is they reflect limited, unidimensional understanding of the mother, totally circumscribed by the reigning emotion of the moment. In this way, there are good and bad introjects; the loved mother (or breast) is separate from the hated mother (or breast). This primitive state is known as the "paranoid-schizoid" position. It is only when the child can *integrate* loving and hateful feelings towards the mother that progression to the "depressive position" is possible. At this stage the child can internalize *whole* objects, in which the mother is understood to be multifaceted, with both good and bad aspects. With this important psychological achievement, the child's recognition of love for the mother can now withstand periodic frustration and anger. The child can remember feeling love for the mother even when angry at her.

While later theorists have criticized Klein's conflation of adult psychopathology and normal infant development as well as her overly concrete emphasis on maternal body parts, the concepts of introjects, part-objects and whole objects have withstood the test of time. It is now widely believed that children do create internal images or schemas of early attachment relationships and that the child's ability to integrate divergent aspects of those relationships into a comprehensive, multifaceted understanding of self and other matures over time. Moreover, in personality pathology, we see regression towards the earlier mode, in which conflicting emotional experiences of the other person are split off from one another. Unable to hold in mind a consistent and integrated understanding of other people, the personality disordered individual alternates (sometimes rapidly) between crudely good and bad perceptions of them. In fact, this kind of *splitting* is characteristic of individuals with borderline personality disorder.

In the 1940s, Ronald Fairbairn, a Scottish psychoanalyst, moved object relations theory further away from Freud's core tenets. He downplayed drive theory, rejected the concept of the death instinct, and grounded the child's psychological development firmly in the real relationship with the real mother. While he retained his own concepts of introjects and of splitting between good and bad objects, he held that, in adulthood, fragmented object representations, i.e., part-objects, were a sign of pathology and not an inevitable result of the infant's libidinal and aggressive drives. In his view, children developed part-objects to defend against painful disappointment from the actual relationship with the mother. In other words, they actively compartmentalized their awareness of good and bad aspects of their mother to manage their own difficult feelings. In this way he conceived of splitting as a *defense* used to manage painful emotions, a phenomenon we frequently see with personality disordered patients. Thus, while Klein showed how adult psychopathology can reflect early developmental failures, Fairbairn showed how a such delayed development can be used defensively, to protect against emotional pain.

Donald Winnicott, another member of the British object relations school, also made important theoretical contributions about the development of interpersonal representations. Specifically, he looked at how the early mother-infant relationship facilitated the *differentiation* of self and other representations. He posited that the infant is born into a subjective "merger" with the mother, not recognizing that she is a different, separate person and outside of the child's control. The recognition of this unbridgeable gulf between self and other is traumatic for children, as if repudiating their longstanding way of seeing their mother is equivalent to destroying the real mother. When children learn that their mother is not the person that they thought she was, i.e. cannot respond with perfect attunement to their every need, it feels as if she has been killed off. However, once children are able to recognize their mother's separate existence, they can *rediscover* her as a distinct individual who can love and relate to her children even if not under their omnipotent control. Winnicott saw the mother's sensitive facilitation of this individuation process as critical for healthy self-development. Importantly we see the relevance of this process in personality disordered individuals, who often cannot acknowledge the separate perspectives and emotional needs of the people in their life. It is only when they can accept and recognize the separate existence of their loved ones that healthy relationships are possible.

Winnicott's concept of the transitional object is a particularly charming and easily observed illustration of his theories (Winnicott, 1971). During the toddler years, children grow increasingly aware of their separation from the mother and their lack of omnipotent control over her. They often latch onto a soft object, such as a stuffed toy or a blanket, as a halfway point between merger and individuation. As an inanimate object, the blanket is physically under their control. Yet, as it is distinct from their own body, it can still provide the child with a sense of being comforted by someone outside the self. We frequently see toddlers intensely attached to a blanket or toy, refusing to let the object out of their sight. Eventually, however, they outgrow their "Binky" and abandon it to a dusty oblivion.

To Winnicott, the abandonment of the transitional object indicates that the soothing behavior of the mother has been sufficiently *internalized* into a mental representation that can successfully regulate the child's own emotions. What does this mean? Initially, it is the mother's job to regulate the child's emotions, to soothe her baby when the child is upset, frightened, hungry, or frustrated. Throughout these experiences, the child builds a *representation* of interactions with the mother, a prototypical memory that serves as a map of the routine. As will be reviewed in relation to attachment theory, at first the child creates a schema of the typical mother-child interaction around various events, including soothing. The child can use this to anticipate the mother's *behavior* and react accordingly. However, Winnicott is referring to something else. When the child can fully internalize the mother's soothing function, the representation of the mother-child interaction is sufficiently consolidated that the child can perform the mother's soothing function him or herself. It is at this point that the child is capable of *self-soothing*. This is a critical notion in the treatment of patients with significant personality pathology as these individuals are unable to self-soothe effectively. And hence they turn to substances, impulsive behaviors or overly intense relationships to regulate their distress. Likewise, patients with borderline personality disorder often describe feeling "empty" inside, as if lacking an internal representation of the soothing other. Of course, the development of such an internal schema depends on the child's actual experience of the mother's soothing behavior. If the mother is abusive, neglectful, or otherwise grossly ineffective at helping the child manage distress, it is very hard to create an internal schema of her that can allow for self-soothing. Thus, Winnicott's work sheds light on the process by which interpersonal representations ultimately serve to regulate emotion, thought, and behavior. Of note, it is the regulation of affect that is seen to be the most central to personality development.

In this vein, Wilfred Bion, another British object relations theorist, made important contributions to our understanding of affective development, of how a child's understanding of emotion develops over time. Perhaps due to his rather arcane and opaque writing style, his work has not received as much attention as Winnicott's. This is unfortunate as his ideas accord very well with modern neuroscience. But let's take a look at what he had to say. Influenced by his experience working with psychotic adults, he became intrigued by primitively organized emotional experience. In other words, he observed how emotional experience can be overpowering and disorganized in psychotic states and concluded that this reflected a regression towards a much earlier state of development. Extrapolating from his work as a therapist, Bion posited that the mother served as "container" for the infant's intense emotions. It was the mother's job to hold or contain the child's overwhelming and disorganizing emotion and then reflect it back in digestible, understandable form so that the child can learn to make sense of it. Central to Bion's work is the assumption that the ability to recognize, label and understand one's own emotional experience is not present at birth but rather develops across childhood. More specifically, the child's subjective experience of emotion is initially experienced as bodily sensations and impulses towards action. Only with development can children recognize their own emotions *as* emotions and then to articulate them in words. As we saw in Chapter 2, this is fully in accord with our phylogenetic history. In the evolution of the human mind/brain, bodily sensations and actions preceded concepts and words.

Importantly, the healthy development of these capacities is dependent upon the empathic responses of early caregivers. If the child's emotions are not well contained by the mother, this will hamper emotional development, resulting in psychopathology in adulthood. This notion was further developed several decades later by Peter Fonagy and Anthony Bateman.

Heinz Kohut, who operated somewhat independently in his Chicago school of self-psychology, focused specifically on the development of *self*-representations. He emphasized the necessity of early parental *mirroring* (a kind of empathic recognition) for the healthy development of a cohesive sense of self. He specifically linked narcissistic pathology in adulthood, a disorder of self-representation, with inadequate or distorted mirroring in childhood.

In sum, Klein, Fairbairn, Bion, Winnicott and Kohut provided theories of how interpersonal representations grow to maturity in the context of the attachment relationship. Perturbations of that relationship, therefore, compromise healthy development of self and other representations. Specifically, Kleinian psychoanalysis highlighted the importance of *integration* and Winnicott the *differentiation* of self and other representations. Bion explored the development of affective experience from bodily-based action to verbal concepts and Kohut the importance of parental recognition or mirroring of children's emotional experience.

By the early 21st century, it is fair to say that all psychoanalytic schools acknowledge the basic premises of object relations. Moreover, at this point, these ideas have spread far outside of the psychoanalytic world and into the broader field of psychology. Additionally, newer developments have provided essential scientific support for this approach. Although psychoanalytic ideas were derived from extensive clinical experience, they were not tested in rigorous empirical research. This changed in the last quarter of the 20th century and continues to progress today. Of note, although many aspects of psychoanalytic theory have not been supported by empirical research and have largely fallen by the wayside (e.g., drive theory, the death instinct, the psychosexual stages, and the primacy of libido and the Oedipal complex), the core notions about interpersonal representations have received robust scientific support, both within and outside of the psychoanalytic camp. Two important bodies of work that grew up outside the psychoanalytic bastion include attachment theory and cognitive behavioral therapy.

Attachment Theory

Attachment theory originally came out of object relations but transferred into the field of developmental psychology with the work of Mary Ainsworth in the 1960s. John Bowlby was a psychoanalyst in the British object relations school who was profoundly affected by his work during WWII with children from disadvantaged backgrounds. In 1951 he published a book on juvenile offenders, in which he noted how many of these adolescents had experienced long separations from their mothers. In large part, his interest in the deleterious effect of parental loss and separation accorded with contemporaneous trends within object relations theory. Yet, he also encountered considerable resistance from psychoanalysts, particularly Melanie Klein, who still prioritized the child's internal fantasies of the mother over her actual behavior.

When Bowlby discovered the new field of ethology in the 1950s, as exemplified by the work of Konrad Lorenz, he found his intellectual home. Ethology is the study of (nonhuman) animal behavior from a Darwinian viewpoint. Thus, Bowlby developed a theory of mother-infant attachment within the context of *evolutionary biology*. In this way, he returned to the notion of instincts, which had so appealed to Freud. However, he understood instincts very differently than Freud did. To Bowlby instincts were not a set of mechanical drives propelled by impersonal energy. Instead, they were goal-oriented behaviors that evolved to promote the animals' survival and reproduction. Specifically, he conceived of the *attachment system* as an inborn, genetically-based drive of the child to seek out closeness to and protection from the mother. When the attachment system is activated, either by threat or separation, the child feels acute distress and seeks out proximity to the mother. The child communicates this need through "proximity-seeking behavior," such as distress cries, reaching, crawling to the mother, etc. When proximity has been accomplished and the child achieves a subjective sense of "felt security," the attachment system deactivates and the child can return to exploratory play. Of note, the Bowlby's notion of attachment instincts dovetails Panksepp's model of the PANIC system, in which juvenile mammals respond to maternal separation with signals of distress. Importantly, Bowlby also introduced the concept of the *internal working model* of attachment, such that the child develops a mental map of the attachment relationship, which then serves to guide attachment-related emotion and behavior.

Mary Ainsworth was hired by Bowlby to work as a researcher at the famed Tavistock Clinic in London. It was Ainsworth who took Bowlby's theory into the laboratory. She also introduced the study of individual differences. Through exhaustive observational studies of a small group of mothers and infants in Uganda and later Baltimore, she not only validated Bowlby's theory of the attachment system, she also identified predictable individual differences in mother-infant pairs. In the late 1960s, she developed "the Strange Situation," a laboratory-based method of measuring year-old infants' reactions to a series of short separations and reunions with their mother in an unfamiliar environment. From their reactions in this experimental paradigm, babies were classified as either securely or insecurely attached. There were three subtypes of insecure attachment, avoidant, ambivalent and disorganized. All of the babies' attachment classifications were associated with maternal behavior at home. Consistently responsive mothers had secure infants, who balanced dependency and autonomy. Predictably unresponsive mothers had avoidant infants, who downplayed their attachment needs and appeared hyper-independent. Unpredictably responsive mothers had ambivalent babies who cranked up their attachment needs and downplayed their autonomous behavior. Abusive or more disturbed mothers had disorganized infants who lacked a consistent strategy to achieve "felt security." Thus, Ainsworth showed that as early as one year of age, children develop an internal working model of the mother-child relationship which serves to guide their behavioral responses. And different kinds of experiences with the caregiver lead to different models of attachment.

In the 1980s, Mary Main extended the study of attachment styles into adulthood. She developed a semi-structured interview in which she looked at how adults speak about attachment. She was more interested in *how* they talked than *what* they said, as she assumed attachment style may not be conscious. Secure adults had direct access to their memories and emotions but could also take distance from them. Their narratives were coherent, and they balanced emotion with thought. They also balanced autonomy with dependency. Dismissing adults, similar to avoidant babies, emphasized autonomy over dependency and thought over emotion. They presented a superficial and unrealistically positive view of their childhood, with few specific memories to back up their generalities. In sum, they took too much distance from their experience. ("Mom was fine. I was happy.") Preoccupied adults, analogous to ambivalent babies, emphasized dependency over autonomy and emotion over thought. Their narratives were overly detailed and emotional, as if caught in the weeds without sufficient perspective. Flooded with specific memories, they could not step back to reflect on them objectively. As such, they took insufficient distance from their experience. Disorganized adults, analogous to disorganized babies, had the most incoherent narratives. Hence, Main highlighted the importance of the *coherence* (or integration) of interpersonal representations as a measure of optimal adaptation. It was the coherent representations that were most effective at regulating thought, affect and behavior.

Notably, Main explicitly references episodic memory. She was particularly interested in the relationship between episodic and semantic memory. Secure mothers balanced both types of information, dismissing mothers privileged semantic, and preoccupied mothers privileged episodic memory. Thus, attachment representations in adulthood are fundamentally linked to episodic memory.

Later attachment researchers have shown particular interest in affect regulation. In the late 1980s, Roger Kobak proposed that attachment styles serve to regulate negative affect in order to maintain a sense of "felt security" in the context of the individual's internal working model of attachment. For example, if mother is consistently unresponsive, a good way to minimize negative affect about unmet attachment needs is to minimize awareness of those needs and emphasize one's own independence. In children, attachment style is reflected in patterns of behavior, how they turn away or turn towards the parent. In adults, it is reflected in their patterns of thought, in how they manage access to specific, emotionally salient memories.

In the four decades since Ainsworth's 1978 publication *Patterns of Attachment*, attachment research has positively exploded. Tens to hundreds of thousands of publications support the importance of attachment security to psychological adjustment from childhood throughout adulthood.[4] Likewise, my own research has shown the correlation between insecure attachment and adult psychopathology, including personality pathology (Cohen et al., 2016b; Hengartner et al., 2015) and even suicidal risk (Cohen et al., 2017). Thus, attachment theory provides robust empirical support for the basic premises of object relations theory. (See Karen (1998) for a review of the history of attachment theory.)

Cognitive Approaches

Cognitive therapists came to the concept of interpersonal representations from a very different vantage point, that of behaviorism. Throughout much of the 20th century, while psychoanalysis held dominance in clinical psychology, behaviorism held sway in academic psychology. While psychoanalysis emphasized the internal workings of the mind to the neglect of the external world, behaviorism privileged the study of observable behavior to the explicit discounting of the mind. Behaviorists quite literally took the mind out of psychology. However, by the 1960s, their anti-mentalism was starting to fray. Even scientists who ran rats in mazes (a frequent subject of behaviorist research) noticed what could only be called mental behavior in their rats. When rats encountered a fork in the path in a maze they had run before, they would often pause, as if stopping to think, before choosing a path to follow. Scientists such as Edward Chase Tolman interpreted this to mean that rats had developed a mental map of the maze and were consulting it when choosing between two options. From insights such as these, a growing interest developed in the step in between perception and behavior. As the mind returned to academic psychology, the "cognitive revolution" was born. Because of this tradition, however, cognitive therapy has emphasized the *cognitive* elements of personality pathology, in contrast to psychodynamic approaches, which focus more upon affect.

As a psychiatrist, Aaron Beck was trained primarily in psychoanalysis but had long harbored doubts about psychoanalytic orthodoxy (Miller, 2012; J. S. Beck, 2011). He critiqued psychoanalytic technique for its excessive emphasis on unconscious processes rather than patients' explicit dysfunctional thoughts as well as its failure to provide practical tools to help patients feel better quickly. While he was never a behaviorist per se, he entered the mental health field just when the cognitive revolution was gaining strength. Influenced by Albert Ellis, the founder of rational emotive therapy in the 1950s, he developed a model of depression that focused primarily on conscious dysfunctional beliefs, such as "I am a loser" and "My situation is hopeless." Beck believed that our cognitive interpretation of events shapes our emotional responses.[5] Hence pessimistic and self-deprecatory beliefs reinforce depressed mood. Out of this paradigm, Beck developed cognitive therapy, which aims to improve emotional adjustment by helping people first become aware of their dysfunctional thoughts and then change them. From the beginning, he was oriented to empirical research, so unlike psychoanalysis, cognitive therapy has always been supported by empirical studies.

Beck recognized that the automatic thoughts and cognitive distortions that drive emotional disorders often derive from more generalized assumptions about the self and other people. He referred to these generalized beliefs as core beliefs or schemas. For example, depressed individuals have core beliefs about the self as worthless and incompetent while anxious individuals have core beliefs about the self as vulnerable and powerless to protect themselves. Such core beliefs are understood to have developed in the context of life experiences, especially in childhood. Various cognitive techniques were developed to challenge these core beliefs, such as checking the evidence to support or contradict these schemas. Thus, in Beck's view, underlying self-schemas give rise to automatic thoughts which then result in depressed mood (or other symptomatology). Note in his clinical formulation, Beck privileged cognition over affect, the reverse of the psychodynamic approach.

Beck's major contribution was to provide a mechanistic analysis of how maladaptive interpersonal schemas actually function. While psychodynamic theory has excelled in analyzing the developmental roots of psychopathology, they have been less successful in identifying the mechanisms that perpetuate it. Beck states that core beliefs about the self and the world, often learned in childhood, bias our cognition towards confirmatory interpretations of events. Thus, when a situation that may be relevant to the core belief presents itself, the core belief or schema is activated. It is triggered. At this point, the person will generate automatic thoughts, filtered through cognitive distortions. This refers to mechanisms such as selective attention, discounting contradictory evidence, or exaggerating confirmatory evidence which bias information processing in ways that conform to the core belief. For example, for someone who feels inherently uninteresting to others, the lack of an immediately returned text will be interpreted as a deliberate rejection, resulting in feelings of dejection, anger, and depression. That the other person is in a particularly demanding period at work will be discounted. In contrast, for someone with a strong sense of self-worth, the delay in returning the text will either be disregarded or attributed to the other person's workload. Accordingly, these different response patterns will have very different effects on each person's general emotional outlook as well as the stability of their relationships.

Jeff Young built on Beck and Ellis's approach but focused more narrowly on interpersonal schemas as his work was geared specifically towards personality pathology. He also made important contributions to a mechanistic understanding of how maladaptive interpersonal representations operate. Young created the Young Schema Questionnaire (YSQ), the latest version of which, developed in 2005, yields scores on 18 different early maladaptive schemas. These include abandonment/instability, mistrust/abuse, emotional deprivation, defectiveness/shame, social isolation/alienation, dependence/incompetence, vulnerability to harm or illness, enmeshment/undeveloped self, failure to achieve, entitlement/grandiosity, insufficient self-control/self-discipline, subjugation, self-sacrifice, approval-seeking/recognition-seeking, negativity/pessimism, emotional inhibition, unrelenting standards/hypercriticalness, and punitiveness (from Schematherapy.com, retrieved 8/30/2019).

Young proposes that children develop early maladaptive schemas (EMSs) in response to detrimental experiences with key attachment figures, such as parents, siblings, and friends. All EMSs derive from core emotional needs, reflecting each child's experience of how such needs were not met. For example, the maladaptive schema of emotional deprivation develops out of frustration of the child's core need for intimacy and affection. Children also develop maladaptive coping mechanisms in response to these schemas, such as surrender, overcompensation or avoidance. They might surrender to the schema (Yes, I'm worthless), overcompensate against the schema (I'm better than that guy!), or strenuously avoid triggering the schema (avoid any performance demand). Like Beck, Young posits that schemas lay dormant until triggered, at which point the individual reacts in "schema mode," resulting in maladaptive ways of engaging with the world.

Of note, Young states that the particular configuration of maladaptive schema and coping mode is influenced by innate temperament. For example, the self-schema of vulnerability to harm or illness might be triggered more frequently in someone with a shy, introverted temperament whereas the schema of insufficient control/self-discipline might be triggered more frequently in someone with an impulsive temperament. Similarly, an introverted person may be more likely to "surrender" to a defectiveness/shame schema while an extraverted person may be more likely to "overcompensate" against it with exaggerated bravado and grandiosity.

Additionally, Young differentiates between "coping modes" (surrender, avoidance, and overcompensation) and "schema modes," which are more general configurations of schemas, coping modes, and emotional states. These are, in effect, self-states, which may be more or less integrated in the individual. To the extent these schema modes are not integrated into a coherent sense of self, the individual will have fragmented or dissociated parts of the self and thereby engage with the world in discontinuous and poorly coordinated ways. The extreme version of this is found in dissociative identity disorder, in which the person's discrete self-states are experienced as different people. This concept is remarkably similar to psychodynamic notions of self-integration. Hence, we see that we have come full circle from behaviorism to the psychodynamic progeny of object relations. This convergence across different theoretical traditions reflects the robust clinical evidence supporting the representational model of personality pathology. Ultimately it is our patients who tell us what is true about their emotional struggles, and it seems that they are giving a consistent message to the many clinicians who try to help them.

Infancy Researchers

One other area of psychological research that has contributed to our understanding of interpersonal representations is the domain of infancy research. Two such researchers, Dan Stern and Beatrice Beebe, have explored how the basic foundations of adult personality were laid down in earliest infancy.

Dan Stern introduced the concept of Representations of Interactions that have been Generalized (RIGs). This is essentially the same concept as interpersonal representations—and by now we've run across quite a number of names for similar concepts, including schema, object representation, introject, and internal working model. Stern, however, was interested in the fundamental processes by which these representations develop in infancy. Stern presumed RIGs to be a type of memory. But a RIG is not a memory of a specific event; rather it is an average account of many similar events. It is a generalized memory of a prototypical interaction. In effect the brain is recognizing a pattern and then encoding the pattern into long term memory. Stern states that the prototype is based on *invariants* across the different individual events. Whatever features of the event are common across all or most individual exemplars is incorporated into the RIG. Parenthetically, as discussed in Chapter 1, the identification of invariant features is emphasized in artificial intelligence.

In the infant, these individual events are initially perceived as nonspecific masses of sensory stimulation. It is only through the repetition of events and identification of invariant features that the infant can make order of the sensory stew and distinguish the different participants in the event. This is mother, that is a chair. Importantly, the initial structure of subjective experience, even before infants can identify distinct objects, is of the almost musical patterning of sensory stimulation. The initial schema is not of a chair per se, but of hardness and sharp corners, thin verticals and broad horizontals, and the thump, thump of the body when placed atop it. In other words, our first understanding of reality involves perception of the changing pattern of sensory activity over time. Stern refers to this as *amodal perception*, recognition of a pattern which generalizes across sensory modalities, coordinating input from vision, hearing, and touch.

Stern then extends this insight to the child's experience of emotion. Here Stern introduces the important notions of *vitality affect* and *affective attunement*. He stipulated that emotion has multiple components to it. The best known is the categorical nature of emotion (which he calls categorical affect), as in sadness, happiness, anger, etc. But there is another element, the musical element, which refers to the patterning of stimulation over time. This might include a sudden crescendo of intensity, a small, steady increase in arousal, or an abrupt decrease in tension. This is what he means by vitality affect.

Like many other theorists, Stern believed that the mother's responses to the infant's affect have long lasting impact on psychological development. Luckily, most mothers automatically and intuitively attune to their children's affect and by so doing teach the child that emotion can be shared. On a fundamental level, the child's subjective world can be known. For Stern affective attunement not only means mirroring back to the child the *categorical* content of the emotion ("I know you're frustrated."). It also means mirroring the vitality affect of the emotion, matching the musical pattern of intensity. ("There, there, baby, don't cry. It's OK, It's OK.") Though Stern does not emphasize this, the mother does not always exactly match the child's vitality affect; sometimes she deliberately increases or decreases the intensity level in an attempt to modulate the child's affective state. As such, affective attunement does more than match the child's affect; it also serves to regulate and contain it (here we have echoes of Bion's earlier work). In this way, the mother's responses to her child *mark* the affect as the child's and not her own. Therefore, at the same time that she is joining the child's affective experience, she is clearly differentiating it from her own. She is standing outside of it. This teaches the child both that affect can be understood and that it is tolerable, that one can take some distance from it. Therefore, our eventual recognition of distinct objects, both animate and inanimate, is built upon an initial schema of rhythmic patterns of activity.

Beatrice Beebe was active in infancy research contemporaneously with Dan Stern and looked at similar issues. She has performed microanalytic studies of mother-infant face to face communication for many decades. She has looked at how nonverbal behaviors such as facial orientation, facial expression, eye contact, vocal tone, and other bodily movements reflect the mutual influence of mother and child on a moment-by-moment basis. Using split cameras, she has looked at how the delicate dance between parent and child in everyday emotional interactions forms the foundation for the child's experience of the interpersonal world. And this in turn forms the basis of personality structure. Likewise, variation in mother-child face to face interaction at 4 months is predictive of later attachment style at age 1 and of cognitive, emotional, and relational development as well as the capacity to manage stress, even as far as 30 years later. Infants whose mothers sensitively and contingently respond to their emotional cues show significantly better psychological adjustment than infants who lack such well attuned caregivers. Thus, as early as 4 months of age, interpersonal representations are being laid down.

What Dan Stern and Beatrice Beebe's work tells us is that in their earliest form, interpersonal representations are *pre-cognitive*. They consist of prototypical memories of sensory-motor and affective arousal patterns. It is only later that these structures will be elaborated into ideas of *people*, of the self in relation to others. In effect, we are dealing with nondeclarative or procedural memory at this point. It is only later that these same kinds of experiences will be encoded in declarative (episodic and semantic) memory. Yet this work tells us that the early forms of representations set the stage for the later ones. Thus, the foundational structures of interpersonal representations, and hence those of personality, derive from primordial psychological functions processed at deeper and older parts of the brain. This becomes relevant when considering how to treat personality pathology in adulthood, as it suggests that true personality change will have to incorporate these older, pre-cognitive processes. We will revisit this notion in Chapter 6 in our discussion of psychotherapy.

Additionally, although the foundations of interpersonal representations manifest as early as four months of age, this does not mean that personality is carved in stone by the first year of life and that later development does not matter. Attachment style is conservative but not immutable and can change during childhood if the environment changes sufficiently. The younger the child, the easier it is to change. Research shows that securely attached children can become insecurely attached if significant misfortune befalls the family and the parents become markedly less available. The converse is also true. Insecure children can become securely attached if family circumstances improve and the parents become more available. It is not until adulthood that personality is truly consolidated. Even so, adults can still change their personality structure, but this is more difficult and generally takes extended and deliberate effort, as in psychotherapy.

SUMMARY

This brings us to the end of our review of the literature on interpersonal representations. Let us summarize the key points as related to the Emergent Systems Theory model of personality and personality pathology.

1. Personality is comprised of both temperament and character, the former largely genetic and the latter largely learned and environmental.
2. Character is composed of a *learned system of interpersonal representations*, that is schemas, maps, or models of how relationships typically proceed derived from memories of key attachment relationships in childhood.
3. Interpersonal representations develop from relative simplicity to greater complexity over time. This development is most marked in early childhood but continues more slowly throughout the lifespan.
4. The nature and organization of children's interpersonal representations is heavily shaped by their parents' day-to-day responses to their emotional experience. Sensitive parenting begets benign and coherent representations; it facilitates development. Insensitive parenting does the opposite.
5. In the adult and the developing child, the entire system of interpersonal representations serves to regulate thought, affect and behavior in a top-down manner.
6. In this context, character pathology in adulthood is defined as *inadequate development of interpersonal representations, producing top-down failures in the regulation of affect, thought and behavior*. This notion will be more fully developed in the next chapter.

SUPPORTING EVIDENCE

The literature reviewed so far has addressed mainly the definition and development of interpersonal representations. However, as it is the basic premise of this book that personality pathology reflects dysfunction at the level of interpersonal representations, it is worthwhile to review literature supporting this specific contention. Is there evidence a) that links dysfunction in interpersonal representations to personality pathology and b) shows this connection to be *specific*, i.e., that it is stronger in personality pathology than in other psychiatric disorders?

Let us first look at the literature on the relative genetic contribution to personality pathology compared to other types of disorders. If personality disorders are based on learned interpersonal representations, then they will have lower genetic heritability than other types of psychopathology. Kenneth Kendler and colleagues have done extensive work on the heritability of a range of psychiatric disorders. Specifically, they used twin studies to estimate heritability across the 10 DSM-IV personality disorders (Kendler et al., 2008). They used a large cohort of fraternal and identical twins, obtained from the health registry in Norway (N=2,796). Heritability estimates for the 10 diagnoses range from 20.5 percent to 40.9 percent with an average value of 29.9

percent. Likewise, environmentality estimates for these same diagnoses range from 59.1 percent to 79.5 percent, with an average value of 70.2 percent. This suggests that on average, personality disorders are about 70 percent environmental and about 30 percent genetic.

In contrast, Wray and Gottesman (2012) conducted a population-based study using the Danish Civil Registration System to assess the heritability for schizophrenia, bipolar disorder, and major depressive disorder by calculating the risk of each disorder in an individual when one or both parents had the same disorder. Their total sample size included 1,278,977 parent-child pairs, comprised of all people born in Denmark between 1969 and 1996 that had available parents at the time of the study. The authors reported a heritability estimate of 67 percent for schizophrenia, 62 percent for bipolar disorder, and 32 percent for major depressive disorder. The lower heritability estimate for major depression is not surprising as this disorder is highly heterogeneous. Depression can be reactive, following a major loss or other stressor, or endogenous, a more biologically-based illness with no external cause. Additionally, depression often occurs as a consequence of personality disorders so the data on depression could be biased by co-occurring personality disorders. What's important here, however, is that both studies use population-based registries and are therefore more reliable than the small sample studies previously reported using data from clinical samples. However, other studies have supported these findings. McGuffin and colleagues calculated an additive genetic contribution of 0.66–0.72 for unipolar depression and 0.80–0.85 for mania (McGuffin et al., 2003) while a meta-analysis of genetic studies of schizophrenia yielded a heritability estimate of 81 percent (Sullivan et al., 2003). In sum, the genetic contribution to personality disorders appears to be at least half that of schizophrenia and bipolar disorder.

Now we should probably step on the brakes a little here and consider the difficulty of distinguishing between genetic vs. environmental etiology. Family studies, as described above, are limited because they do not address specific genes or the interactions between the genes and they can only crudely assess the proportion of shared genes across research subjects (50 percent for full siblings, 25 percent for half siblings, etc.). Also, they have even less ability to measure the effect of environment. Still, that we are comparing studies using similar methodology suggests we can draw conclusions about the *relative* heritability of different disorders in comparison with one another. These days, due to technological advances, genome wide association studies (GWA) are often considered more precise than family studies. GWA studies allow for whole genome assessments, capturing all genes on the human genome and their intercorrelations (Zwir et al., 2020). However, given the extraordinary complexity of genetic processes, GWA are likely to miss out on more complex interactions or on the cumulative effect of very small genetic influences. In this regard family studies can give us a different view of the actual outcome, of how the pie turns out, if not of all the ingredients going in. In sum, the science of human genetics is in its infancy and much more research is needed before we can make any final conclusions about the genetic vs. environmental etiology (c.f. Fox & Kalin, 2014). Nonetheless, early data about the largely environmental vs. genetic influence on personality pathology compared to that of other major mental illnesses is intriguing and consistent with other clinical information.

Likewise, there is strong evidence of the role of *environment* in the development of personality pathology. Important support for the environmental etiology of personality pathology comes from the robust findings of its association with childhood maltreatment. In my own research we found that multiple types of childhood maltreatment were strongly associated with overall personality pathology. Specifically, in a sample of 156 psychiatric inpatients, those who scored in the top half of the sample on measures of childhood neglect, physical, emotional or sexual abuse were approximately 1.5–3.5 times more likely to score in the top half of the sample on total personality disorder traits. Moreover, the relationship was stronger when looking at more extreme ends of the continuum. Subjects with high levels of childhood trauma were approximately 2.5 to 5.5 times more likely to score in the top vs. bottom third of the sample on personality disorder traits (Cohen et al., 2013).

A related study tested the hypothesis that maladaptive interpersonal schemas are strongly related to personality disorders but largely unrelated to mood and psychotic disorders (Cohen et al., 2016c). In a different sample of 100 psychiatric inpatients, study participants with scores in the top half on each of 5 general schema domains from the YSQ-S2 (earlier version of the Young Schema Questionnaire) were between 2 and 9 times as likely to have a diagnosis of borderline personality disorder as those with scores in the bottom half. The domains included disconnection/rejection, impaired autonomy, impaired limits, other directedness, and over-vigilance and inhibition, in descending order of relation to borderline diagnosis. However, high scorers on all these domains were no more likely to have bipolar disorder, schizophrenia, or major depressive disorder after controlling for comorbid personality disorders. Thus, maladaptive interpersonal schemas were strongly associated with borderline personality disorder but unrelated to other severe mental disorders. Similar findings were reported in a study comparing YSQ scores in patients with borderline personality vs. bipolar disorder (Kahr Nilsson et al., 2010).

NEUROBIOLOGICAL SUBSTRATES

Now that we have reviewed the literature on interpersonal representations and their relevance to personality pathology, we will shift our focus back to neuroanatomy. As mentioned before, it is a core premise of this book to locate personality pathology at the level of interpersonal representations within the hierarchical structure of the mind/brain. This higher-level system serves to regulate thought, affect and behavior located at lower levels of the mind/brain in a top-down manner. Thus, it is important to consider what parts of the brain may be centrally involved in these systems. I propose that interpersonal representations are largely mediated by medial (i.e., inner) regions of the neocortex, particularly within the frontal lobe. In addition, there may be involvement of older parts of the cortex, also known as the limbic lobe. (You can refer back to Figures 2.1 and 2.2 for a diagram of the brain regions.) This is consistent with MacLean's neo-mammalian brain but also overlaps with parts of his paleo-mammalian brain. Likewise, it is consistent with Panksepp's tertiary emotional system, in which conceptual systems in the higher cortical areas mediate core emotional processes from the lower and older regions of the brain.

Locating the substrates of interpersonal representations in these regions makes sense for a number of reasons. For one, these representations are concepts; they are ideas held in mind when the immediate object of the idea is distant in time and space. Concepts are processed in the neocortex. Secondly, the level of complexity in human personality far outstrips that found in other animals. Hence, we would expect the building blocks of human personality to rely upon the areas of the brain more advanced in humans than in other animals. Thirdly, the medial regions of the cortex are excellently placed to interact both with the lower brain regions involved in basic emotional processing and the higher cortical regions associated with complex thought and language.

So, what does the literature have to say about this? There is a fairly large and growing neurobiological literature on related domains, if not on interpersonal representations per se. Allan Schore (2003, 1994) is a psychoanalytically-oriented psychiatrist who has written a number of books about the neurological substrates of personality, as understood from a psychodynamic perspective. He notes that he comes out of the attachment, object relations and developmental psychopathology tradition. This has led him to focus upon interpersonal representations and affect regulation, specifically how interpersonal representations serve to regulate both negative and positive affect. He puts forth that the right orbital frontal cortex (OFC), a lower, medial (inner) region of the frontal lobe, located just above the eye sockets, is a central node for these personality functions. The OFC is involved in impulse control, learning from punishment and the general integration of thought, emotion, memory, and behavior. Schore also states that the OFC is central to inferring emotional states in the self and others. Likewise, the right hemisphere is more strongly associated with emotional processing than the left hemisphere, and is known to mediate recognition of emotional facial expression and intonation of speech. It is also more dominant than the left hemisphere in regulating autonomic arousal. Of particular relevance to the issue of interpersonal representations, the right hemisphere mediates empathic cognition and the perception of emotional states in other people. Further, the right OFC is uniquely well located to integrate cortical and subcortical circuitry as it is one of the most widely connected regions of the whole brain, giving and receiving direct input to areas involved with sensory, motor, emotional, visceral and arousal functions. Specifically, it has the richest connections with the limbic forebrain of any part of the frontal lobe.

George Northoff and colleagues (including Jaak Panksepp) addressed similar constructs but from a slightly different vantage point. They were interested in self-related mental processes and reviewed brain imaging findings on a range of relevant psychological tasks, such as verbal labeling of the self and viewing emotional pictures. These tasks utilized multiple processing modalities, such as verbal, facial, spatial, memory, motor, social, and emotional domains (Northoff et al., 2006). The findings pointed to a group of brain regions termed the cortical midline structures (CMS) which were preferentially involved with self-related processes regardless of the source of the information (i.e., verbal, spatial). If you draw a line from the back to the front of the brain, splitting the brain into two equal halves, the CMS lie along that line but deeper inside the brain, below the outer surface of the cortex. Additional analyses suggested three distinct areas of the CMS are involved in self-related processes, the ventral part (a lower, frontal region, close to the orbitofrontal cortex favored by Schore), the dorsal part (a higher region of the frontal lobe, close to the middle of the brain) and the posterior part (towards the back of the brain). These authors speculate that the ventral part of the CMS links information from inside the body (including the emotions) and the outside world into a coherent self-representation. The dorsal part of the CMS could be involved with the cognitive evaluation of self-related information. The posterior part could be involved with autobiographical memory, putting self-related information in the context of memory.

Another critical area of research involves the default mode network (DMN). The DMN was actually discovered accidentally. Early brain imaging studies sought to identify brain regions activated during various psychological tasks, for example when reading particular words from a list. But to do this they needed a control condition, something to compare the experimental condition against. Typically, this consisted of asking the subjects to lie in the scanner and do "nothing." However, over time it became clear that the control condition was far from neutral. Specific regions of the brain consistently lit up when subjects lay in the scanner "doing nothing." These brain regions, now referred to as the DMN, included the inner regions of the neocortex and the limbic lobe, specifically the dorsal and ventral medial prefrontal cortex, posterior cingulate, precuneus, and broader hippocampal regions, plus parts of the temporal and parietal lobes (Kluetsch et al., 2012). Of course, the subjects were not doing nothing. Although not engaged in goal-oriented mental work, subjects would let their mind wander, reminisce, plan ahead or generally think about issues relevant to themselves. Because of this, the DMN was considered to be involved in self-relevant processing. Some authors see the CMS as part of the DMN. Moreover, a study by Kluetsch and colleagues (2012) showed abnormal DMN connectivity during pain processing in patients with borderline personality disorder, supporting the DMN's involvement in personality pathology. Interestingly, there seems to be a complementary network known as the task positive network (TPN), which is activated when the person is not focused internally but rather on the external environment and the task at hand. This network includes lateral (outer rather than inner) prefrontal regions associated with complex thought plus areas of the parietal cortex involved in attention. Moreover, brain imaging studies have shown that activation of The TPN is associated with deactivation of the DMN and vice versa (Di & Biswal, 2014; Hamilton et al., 2011).

Additionally, research on the neurobiological substrates of empathy is also of interest. There appear to be two distinct components of empathy, the first involving a shared subjective experience of the other's state, which in turn involves emotional, somatosensory, and motor components. When empathizing with someone, we actually feel some of the same sensations and emotions as the other person. The second involves a cognitive component, in which the empathizer deliberately takes the other person's perspective. The first component recruits the same brain areas involved in the actual experience of pain, sadness, banging the hand against the wall, being touched, etc. Specifically, the insula and anterior cingulate, located, respectively, in the inner cortex and limbic lobe, are activated when observing other people feeling physical pain. The second, cognitive component of empathy has been linked to theory of mind, perspective taking and mentalizing and involves the medial prefrontal regions, precuneus, and temporo-parietal junction (Lamm & Majdandzic, 2015).

Finally, a fascinating new line of research looks at the role of the hippocampus in navigating social space (Schafer & Schiller, 2018). As noted in

Chapter 2, the hippocampus supports place memory for many species. It helps them recall the spatial location of important aspects of their environment. The authors investigated whether the spatial features of important social relations were also encoded by the hippocampus. They found that, indeed, the spatial features of social power and affiliative relations are mediated by hippocampal regions. This helps us track the location of people who have social significance for us, sort of like the location features on certain social media platforms.

Thus, we see a converging body of literature pointing to involvement of the inner cortex, particularly the medial frontal cortex, as well as the limbic lobe in interpersonal representations and personality structure. This supports the location of personality pathology at a relatively high level of organization in the human mind/brain, which has significant implications for differential diagnosis, that is for distinguishing between personality pathology and psychopathology located at a lower, subcortical level of the mind/brain. This will be examined in greater depth in Chapter 5. In our next chapter, however, we will address the nature of personality *pathology*. What exactly happens when personality development goes awry?

NOTES

1. In everyday language character often has moral connotations, but here we are using a more specific meaning strictly relating to personality.
2. The Diagnostic and Statistical Manual of Mental Disorders is the official diagnostic manual for the mental health field. It is in effect the diagnostic bible. The 5th edition (DSM-5) was published in 2013.
3. Panksepp capitalized these terms to differentiate them from their colloquial meanings.
4. A quick search for "attachment theory" on Google Scholar yielded 194,000 hits.
5. This notion is a cornerstone of the ancient philosophy of the Greek Stoics, whom Beck explicitly credits.

Chapter Four

Describing Personality Pathology

In the last chapter, we explored the concept of interpersonal representations. In this chapter we will look at personality *pathology*, what personality looks like when development goes awry. And we will consider it in the context of Emergent Systems Theory. Chapter 3 introduced Robert Cloninger's definition of personality as consisting of both temperament and character, the former a set of largely genetic traits and the latter a learned system of concepts about the self in the world. In this chapter we will focus upon character, putting temperament to the side, at least for now. Thus, in this chapter, we use the terms character and personality interchangeably. To further clarify, we will only consider personality pathology in adulthood. It is tricky to speak of this kind of pathology in children or adolescents as their personality has not fully consolidated.

Defining Personality Pathology

So now we can ask, what is actual personality pathology? What does it look like, both in clinical settings and in daily life? In the previous chapter, we defined character pathology as an *inadequate development of interpersonal representations, producing top-down failures in the regulation of affect, thought and behavior*. I will add that pathology of interpersonal representations manifests in maladaptive *form* and *content*. Form refers to the organizational structure of the representations, namely that they remain simplistic and crude rather than well integrated and differentiated—this will be discussed in detail later in the chapter. Content refers to the "what" of the representations. How do people see themselves and other people? For example, do people see themselves as capable or incompetent, as loveable or unworthy? Likewise, do they see other people as malevolent or benevolent, as trustworthy or unreliable? This also will be elaborated below.

But first let us look at how personality disorders are defined in DSM-5, the official diagnostic manual of the mental health field. The DSM system lists categorical diagnoses; you either have them or you don't. In psychotherapy, we work more on a continuum; patients have varying degrees of personality pathology. Nonetheless, the authors of the DSM elected to use diagnostic categories as they believe it enhances communication across the mental health field and facilitates decision making.

In DSM-5, personality disorders are defined as problems in affect, thought, impulse control and interpersonal functioning that have been evident since adolescence or early adulthood, are consistent across time and situation, and cause dysfunction and distress to the individual. These problems are not due to another diagnosis, such as a mood or psychotic disorder. Moreover, they are abnormal for the person's culture or subculture. Ten specific personality disorders are grouped into 3 clusters. Cluster A, the "odd cluster," refers to disorders characterized by distortions of thought. Paranoid personality disorder is characterized by suspiciousness; schizoid by avoidance of social relations coupled with odd thoughts and behavior; and schizotypal by particularly peculiar thoughts and behavior in the absence of psychosis per se. Cluster B, the "dramatic cluster," is characterized by dramatic and impulsive behavior. Histrionic personality disorder is characterized by a volatile but shallow and performative emotionality; narcissistic by grandiosity, an excessive need for admiration and lack of empathy; borderline by emotional volatility, impulsive behavior, intense and unstable relationships, diffuse identity, and suicidal gestures; and antisocial by gross lack of empathy, illegal behavior, and the exploitation and manipulation of others. Cluster C is known as the "anxious cluster." Avoidant personality disorder is characterized by intense harm avoidance and social anxiety; obsessive-compulsive by an excessive need for control and order; and dependent by over-dependence on others for daily functioning.

While the DSM system has a considerable amount of empirical support—it is predictive of numerous social, mental, and even physical outcomes and shows strong inter-rater reliability (i.e., can be diagnosed consistently by different clinicians)—it has been criticized on a number of fronts. For one, it is far from comprehensive and many patients with personality pathology simply don't fit into any of the 10 categories; most patients have traits of more than one diagnosis; and many do not meet full criteria for any of them. Finally, the categorical system does not account for severity, which is probably more important in terms of how the person functions in the world than the discrete type of personality disorder.

Because of these limitations, the task force for personality disorders for DSM-5 tried to come up with an alternative diagnostic system before the 5th edition of DSM was published in 2013. This system highlighted self and interpersonal functioning, making moderate to severe impairment in either of these domains the gateway criterion for a personality disorder. Specifically, this included difficulties with identity, self-direction, empathy and/or intimacy. Then to refine the diagnosis, the patient could be described in terms of the 5-factor model as translated into pathological rather than normal personality traits. These included negative affectivity (vs. emotional stability), detachment (vs. extraversion), antagonism (vs. agreeableness), disinhibition (vs. conscientiousness), and psychoticism (vs. lucidity). There were an additional 26 traits to refine these dimensions. Further 6 out of the original 10 DSM diagnoses were retained. Ultimately, this new system was deemed too complex and lacking sufficient research support for an official diagnostic system. It was therefore included in the manual as provisional and in need of further research.

In my mind, the take-home message from this endeavor is two-fold. One, that it is extremely difficult to encapsulate all of personality pathology in any one diagnostic system. Possibly, this is because of its environmental etiology. If there are infinite varieties of life experience, there will be infinite varieties of personality pathology—although they may well cluster into a finite number of groups. The second take home message is that self and interpersonal representations are central to the definition of personality pathology.

DYSREGULATION OF THOUGHT, AFFECT AND BEHAVIOR

Within the framework of Emergent Systems Theory, interpersonal representations are seen as a higher-order system that regulates the subsystems of thought, affect and behavior. Although the pathology *stems* from interpersonal representations, however, it is most *detectable* through its downstream impact on subjective experience and actual behavior. In fact, the underlying interpersonal representations are not always evident and often take considerable work to uncover. Therefore, it is the problematic emotions, thoughts and behaviors that provide our entry point into the individual's personality. Nonetheless, while these symptoms offer the most visible signs of pathology, their diagnostic significance is not always clear. For example, the symptoms of borderline personality disorder can mimic those of bipolar disorder. Likewise, the symptoms of narcissistic personality disorder may overlap with those of hypomania and paranoid personality disorder may be mistaken for delusional disorder. These questions of differential diagnosis, however, will be covered in the next chapter.

So, let us now look at how dysregulation of thought, affect, and behavior can present in personality disordered patients. Although we will consider these domains separately, they are generally intertwined. For example, thoughts can set off affect which can set off behavior, which can then route back to thoughts. In this way interactions between these subsystems can create positive feedback loops. Still, it is helpful to first consider each subsystem in isolation.

In general, at the level of each subsystem, we're looking at *regulatory failures*. This refers to the failure to flexibly modulate psychological functions in order to best adapt to the environment. A psychological function is adaptive when it promotes and protects the individual's wellbeing in the context of the (typically interpersonal) environment. It is pathological when it causes unnecessary distress or impedes adaptation to the environment. Keep in mind as well that pathology can range in severity from the subtle and even questionably pathological to the severe and unmistakably disturbed.

Dysregulation of Behavior

Let us start with the regulation of behavior. In general, there can be problems with disinhibition (under-controlled behavior) or excessive inhibition (over-controlled or constricted behavior). Disinhibited behavior is impulsive and rash and can include getting into bar fights, spending too much money, quitting a job with no back up plan, binge eating, or unsafe sex. Addictive behavior (e.g., alcoholism, drug abuse, gambling, compulsive sexual behavior) and self-destructive behavior (e.g., suicidal threats and gestures or non-suicidal cutting) also count as inhibitory failures. These kinds of behavior are most common in Cluster B personality disorders.

Excessively inhibited behavior frequently involves some type of avoidance of an anxiety-producing situation. Alternatively, people can fail to act due to impoverished motivation or initiative. They are not avoidant so much as lacking the desire to pursue a goal. In milder cases, people might avoid confrontations with other people, public speaking or pursuing a romantic possibility. In more extreme cases, people can be housebound for years, refuse to look for a job, or become intensely socially isolated. People may also fail to follow through on necessary activities, such as medical care or paying rent.

Additionally, people might demonstrate compulsive behavior. This refers to driven, effortful behavior that is performed in order to avoid some kind of perceived harm. This becomes pathological when it causes more harm than benefit, for example with workaholic behavior or compulsive exercise. For more discussion about the different types of behavioral dysregulation, see Stein et al. (2000) and Cohen (2015).

Let us now consider some clinical examples. I have drawn these primarily from my clinical experience but also from other aspects of life. Because of the need for confidentiality, I have changed all identifying information and combined different people's stories into composite case examples.

***Sarah*:**

Sarah provides an example of grossly disinhibited behavior. She is a 27-year-old female who works in a high-end art gallery. Her parents divorced when she was 6 years old. Her father lived nearby and was involved with her life, but the bulk of her upbringing lay with her mother. Her father did not significantly interfere. Although he drank too much, he was otherwise reasonably stable. However, her mother was far from that. She had bipolar disorder coupled with polysubstance abuse and was highly erratic and often abusive. While Sarah was able to obtain a college education and to maintain a meaningful job, daily life for her was a continual struggle. She was extremely dependent on her boyfriends and often made poor choices, turning to emotionally and even physically abusive men who also abused drugs. One night after a particularly long and intense fight, in which her boyfriend berated her mercilessly, she took off for a casino in Connecticut, where she gambled, drank, and smoked cigarettes until the next morning. She was sick in her hotel room, vomiting repeatedly, and returned home thousands of dollars in debt. Such episodes occurred repeatedly, perhaps several times a year.

***George*:**

George provides an example of excessively inhibited behavior. He is a 42-year-old male who was raised in an upper middle-class suburb with parents whose financial fortune fluctuated widely. For most of his adolescence his father did quite well financially, but his fortunes reversed when George was a young man. Throughout his childhood, George had been irresponsible. He had high native intelligence but was loathe to study. He liked to make money but was quick to leave jobs. Most of the time, when he ran into trouble, his parents came to the rescue. However, this abruptly stopped when George was in his mid-20s. At this point, George did succeed in obtaining a good job in real estate sales. For a while, he was quite successful, but when the company changed management, George did not get along as well with the new owners. Eventually he quit, stating that he would take some time to relax before looking for new job. He had amassed a fair amount of savings and could live off of that for some time. But one year turned into two. Two years turned into ten. Effectively, George sat passively, smoking pot and surfing the internet until all his savings ran out. By this point, his father had died of cancer and his mother could not afford to help him. Still, he failed to mobilize himself to find a new job. Eventually, he needed to go on welfare and move to a much smaller apartment in a high-crime area.

He did finally obtain a new job, but it paid much less and afforded a drastically reduced quality of life.

***Jennifer*:**

Jennifer provides an example of compulsive behavior. Jennifer is a 56-year-old divorced woman who works as a secretary in a finance firm. She was raised in poverty by a single mother. Her mother was an alcoholic, who was frequently absent, leaving Jennifer to care for her younger siblings. She often spent time with her grandparents, who, although more stable than her mother, were very religious and extremely strict. Her grandfather was quick with the strap, frequently utilizing corporal punishment. From age 8 to age 12, she was sexually abused by one of her mother's boyfriends. When she told her mother about this at age 12, her mother kicked the boyfriend out and initially pressed charges. But she soon dropped the charges and a few years later relented and let him move back in, convincing herself that Jennifer was lying. Within a few years, she married him. Although he never again molested her, Jennifer harbored an enormous sense of betrayal and deep grief at not having been believed by her mother. As an adult, she had a difficult time listening to the needs of her own body. As a worker, she was tireless. She would always work through lunch, never taking a break even to sit down and rest for 10 minutes. She became very tired and had medical problems that demanded rest but she would not stop working. Her legs swelled up but still she would not rest. She would say that she wanted to prove that she was a good worker so that no one could criticize her. She also could not tolerate her work being left undone at the end of the day and would become enraged at what she perceived to be other people's carelessness. Eventually she was forced to retire early on disability due to neglect of her medical problems.

***Martin*:**

While these last three case examples present severe personality pathology, many of our patients are not so disturbed. Martin provides an example of a patient with much less severe characterological difficulties. Nonetheless, his dysregulated behavior causes him distress and interferes with his functioning. Martin is a 62-year-old married man with 3 grown children. He was born to an intact family with one brother, 5 years younger. Martin's early years were happy but when he was 8 and his brother 3, the family fortunes changed. His father was badly injured in a construction accident and his mother slipped into a depression from which she never fully recovered. With financial support from the extended family, they got by but Martin's mother became increasingly emotionally dependent on him. His brother, who lost out on maternal attention at a much younger age than he, later came to resent him, feeling that Martin had been favored by their parents. Nonetheless, Martin has done very well in life. He owns a successful contracting business which he built up himself over 3 decades. He has a solid marriage, and his adult children are doing well. However, he has considerable difficulty managing his finances. He has a particularly hard time putting together his invoices and procrastinates for months before billing his clients. This leads to considerable stress about unpaid bills and to frequent arguments with his wife. Sometimes he loses money as he has not adequately documented the work he has done. When pushed, he reports that he is aware that he is only hurting himself by procrastinating but still cannot force himself to behave otherwise. More frequently he dismisses the relevance of his procrastination, insisting his financial stresses are due to external causes and a difficult financial climate.

Dysregulation of Affect

Dysregulated affect is often the hallmark of personality pathology. It is a critical target of treatment as it is typically the impetus for dysregulated behavior, including suicide attempts or violent outbursts. As with behavior, affective dysregulation can manifest in either insufficient or excessive control as well as alternation between both extremes. Insufficient control includes affective volatility and extreme emotional reactions. Individuals can have intense rage episodes, profound bouts of despair, or paroxysms of fear, all in response to triggers that would not elicit such reactions in most people. They can also have excessively positive emotional reactions. This causes problems when it results in poor judgment, for example when moving in with a new romantic partner after only two weeks. Excessive emotional control can manifest in dissociated responses, emotional blunting, or alexithymia, where the people have no subjective awareness of what they are feeling. People can also swing between both states, suppressing their distress until they reach a critical threshold and explode. Let us now return to our four case examples and see how dysregulated affect plays out in each of them.

***Sarah*:**
Sarah has great difficulty in modulating her emotions. She is aware that her choice of boyfriends is problematic and that their verbal and even physical abuse cause her great distress. But she is unable to tolerate being alone for any length of time. After she initially breaks up with an abusive boyfriend, she feels liberated and proud of herself. But soon she becomes restless and a great gaping emptiness opens up inside her. She feels incredible loneliness and despair, which she describes as a black hole of sadness. This in turn makes her anxious and at any sign of these profoundly painful feelings, she feels an onset of panic and immediately turns to action to distract from her emotional pain.

***George*:**
George suffers from inadequate control of negative emotions and notable constriction of positive emotions. He frequently feels a heaviness and dark lack of joy in life. There is little that he looks forward to. Most of the time he is smothered in shame, feeling that he is worthless and a complete failure. These

feelings alternate, however, with occasional bursts of energy and enthusiasm and a gleeful sense of superiority over others. When he feels he has found an arena in which to succeed or to meet his exalted expectations of himself, he becomes exhilarated as if filled with power and triumph. However, he is also prone to a brooding anger and resentment, particularly when he feels humiliated or put down by others. Unfortunately, it takes very little provocation for him to feel demeaned, creating a propensity towards humiliation and rage as well as a tense hypervigilance for possible threats to his self-esteem.

***Jennifer*:**
Jennifer alternates between extremes of affective suppression and volatility. When working compulsively, she is unaware of anger, anxiety or any sense of sadness. Nor does she feel particular joy or pleasure in her work, only a mild sense of grim satisfaction that she is completing the tasks she feels obligated to do. She does feel irritation at coworkers when they behave in what she considers irresponsible ways. This can erupt into rage, particularly if she feels unfairly criticized or blamed at work. Her rage soon subsides into a childlike tearfulness, however, as if exaggerating her defenselessness before towering and punitive adults. Her employers tolerate her erratic emotional responses because of her effectiveness on the one hand and her otherwise caring and sympathetic manner on the other.

***Martin*:**
Although Martin's difficulty with emotion is less crippling than the others, he still suffers unnecessarily. Martin often feels a blanket of anxiety around him relating to financial stress. He constantly worries that he will run out of money and miss payments on his own or family's expenses. Yet he experiences this as solely related to the level of work coming in, constantly feeling pressure to work harder. When it comes to sending out his invoices, however, he does not consciously feel anxiety or resentment; rather he continues to forget these tasks on his to-do list as if they simply slip his mind.

Dysregulation of Cognition

Dysregulation of cognition is an important part of personality pathology, as explored in detail by the cognitive therapists (See Chapter 3). However, the relationship between cognition and interpersonal representations is complex. Higher-order cognition, that is the more complex forms of cognition, are largely independent of interpersonal representations and in fact can be placed at a higher level of organization in the mind/brain, involving the dorsolateral frontal cortex. Our ability to perform advanced math, to diagnose a car's mechanical problems, or to understand political theory has little direct connection with core personality structure. We can therefore speculate that complex and abstract thought arose later in human evolution than did interpersonal representations. Certainly, these intellectual capacities emerge later in human development, well into the teenage years if not later.

However, the more fundamental components of cognition, such as attention, memory, concentration, and simple reasoning, arise earlier in human development. As discussed in Chapter 2, they emerged earlier in human evolution as well. Unquestionably, they are influenced by our emotional state as well as our basic assumptions about self in world. What we pay attention to, enter into our memory and perceive to be true are deeply affected by our emotional state and self-perception (Ask & Granhag, 2007). In effect, we bias our cognition to process information in a way that is consistent with our frame of mind. As such, we can say that our interpersonal representations regulate these simpler forms of cognition in a top-down manner. However, we can add that our representations regulate more complex cognitive processes in a bottom-up manner, to the extent that our more complex cognition is also biased by our pre-set view of the world.

So let us consider how cognition is compromised in the context of personality pathology. What does this look like? I will propose three interrelated aspects of cognition impacted by personality pathology: filtering, evaluation and flexibility. Cognitive *filtering* refers to the utilization of attention, memory and concentration to regulate the level of emotionally stimulating information taken in at any given time. This concept is similar to the psychoanalytic concept of defense mechanisms as detailed in Anna Freud's classic work on the mechanisms of defense (1966). Inadequate filtering leads the person to become overwhelmed by emotionally stimulating information. There may be rumination about unpleasant situations or preoccupation with perceived problems or desired goals. Obsessional thought also counts as a failure of filtering. In contrast, excessive filtering stops uncomfortable information from getting in. There may be flat out denial of a reality that is obvious to everyone else or the reality may be acknowledged but then rationalized so that it is more tolerable. There may also be dissociated responses, in which attention and awareness are altered to keep the person unaware of specific circumstances, as if disconnected from their environment.

Evaluation refers to the continuous task of making sense of our environment. We have to evaluate and interpret all events we experience, both our own actions and those of objects and people we do not control. This is a reasoning process in which we identify a sequence of events and the relationships among them. We attribute causation to events. What just happened and how did it happen? In personality pathology, the person's reasoning about events may become highly distorted. It can be overly positive, overly negative, highly egocentric or frankly illogical.

Finally, cognitive *flexibility* refers to the ability to change cognitive set in the context of new information. Can you change your mind when new evidence shows that you might have been wrong? Or that the old belief system is no longer adaptive? Alternatively, are you too quick to change your mind, shifting beliefs with the changing fashions? People with personality pathology can show either cognitive rigidity or excessive flexibility and often show both.

***Sarah*:**
Sarah demonstrated marked impairment in all three cognitive functions. Although her boyfriends were repeatedly abusive, always verbally and not infrequently physically, each time it happened she was caught by surprise. It was if it had never happened before. She could not or would not learn from experience. She would accept at face value her boyfriends' promises to change. Alternatively, she would insist that from now on she would have the upper hand because of some minor concession she was able to extract. Thus, her understanding of her boyfriends' behavior rapidly fluctuated from condemnation to facile belief in their excuses. These cognitive distortions were fueled by a profound desire to repair a broken relationship, just as she had so longed to fix her childhood relationship with her mentally ill mother. In other words, her intense wish to fix the unfixable led her to distort reality.

***George*:**
George similarly showed significant disturbances in cognition. Although later in his life he mostly perceived himself as an extreme failure, as a young man he maintained a dramatically unrealistic view of his own superiority. As an undergraduate, he believed himself to be the most intelligent student in his class and his papers the most insightful and sophisticated. Although his grades did not reflect this as he maintained a B average—acceptable though hardly stellar—his aggrandized view of himself did not change. Factual information did not impact his evaluation of his standing vis a vis other people.

***Jennifer*:**
Jennifer's difficulty primarily involved inadequate filtering. She was not able to distract herself from her perfectionism and a compulsive need to complete all tasks. Simultaneously, her disregard of her own health reflected excessive filtering; the information about her physical needs simply did not get through. Preoccupied with the minute details of each task, she was unable to step back and see the larger picture, to recognize what was and was not important. In this way her evaluation of the situation was distorted; she missed the forest while fixating on the trees. Additionally, her inability to shift her attention away from her work and to appreciate the cost to her health demonstrated profound cognitive rigidity.

***Martin*:**

While Martin's difficulties were less extreme than the others, he still demonstrated maladaptive cognitive processes, including faulty filtering and distorted evaluation. He was highly lax about his accounting and avoided completing his invoices, maintaining a remarkable lack of anxiety about these delays. If asked, he would minimize the importance of his own accounting, saying "I'll get to it. I'll get to it." Though he was preoccupied with concerns about his general financial wellbeing, it was almost exclusively focused on factors outside of his own behavior. He constantly worried that his business leads would dry up and he would not have enough customers coming in. Eventually, he would recognize the need to catch up on his billing and would do so in order to pay his bills; hence his actual financial situation was fairly stable. In this way he differed from the other three case examples, as he was able to maintain a high level of functioning. Yet he experienced a constant state of tension, the source of which he continually misinterpreted to lie outside his control.

Dysregulation of Interpersonal and Self-Functioning

Given the centrality of interpersonal representations in personality pathology, we also see direct dysregulation of both interpersonal and self-related behavior. With regard to interpersonal functioning, there can be notable impairment in the capacity for intimacy, empathy, and conflict negotiation, as well as the stability of relationships.

With Sarah we can see how her choice of partners and ineffective conflict resolution strategies powerfully impact her functioning. We also see how deeply impaired George is in the interpersonal realm. His hypersensitivity to feeling demeaned and humiliated by others results in a paranoid hostility that eventually drove all his friends and family away from him. Jennifer was also socially isolated. Though she had a warm and nurturing side, developed as a child when caring for her younger siblings, this was compromised by her irritability and unrealistically exacting standards. Perhaps more importantly, a general fear of depending on others led her to maintain considerable distance from other people. She would not let anyone get too close. Of the four, Martin is the least impaired in social relations, though his chronic state of anxiety leads to an unnecessary level of irritability and resulting family conflict.

With regard to self-functioning, individuals with personality pathology often have problems regulating self-esteem, self-confidence, assertiveness, and/or entitlement. Sarah's tolerance of abusive behavior in her partners betrays a deeply degraded sense of self and a tragic lack of healthy entitlement. She simply does not believe she deserves better. George's grandiose sense of self is essentially the root of his problems, as is characteristic of narcissistic personality disorder. His inability to live up to his own unrealistically elevated expectations of himself paralyzes him; he cannot tolerate being anything but the best. This of course only reinforces his sense of failure. Jennifer's behavior, like Sarah's, betrays a profound lack of self-worth and a deeply deficient sense of healthy entitlement. Her relationship with her body is particularly disturbed, as can happen with sexual abuse survivors. She cannot recognize her right to take care of her own body. Martin's difficulty with self-functioning is not as obvious as he can come across as highly dominant and self-confident. However, his difficulty billing his clients stems from a deep sense of guilt at taking from others, at getting more than another person. This is related to his excessive sense of obligation to his depressed mother as well as his guilt at feeling preferred by his mother compared to his younger brother. Thus, he lacks a sufficient sense of entitlement.

Interpersonal Representations

Now that we have looked at how personality pathology can manifest in dysregulated affect, cognition and behavior, let's go back to the source of the Nile, namely maladaptive interpersonal representations. As mentioned above, personality pathology stems both from the *content* and *form* of interpersonal representations. Let us first consider content. As discussed in Chapter 3, interpersonal representations are prototypical memories of self and other in relationship with one another. The lived experience becomes condensed into a schema or map of how people interact and the representation of self and other are abstracted from this narrative.

The 18 maladaptive schemas from the most recent version of the Young Schema Questionnaire (YSQ-S3) provide a pretty comprehensive sample of maladaptive schema content. These include: Abandonment/Instability, Mistrust/Abuse, Emotional Deprivation, Defectiveness/Shame, Social Isolation/Alienation, Dependence/Incompetence, Vulnerability to Harm or Illness, Enmeshment/Undeveloped Self, Failure to Achieve, Entitlement/Grandiosity, Insufficient Self-Control/Self-Discipline, Subjugation, Self-Sacrifice, Approval-Seeking/Recognition-Seeking, Negativity/Pessimism, Emotional Inhibition, Unrelenting Standards/Hypercriticalness, and Punitiveness (http://www.schematherapy.com/id73.htm, retrieved October 31, 2019).

While these 18 maladaptive schemas are extensive, they are not and probably cannot be exhaustive. In as much as there are an infinite amount of possible life experiences, there are likely an infinite number of interpersonal schemas. We must also emphasize that most of the time these representations are implicit and not conscious. Therapy aims to make them more explicit to the patient, which provides the opportunity to rework them into a healthier and more flexible view of self and world.

Now let's return to our four patients. How can we understand the *content* of their representations of self and other?

***Sarah*:**

With her history of severe abuse and neglect, Sarah sees relationships as characterized by rejection, volatility, and abuse. That to her means love. This is not conscious—rather she simply believes that such relationships are normal, or that they are all that she can realistically hope for. As such, she believes herself incapable of attracting anyone who would treat her well, that she is not worthy of a genuinely caring and reciprocal relationship. While she feels powerless to find and maintain a relationship with a truly loving partner, she also harbors an exaggerated sense of her own power—that if she tries hard enough, she will be able to change these men and turn them into the people she wants them to be. Thus, the content of her representations contains highly contradictory elements.

***George*:**

George holds an exaggerated view of his own worth. He feels that he is inherently superior to others, more intelligent, talented, witty, etc. That he has not attained the success he believes to be his due is attributed to the malicious efforts of others to sabotage him. Therefore, he assumes other people to be envious, competitive and malevolently intentioned. But, as with Sarah, there is another side to this self-representation; if he cannot meet his own elevated expectations, then he must be a complete failure, a shameful ruin of a man with no redeeming qualities. Thus, he lives in continual fear of exposure as a sham. Using a paranoid defense, he projects his fears of how others might perceive him outward onto the world. He attributes to other people all sorts of demeaning and malevolent attitudes towards him that have little to do with their actual thoughts.

***Jennifer*:**

Jennifer often sees other people as towering and harshly punitive authority figures that she has to appease. Likewise, she perceives herself to be largely powerless in this world and subject to extremely exacting demands that she cannot and does not question. She feels the only control she has in her life is to ensure that she lives up to these standards. Further, her sense of self-worth is deeply damaged. She does not experience her body as belonging to herself nor as deserving of care and protection. Here we can see how she has internalized her relationship with her authoritarian grandfather as well her experiences with both her neglectful mother and sexually abusive step-father. Her workaholic behavior seems to pertain most to her grandfather, although her neglect of her own medical conditions can be traced to the treatment she received from her mother and step-father.

***Martin*:**

Martin's maladaptive representations are less easily inferred from his area of problematic behavior. Nonetheless, they still exert a strong influence on him.

> At base, Martin perceives himself as unfairly privileged and therefore obligated to provide for others. Because others are so much more deprived or in need than him, his own needs are less important. Therefore, any claims he makes on others are illegitimate and indicative of an excessive sense of entitlement. He feels significant guilt whenever he tries to put himself first. Hence, he avoids billing his clients as he fears exposing himself to moral judgement. However, there is also a rebellious part of him which reacts with anger to this excessive sense of obligation. But this anger only reinforces his guilt, fueling a vicious, self-perpetuating cycle.

THE STRUCTURE OF INTERPERSONAL REPRESENTATIONS

Now that we have addressed content, we will turn to the question of structure. The formal structure of individuals' interpersonal representations, that is the way that they are organized, is a central component of their personality. As such, a hallmark of personality pathology is the relatively crude organization of interpersonal representations. But before we go further, let us revisit the principles of Emergent Systems Theory presented in Chapter 1. As discussed in Chapter 1, complex systems generally develop from a state of general simplicity to one of greater complexity. The same is true for interpersonal representations. As such, personality pathology reflects the failure of these structures to develop to an *adequate state of complexity*. At its essence, therefore, personality pathology reflects a failure of psychological development.

To briefly recap, we define a system as a whole that is defined by the interactions of its component parts. Systems interact with one another to form higher level systems, which in turn serve as component parts of even higher-level systems. In this way, systems form hierarchical structures. And in so doing, they develop from relative simplicity to relative complexity. In this book, the human mind/brain is seen as just such a hierarchically organized system and interpersonal representations as a *subsystem* of the larger mind/brain. Moreover, as discussed above, affect, behavior, and simple thought processes are seen as subsystems of interpersonal representations. They operate on a lower level of the mind/brain and are regulated by interpersonal representations in a top-down manner (with exceptions for complex cognition as noted above).

In living organisms, complexity provides many advantages. It allows for greater flexibility, a broader behavioral repertoire and improved adaptability to changing conditions. In particular, the higher levels of system organization can direct and control the lower levels, much as a CEO directs the operations of all the company's departments. This centralized control is extremely powerful as it creates efficient coordination across subsystems. Likewise, complexity at the level of interpersonal representations allows for more powerful, efficient, and flexible regulation of affect, cognition, and behavior. Thus, individuals with maturely organized interpersonal representations can regulate their thought, emotion, and behavior more effectively. Consider the self-regulation of an adult compared to a 2-year-old child. The child is all impulse and no foresight—the slightest frustration can lead to a complete melt down. Children are therefore highly dependent upon adults to help them regulate affect and behavior as they are not yet capable of it.

Integration, Differentiation and Articulation

As detailed in Chapter 1, there are three component processes to system development. These inter-related processes: *integration*, *differentiation,* and *articulation*, are key mechanisms by which systems develop to higher levels of complexity. Integration refers to the coordination between two component subsystems; two parts interact to form a larger whole. Differentiation refers to the separation of two parts out of a larger whole. What was one becomes two. Articulation is another side of differentiation. It refers to the creation of variation in a previously homogenous whole. What was uniform becomes multi-faceted.

As presented in Chapter 2, there are numerous examples of this in biology. Across billions of years, single cell organisms evolved into cell colonies and then into multi-celled organisms whose cells differentiated to form distinct functional units, such as organs, legs, and eyes. Simultaneously, these distinct body parts coordinated with one another to create an integrated, multi-faceted organism with a much broader range of behavioral responses to the environment than is found in simpler life forms. In this way, the extraordinarily complex species of homo sapiens (i.e., human beings) has evolved out of the simplest of bacteria (or archaea).

The same processes are central to the development of interpersonal representations. Across infancy and childhood, the child's representations of self in relation to others becomes more integrated, differentiated, and articulated. In other words, as children mature, their view of self in world becomes increasingly complex. This is dependent upon contemporaneous neurological development. Increased synaptic connections allow for greater connection between neurons. This permits greater integration and subsequently greater differentiation and articulation of brain networks. Moreover, the myelination of axon fibers allows for more rapid and therefore more frequent communication among different neurons. The subcortical areas of the brain myelinate before the cortex. In fact, the myelination of the frontal lobe does not complete until the third decade of life. Thus, development of cortically mediated concepts, including interpersonal representations, occurs much later than that of core emotions or basic physiological processes.

That psychopathology reflects inadequate levels of integration and differentiation of self and other representations is not a new idea. In fact, it is found throughout psychoanalytic writings. We saw in Chapter 3 how Melanie Klein described the integration of early "part-objects" into a fuller, multi-faceted view of the caregiver. Likewise, Donald Winnicott described how the young child grapples with self-other differentiation. These concepts are implicit in much of cognitive therapy as well, as shown in the focus upon cognitive distortions and erroneous thinking (as discussed below). However, here we will focus our discussion on the work of Irene Fast, a psychoanalytic theorist who explicitly addresses this topic in her work on Event Theory (Fast, 1985; Fast et al., 1996).

Irene Fast aimed to synthesize the contributions of Sigmund Freud and Jean Piaget, the Swiss psychologist famous for his work on cognitive development. She believed that Piaget offered the best framework to account for the clinical phenomenon of primitive thought processes, in which the patient's understanding of the world regresses to a disorganized, immature, or even bizarre state. According to Event Theory, the most fundamental unit of knowledge is of the *event*.[1] The infant creates a schema or representation of a typical class of lived events, such as crying, nursing, playing with a rattle, etc. Initially, the participants in the event schema are *embedded* in the event; they are not differentiated out of it, and they have no independent identity outside of the event. Moreover, each event schema is self-contained; there is no continuity between distinct events. The mother of peaceful nursing and the mother of wailing hunger are not connected with one another. They are essentially different mothers. We know now that this lack of differentiation is never complete. As Dan Stern discussed in his 1986 book, there are inborn organizing properties of the brain that ensure some primordial awareness of the connection between events and the difference between self and non-self from earliest infancy. Nonetheless, compared to adults, children have dramatically less differentiated and integrated representations of their world. Fast uses the term *event-bound* to refer to the child's perception of objects and people as embedded within the event in which they are encountered.

Piaget's concept of object permanence provides a beautiful example of event-bound thinking (Piaget, 1954). Piaget's initial research was conducted on his own children. He closely observed their behavior under a range of natural conditions. When the children were infants, he engaged their attention with various objects (e.g., a pencil, rattle, or watch). Then he observed their behavior as he removed the object. Initially, the babies would watch the object as long as it was in their line of vision but quickly lose interest once it was removed. If the object was out of sight, it was out of mind. A few months later, they would follow the object with their eyes as it disappeared from sight but showed no searching behavior after it was removed. However, by the age of 8 months (give or take), his children exhibited searching behavior. If he put the object behind a pillow and then removed his hand without it, the children would move the pillow to search for the toy. This showed that they had differentiated their representation of the toy from the immediate event of seeing it; the representation of the toy was no longer event-bound.

Once children are old enough to talk, their speech can offer a wonderful window into their event-bound thought processes. Vanessa at two years old was a very verbal little girl. When her parents took her to visit her extended family in another city, her aunt and uncle were excited to explain their relationship to her. "Vanessa," her uncle told her, "Marie is Julie's *sister*." (Julie was Vanessa's mother.) Daniel is Julie's *brother*." Vanessa looked utterly confused by this so her aunt pressed on. "Julie is Marie and Daniel's sister." Suddenly Vanessa caught on. But she didn't like what she was hearing. "Julie is MYYYYY mother!" Vanessa shouted and then repeated about five times. "Julie is MYYYYY mother! Julie is MYYYYY Mother!" Vanessa could not grasp that Julie had any relationships outside of that between the two of them. As such, her representation of her mother was not *differentiated* from that of their relationship. Likewise, Vanessa could not *integrate* Julie's role as mother with that as sister. In Vanessa's mind, her mother could only have one identity. If she was sister to her siblings, she could not be mother to Vanessa. And if a choice had to be made, it was clear what that choice would be!

Later in the same trip, Vanessa joined the family at the breakfast table. "My, Vanessa, don't you look cute today, with your hair in ponytails," her grandfather said to her. In response, Vanessa stuck out her round belly and loudly asserted "Baba is MYYYY grandfather and MYYYY granddaughter!" Here we see a perfect example of event-bound thinking. As grandfather and granddaughter are both wholly defined by their relationship with one another, their roles are essentially interchangeable. Vanessa's assertive possessiveness is also notable, and can be seen as an initial stage in the development of a differentiated self-concept. At two years old she has discovered that not only does she have a self that is distinct from others, but that self can *own* things and therefore relate to the world through the process of possession.

Thus, we see how event-bound thinking characterizes the early development of interpersonal representations. Now let us consider some important implications of this kind of thinking. For one, event-bound thinking lacks a *temporal context*. The person lives in a perpetual now. If there is no connection between different events, then there can be no sense of past or future; there can only be now. This is what underlies the delightful purity of children's joy but also the stark terror of their fear and the unmodulated nature of their aggression. The child cannot reduce the emotional impact of the present by understanding it within a larger temporal context, by considering what has happened in the past and what will happen in the future. Secondly, event-bound thinking distorts *causality*. If one cannot see the connection between events, it is not possible to understand how one event can affect the subsequent event. Instead, the behavior of the participants in the event can only be explained by their co-existence *in* the event. This is what underlies children's egocentricity, which renders them vulnerable to long lasting psychological damage in the context of maltreatment. Things happen when I'm watching them, therefore I must have caused them. Daddy left because I didn't make my bed. Mommy hits me because I'm bad. The child cannot understand that Daddy left because the marriage broke up, which had nothing to do with the children. Likewise, there is no separation of the child's sense of self-worth from the mother's abusive behavior.

Thirdly, in event-bound thinking, there is no differentiation between the child's subjective experience and the external, objective reality. The object and the child's subjective perception of the object are embedded in the event of seeing the object. This is the basis of *solipsism*, the idea that one's thoughts create external reality. (I think therefore you are.) It also underlies the young child's difficulty distinguishing fantasy from reality, such that harmless clothes in the closet can become monsters after dark. Objects and people are controlled by the child's imagination not by impersonal, objective laws of cause and effect.

Event-bound Thinking in Adult Psychopathology

Importantly, we see all these features of event-bound thinking in the interpersonal representations of personality disordered adults. Thus, in personality pathology, the representations of self and other are insufficiently integrated, differentiated and articulated, with resulting disturbances in perception of temporal context, causality and subjective vs. objective reality. Let's consider some examples commonly seen in clinical work.

Splitting, which is a characteristic of borderline personality disorder, involves seeing people as either all good or all bad. Either one's view of another person can alternate from all good to all bad, as in the rapid idealization and devaluation of others listed as a diagnostic criterion for borderline personality disorder in DSM-5, or one person is seen as all good and another as all bad. These representations lack articulation as people are perceived as uniformly one way or another, with no nuance or complexity. Likewise, there is a failure to integrate the different aspects of the person into a multi-faceted portrayal. Instead, whatever does not fit into the simplistic portrayal is simply disregarded.

The self-absorption characteristic of narcissistic personality disorder reflects failure of self-other differentiation. Other people are not seen as separate individuals with their own motivations, histories, and perspectives. Rather, they are seen as extensions of the self, entirely embedded in the self's own subjective experience. Their subjective life is not *differentiated* from the self's own mental life. Other people's subjective experience may be seen as complementary to that of the self, serving either to boost or threaten self-esteem. Alternatively, other people's mental life may be entirely disregarded, so that they are seen more as objects to be used or discarded rather than independent sentient beings.

The lack of temporal context is a frequent problem in clinical work. Personality disordered people can become so overwhelmed by their dysregulated emotion that they lose perspective. They cannot remember that these emotions did not exist last week and will likely be gone by next week. The emotional state feels like a perpetual now; it has always been this way and always will be. It is in these states that people act out impulsively, as if their current emotional state is the only one to consider. Likewise, people cannot think through the future consequences of their action. Tomorrow is another lifetime. Why worry about it now?

The confusion between internal/subjective vs. external/objective reality is also a frequent problem in clinical work. While we rarely see outright delusions, we frequently see wishful thinking that approaches delusional thinking. Likewise, it is very difficult for anyone in a highly charged emotional state to filter out their emotional biases. For personality disordered people this is particularly hard, given their difficulty with emotion regulation. This harkens back to the work of Feinberg and Mallat discussed in Chapter 2. These neuroscientists noted that emotions reflect a kind of consciousness that is not located in space. This is in contrast to two other types of consciousness, exteroceptive and interoceptive consciousness. Exteroceptive consciousness pertains to sensory/perceptual information about the external world and is experienced as "out there." Interoceptive consciousness involves perceptions about the body's internal state which are experienced as "in here." However, as emotions, or "affective consciousness," are not located in space, it is very easy to get confused about where the emotions come from, especially in an affectively aroused state when cognition is compromised. In this way, people can think that emotions coming from inside the self are really located on the outside, or at least wholly caused by another person's behavior.

The work of Peter Fonagy and colleagues on mentalization represents a relatively recent advance in psychodynamic theory (c.f. Bateman & Fonagy,

2019) and ties in quite nicely with Fast's event theory. Fonagy and colleagues have largely focused upon borderline personality disorder with special attention to distortions in these patients' interpersonal representations. They attribute these problems to difficulties with *mentalization*, the ability to make sense of mental processes in both the self and others. Specifically, they address three types of disturbances in mentalization, the psychic equivalence mode, the pretend mode and the teleological mode. In the psychic equivalence mode, individuals fail to differentiate between their own subjective experience, particularly their own emotionally charged perceptions, and the outside world. If I *feel* that you hate me, you must hate me, regardless of any factual evidence that contradicts my feelings. The pretend mode is the inverse of psychic equivalence. Whereas in psychic equivalence the internal experience is too real, in the pretend mode it is not real enough. People can be dissociated from their internal experience or they can have an intellectualized understanding of what they are feeling without actually experiencing the feelings as real. While they can give a coherent explanation of their psychic life, to the listener it does not feel genuine or truly lived in. Thus, in pretend mode, people fail to integrate their cognitive analysis with their internal, emotional experience. In the teleological mode, behavior is privileged over internal experience. Emotional life is only real if it manifests in behavior; one cannot feel an emotion unless the related behavior is displayed. If you do not hug me, you do not care about me. If I am not shouting, I am not angry. In the teleological mode, there is no differentiation between emotion and behavior.

Many of the cognitive distortions listed by the cognitive therapist David Burns (c.f. Burns, 2000) are also characterized by event-bound thinking. Cognitive distortions reflect common cognitive biases that perpetuate depression and low self-esteem. For example, "all or nothing thinking," in which people see the world entirely in black and white with no gray, reflects a lack of articulation. People and situations are seen as globally bad or good, a failure or a success. "Labeling," in which a pattern of behavior is generalized to the person's entire character, also reflects global thinking with inadequate articulation. If I failed a test, it's not that I didn't study, it's that I'm stupid. "Emotional reasoning," like psychic equivalence, reflects failure to differentiate internal emotional responses from external reality. The person's emotional reactions are treated as facts about the external world. If I feel insecure, there must be a real threat. Additionally, "disqualifying the positive," in which only negative information is treated as true, reflects a lack of integration of positive and negative information. Finally, distortion of temporal context is reflected in "predicting the future," in which a prediction of future events is taken as established fact, and "overgeneralization," in which a single negative event is assumed to reflect all future events.

So, we see here how event-bound thinking permeates clinical phenomena. Let us now return to our four case examples and see how event-bound thinking is reflected in their interpersonal representations.

***Sarah*:**
Sarah fails to integrate the "bad boyfriend" with the "good boyfriend." As soon as the abusive episodes pass and her boyfriends exhibit some supportive or prosocial behavior, she puts the memory of the abusive behavior out of mind. Hence, she is continually surprised when it returns. Moreover, she does not differentiate her sense of self from her mother's mistreatment of her in childhood. If her mother abused her, it must be what she deserved. In this way, her representations of relationships are entirely event-bound. Her perceived capacity for relationships and the men she feels compelled to choose are thoroughly defined by her childhood relationship with her mother. Her past stays alive in a continual present.

***George*:**
George's perception of himself as either wholly superior, better than all around him, or as a complete failure, without any redeeming features, reflects the lack of articulation of his self-representation. His view of himself is extremely global; he is either all good or all bad. Moreover, he fails to differentiate other people's thoughts and feelings from his own damaged self-esteem. If he feels shamefully inadequate, they must be mocking him. There is no sense that other people have their own point of view, entirely unrelated to his self-perceptions.

***Jennifer*:**
Jennifer fails to differentiate her own attitude towards her body from the behavior of her step-father and mother. If they objectified her and failed to protect her from physical harm, then she must do the same. Similarly, she fails to differentiate the demands of her current employer from those of her grandfather. All authority figures are the same. In effect, they are interchangeable. Moreover, her understanding of responsibility is remarkably global. There is no room for imperfection. She is either completely flawless or completely flawed.

***Martin*:**
Martin fails to connect his anxiety about finances with his avoidance of billing his clients. This failure of integration prevents him from recognizing cause and effect. On a deeper level, he fails to differentiate his own desires from his mother's neediness and his brother's sense of deprivation. It is not his fault that his mother was a competent parent for more of his childhood than his brother's and it helps neither mother nor brother for him to deprive himself of his properly earned revenues. His self-deprivation exemplifies event-bound thinking—if his brother was deprived relative to him in childhood, his self-sacrifice in adulthood will rectify the imbalance. His behavior in the present will somehow change

the past. Thus, we see how event-bound thinking exists outside of a temporal context. The past is never past; it remains a continual present.

We have now finished our exploration of interpersonal representations in personality pathology. We have seen here how maladaptive form and content in the perceptions of self and others impedes the smooth regulation of thought, affect and behavior. In the next chapter, we will pull together the prior four chapters to broach the topic of differential diagnosis. We will synthesize our discussion of Emergent Systems Theory, the evolution of the human mind/brain and the role of interpersonal representations in personality pathology to ask the following questions. How does personality pathology fit into the larger system of the mind/brain and how does it relate to other types of psychopathology?

NOTE

1. Fast's view, like that of many other psychodynamic thinkers, implicitly assumes the capacity for episodic memory. However, it is not clear how episodic memory might manifest in infants nor to what extent episodic memory in human infants is either similar to or different from that of animals with smaller, less developed neocortices. Hopefully, future research will shine light on this question.

Chapter Five

Differential Diagnosis

In this chapter we are finally going to pull together the topics discussed in the preceding four chapters. We are going to see how they all fit together. In the next few pages, I will present a model of the hierarchical structure of the human mind/brain. More specifically, I will identify the specific neuroanatomical regions and psychological functions associated with each level of the hierarchy. Think about it like a large office building. We will first map all the floors of the building and then identify the businesses located on each floor. We will of course consider the floor where personality pathology has its offices, but we will not stop there. We are also interested in the levels associated with *other* forms of psychopathology. In this way, we will consider the question of *differential diagnosis*. How do we understand the distinction between psychopathology that is and is not attributable to personality? We will also look at how the different psychological levels interact with one another to form the complex comorbidities that are so common in clinical practice.

Before we outline the specific levels, it is necessary to recap some key points from Chapter 2, where we reviewed the evolutionary history of the human mind/brain. As a hierarchically organized, emergent system, the mind/brain evolved over hundreds of millions of years. Newer structures grew on top of older structures and integrated with them to form layered systems of great complexity. In general, our brain evolved from back to front and from bottom to top. (See Figures 2.1 and 2.2 for diagrams of the brain.) The lowest levels are the oldest, the most conserved across evolution. They are the least complex but also the most fundamental. They are necessary for the whole system to run—for example, heart rate and respiration are controlled by the brain stem. When these levels break down, the whole system collapses. The person dies.

The newest and most sophisticated regions of the brain are found in the upper and outer layers of the cortex. Both anatomically and functionally, they are the most complex. These levels are necessary for the whole system to run *well* and to survive over time but not necessarily to sustain life in the near-term. They allow for flexible, coordinated, and sophisticated adaptations to the environment. For example, if it's not too big, a stroke in your left cerebral hemisphere may impair your speech but it probably won't kill you.

As described by Stephen Jay Gould (See Chapter 2), the oldest systems are the most conserved across evolution and appear earliest in embryonic development because they are the most fundamental. As the rest of the edifice rests upon these fundamental structures, a problematic change at these levels poses real risk of destroying the whole organism. Returning to our metaphor of an office building, it is far more dangerous to knock out the walls and supporting pillars of the ground floor than those of the top floor. The top floor can afford to make mistakes. That is why we see such variation across species in the evolutionarily newer sections of an organism. Evolution can afford to experiment as there is far less danger of wiping out the whole organism. Now, to clarify, this does not mean that there has been no evolutionary change in the lower-level systems in humans, but that the earlier the system develops in utero and the more fundamental to the overall structure, the more conserved it is across evolution.

In sum, our mind/brain contains different psychological processes that evolved at very different times. The older levels are shared with many other species. As we go up the hierarchy, however, our psychological processes become more distinctly human. And it is in the interplay between these older and newer systems where psychotherapy does its work.

The 5-Level Model of the Mind/Brain

Building on this history, I will now present a model of the hierarchical structure of the mind/brain as is most pertinent to clinical diagnosis. This model proposes a five-level structure, which represents a section of the larger human hierarchical system. These five levels constitute the purely *psychological* levels of the human system. They lie above the physiological levels (e.g., respiration, heart rate) and below the socio-cultural levels (e.g., ethnicity, religion, group identity) (See Figure 1.2 for a diagram of the larger human systems).

A summary of our five-level model can be found in Tables 5.1 and 5.2. The specific levels are listed in the first column of each table. Table 5.1 also includes the relevant brain areas and approximate phylogenetic age of each level plus the corresponding levels of both Jaak Panksepp's and Paul MacLean's models of brain evolution. Table 5.2 addresses the psychologi-

Table 5.1. Five Levels of the Mind/Brain: Evolutionary Context

Mind/Brain Level	*Time of Emergence*	*First Animal at this Stage*	*Brain Regions Involved*	*Panksepp's Nested BrainMind Hierarchy*	*MacLean Complex*
Verbal Conceptual	1 mya – 200 kya	Non-ape Hominins	Forebrain: neocortex, left hemisphere language regions, dorsolateral pre-frontal cortex	Tertiary Emotions	Neo-Mammalian
Basic Conceptual	14 mya	Great Apes	Forebrain: medial cortical areas, limbic lobe (hippocampal regions, cingulate)	Tertiary Emotions	Neo-Mammalian
Pre-conceptual Learning	200 mya	Mammals	Forebrain: ventral telencephalon (nucleus accumbens, basal ganglia, amygdala)	Secondary Emotions	Paleo-Mammalian
Unlearned Core: Social	200 mya	Mammals	Forebrain: ventral telencephalon, diencephalon, Midbrain: periaqueductal gray Hindbrain: brain stem	Primary Emotions: CARE, PANIC, PLAY	Reptilian
Unlearned Core: Survival	300-500 mya	Reptiles or Fish	Forebrain: diencephalon Midbrain: periaqueductal gray, ventral tegmental area Hindbrain: brain stem, raphe nuclei, locus coeruleus	Primary Emotions: SEEKING, RAGE, FEAR, LUST	Reptilian

Table 5.2. Clinical Significance of the Five Mind/Brain Levels

Mind/Brain Level		*Psychological Processes*	*Primary Etiology*	*Psychological Disorders*
Level 5	Verbal Conceptual	Language, Reasoning Capacity, High Level Cognition	Verbal Learning	Cognitive Disorders, Learning Disabilities, Poor Coping Skills
Level 4	Basic Conceptual	Interpersonal Representations, Self-Conscious Emotions	Experiential Learning	Character Pathology, Insecure Attachment
Level 3	Pre-conceptual Learning	Cue-Based Learning	Classical or Operant Conditioning	Anxiety Disorders, OCD, Addictions, Hyperreactive Stress Response, Impaired Impulse Control, Emotional Volatility from Personality Pathology
Level 2	Unlearned Core: Social	CARE/nurturance, PANIC/sadness, and PLAY systems, Temperament	Genetic	Mood and Psychotic Disorders
Level 1	Unlearned Core: Survival	SEEKING, FEAR, RAGE, & LUST systems, Temperament	Genetic	Mood and Psychotic Disorders

cal processes and clinical disorders associated with each level. Figure 5.1 presents a visual diagram of the brain regions associated with each of the five levels.

The first and lowest two levels of our 5-level model together comprise the *Unlearned Core*. The first level, *Unlearned Core: Survival*, dates back about 300 to 500 million years. The second level, *Unlearned Core: Social*, dates back about 200 million years. These levels encompass the lowest and oldest parts of the brain and control instinctual emotional behaviors that we share with many other animal species. The third level is termed *Pre-conceptual Learning* and dates back about 200 million years. It links emotions with simple learning and memory. The next two levels comprise *Conceptual Learning*. Here we introduce the notion of "ideas," the ability to think about events when they are not occurring. The fourth level, the *Basic Conceptual level,* dates back about 14 million years. At this level we locate interpersonal representations and the core of personality pathology. Finally, the fifth level is termed the *Verbal Conceptual Level*. This is the most uniquely human level, dating back 1 million to 200 thousand years. This is where language and complex cognition enter the picture.

I want to emphasize here that this represents a *model*. It is not intended to be a definitive statement about brain anatomy or function but rather a heuristic scheme, based on extant science, that can guide clinical practice. Undoubtedly, some of the details are wrong and hopefully future research will allow for refinement of this model. Nonetheless, I believe the general concepts will prove to be quite durable. The primary intention here is to adapt and extend the hierarchical view of the brain from neuroscience into the domain of clinical psychology.

LEVELS 1 & 2: THE UNLEARNED CORE

Let us now consider this model in more detail. We will start with the Unlearned Core, the lowest general level of the mind/brain. It involves the oldest parts of the brain: the hindbrain (specifically the brainstem), the midbrain, and the oldest parts of the forebrain (the diencephalon and ventral telencephalon). (See Figure 5.1.) This level of the mind/brain aligns with Panksepp's primary emotional systems and MacLean's reptilian brain. The Unlearned Core is further divided into two sections, the Survival and Social levels (Levels 1 and 2, respectively).

The psychological processes mediated at these levels form the foundations of our emotional life. These coordinated emotional systems combine subjective experience, physiological response, and motor behavior into distinct modes of engaging with the environment. At the Unlearned Core, we find the most primitive and also the most powerful elements of our emotional life. This is sheer animal emotion, separate from any cognitive influence. In fact, when people are stimulated in sections of the periaqueductal gray, a critical midbrain structure in the Unlearned Core, they experience pure, unadulterated terror or rage, depending on the brain area stimulated (Panksepp & Biven, 2012). Importantly, these emotional-behavioral patterns are unlearned—they are largely fixed responses to set stimuli. It is only at the higher levels of the mind/brain that our emotions are modified by learning and memory. Therefore, to a large extent, individual variation at this level is genetically determined.[1]

The Survival level is the oldest of the two levels of the Unlearned Core. It likely dates back perhaps half a billion years to the time of the first vertebrates as the periaqueductal gray is found across vertebrate species (Linnman et al., 2012) and we see related behavior in fish, the oldest form of vertebrate

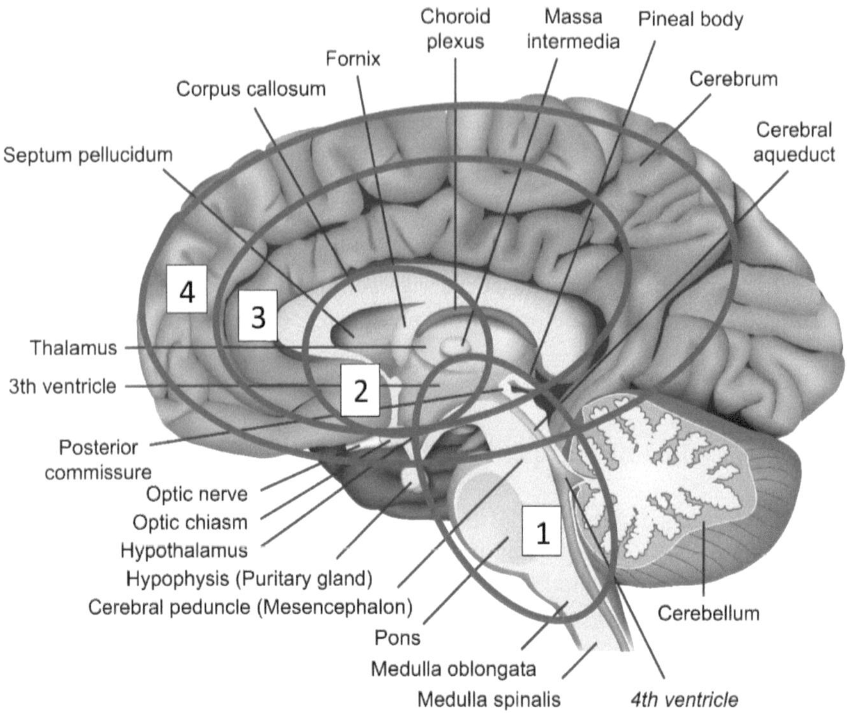

Figure 5.1. Approximate anatomical regions corresponding to the 5 levels of the Mind/Brain. 1. The *Unlearned Core* (both Survival and Social levels) includes the brain stem, midbrain and areas of the ventral (lower) forebrain, such as the hypothalamus. 2. The *Pre-conceptual level* includes subcortical regions such as the amygdala, septal nuclei, nucleus accumbens and other areas of the basal ganglia. 3. The *Basic Conceptual level* includes the medial (inner) cortex and the limbic lobe (cingulate cortex and hippocampal regions). 4. The *Verbal Conceptual level* includes the outer regions of the neocortex, centrally the frontal lobe. Medicalstocks. Shutterstock. Image modified by Lisa J. Cohen.

(Huntingford, 1976). Borrowing from Panksepp's model, the Survival level would include the SEEKING, FEAR, RAGE/Anger and LUST primary emotional systems.[2] SEEKING is the all-purpose motivation machine that stimulates animals to seek out rewarding stimuli. In its most primitive form, this is restricted to food and sex but in humans it underlies any type of enjoyable activity, for example shopping, engaging in sports, or even visiting art museums. RAGE/Anger and FEAR pertain to the fight/flight response, our core responses to danger. Predatory aggression, as we see in hunting, likely does not fall under the RAGE/Anger system but rather is mediated by the SEEKING system. The LUST system pertains to our sexual arousal patterns.[3]

The Social level includes core emotional systems related to *attachment* and likely dates back to the evolution of mammals, about 200 mya. Based again on Panksepp's model, the Social level would include CARE/Nurturance, PANIC/Sadness, and PLAY systems which refer, respectively, to the deep sense of nurturance of a mother to her infant, the powerful attachment of the infant to the mother as evidenced in separation distress, and the enjoyable desire for playful interactions with peers. In most mammals, PLAY diminishes with maturity. In humans, however, it remains active throughout the life span, an example of how our evolution was shaped by the retention of juvenile characteristics into adulthood, a process known as pedomorphy (See Chapter 2).

Mood and Psychotic Disorders and the Unlearned Core

Now let us consider the psychological disorders based in the level of the Unlearned Core. But before we do so, it is critical to take a moment to consider the issue of brain localization. The practice of localizing particular psychological functions to specific areas of the brain has a long and contentious history. There is no question that certain areas of the brain are central to specific psychological functions; the after-effects of strokes or other types of brain damage show this quite dramatically. Yet, we must be careful when we speak of "locating" any psychological function in any particular brain region. The brain operates as an integrated system and complex psychological functions typically involve widely distributed neuronal circuits. Few if any psychological functions can be entirely localized to a single region. Nevertheless, it is the basic contention of this book that many clinically-relevant psychological processes are *preferentially dependent upon and emergent from* the activity of specific areas of the brain. Further, the brain regions involved tell us something meaningful about the evolutionary history of our species

Likewise, current trends in brain imaging research target coordinated activity across different brain regions, aiming to identify the network of brain regions involved in specific psychological tasks or conditions (c.f. Fox et al., 2015). I would argue, however, that such findings reflect *vertical integration*, involving circuits that cut across all levels of the mind/brain, from the evolutionarily oldest to the most recent. This tells us how the brain functions *now*, as a complex integrated system. But it does not address the *history* of the mind/brain as our species evolved over millions of years. In contrast, this book takes a *horizontal* approach, emphasizing horizontal differentiation rather than vertical integration. As such, we distinguish between the different layers of the mind/brain that arose at distinct periods across the evolution of our species as well as their corresponding psychological processes. I propose that this allows us to enhance differential diagnosis and thereby identify the most appropriate treatments for our patients.

With this in mind, I propose that the major mood and psychotic disorders, including bipolar disorder, schizophrenia, schizoaffective disorder, and the more genetically-based form of depression, are located at the level of the Unlearned Core. These are among the most debilitating forms of mental illness and account for the majority of admissions to inpatient psychiatric services. Of critical importance, these disorders are placed at a different level of the mind/brain than are personality disorders, underscoring the necessary distinction between these two types of disorders. Although they often produce similar symptoms, the two groups of disorders are very different animals with very different etiologies. As such, I propose that they operate on different levels of the mind/brain. Bipolar disorder, once known as manic-depressive disorder, involves intense mood swings from deep, deep depression to a hyperactivated state known as mania. This is a severe disorder, to be distinguished from the normal mood swings many people experience. Schizophrenia is characterized by positive psychotic symptoms such as auditory hallucinations and delusions, as well as negative symptoms such as lack of motivation, emotional expression, and interest in the outside world. Schizoaffective disorder shares all these symptoms but is also characterized by distinct and frequent mood episodes.

Supporting Evidence

So now we can ask: What evidence supports basing the major mood and psychotic disorders at the Unlearned Core? As most imaging studies of patients with these disorders show activation of the whole brain and clear abnormalities at cortical levels, what basis is there for anchoring these disorders at such a low level of the mind/brain? I will go into this in some detail as it underlines the important distinction between this group of disorders and personality pathology, a distinction that is not universally recognized.

For one, as discussed in Chapter 3, family studies point to a higher genetic loading in these disorders than in personality pathology, perhaps twice as high with regard to bipolar disorder and schizophrenia.

Secondly, we can map Panksepp's seven primary emotional systems directly onto these disorders, especially the mood disorders. With regard to mania, we can see how the characteristic symptoms of this condition reflect hyperactivation of the SEEKING and LUST systems with concomitant suppression of the FEAR system. Hyperactivation of the SEEKING system manifests in excessive involvement with the environment and unmodulated pursuit of rewarding stimuli. People in the throes of mania often have unbridled enthusiasm about new projects and engage in pleasurable activities in reckless ways. They commonly spend far more money than they can afford, purchasing whatever goods appeal to them in the moment. Hyperactivation of the LUST system is reflected in manic hypersexuality, such that there may be multiple and problematic sexual encounters. Suppression of the FEAR system is seen in the failure to inhibit reckless behavior. Manic individuals are not afraid when they should be. There is little consideration of consequences and people's perception of their ability to achieve their own ends is exaggeratedly optimistic. Additionally, when manic people get irritable, they can become violent, reflecting overactivation of the RAGE/Anger system. Finally, mania also involves hyperactivity of the PLAY system. Manic people are often very playful; their speech is marked by word play and their affect can be euphoric and expansive, in that they make other people feel good to be around them. For example, in the midst of a manic episode, a 48-year-old woman tried to sell the family house without bothering to tell her husband. She had abruptly decided to move to Los Angeles to start a film career. Similarly, a 32-year-old man was hospitalized after he dragged all the chairs in a classroom onto the roof of a college building. His goal was to start a school for children on the roof.

Depression is the inverse of mania. In depression, we see *suppression* of the SEEKING and LUST systems and frequently *over*-activation of the FEAR system. People have diminished interest in pleasurable activities and commonly lose their sex drive. They have little motivation to engage with the world, such that any activity feels enormously effortful. They may lie in bed all day. Rather than disregarding the possible negative outcome of their actions, they may ruminate over any potential problem. Their outlook is irrationally pessimistic. Depression also reflects disturbance of the PANIC/sadness system as related to attachment. People frequently become depressed after the loss of an attachment figure, such that romantic loss is one of the most common triggers for depression and even suicidal behavior. In fact, the state of bereavement following the death of a loved one is often indistinguishable from major depression. Additionally, depression reflects suppression of the PLAY system. One of the first things to disappear in depression is a sense of playfulness.

Let us consider a case example.

> Rich was a 28-year-old man with an 8-year history of major depressive disorder. He was a lively, gregarious and ambitious young man when not depressed. Unfortunately, following a romantic rejection he slipped into a deep depression. He felt that his life had no purpose and lost interest in socializing or any of his hobbies. He had no energy to attend to his job and subsequently took a medical leave. He ruminated continuously about the futility of his life and his own inadequacies. Eventually, he took to his bed perhaps 16 hours a day and started

to consider means of suicide. His depressive episode only abated after a course of electro-convulsive therapy (ECT).

Importantly, depression presents a more complicated diagnostic picture than mania. Depression is complex because it is highly heterogeneous. There are many types of depression. While depression can be a chronic and debilitating disease with a strong genetic basis, it can also be a transitory and fairly mild reaction to a loss or stressor. This type of depression has been termed reactive depression. Further, depression can result from personality pathology. This kind of depression often involves low self-esteem or inner feelings of emptiness. Likewise, different types of depression respond differently to treatment. I propose that it is the more genetically-based form of major depressive disorder, what used to be called endogenous depression (as it was not caused by external circumstances), that is located at the Unlearned Core. The other types of depression are more appropriately anchored at higher levels of the mind/brain.

Now let us consider schizophrenia and related disorders. The primary symptoms of schizophrenia can be grouped into positive and negative symptoms. The positive symptoms include delusions (fixed false beliefs), hallucinations (false sensory perceptions), disorganized speech, and grossly disorganized or catatonic behavior. The negative symptoms include blunted affect, lack of motivation, lack of initiative and social withdrawal. Cognitive deficits (reduced concentration, memory, and complex intellectual functions) are also common in schizophrenia.

For example, consider the case of Jimmy, a 19-year-old man. He had been a fairly healthy person into his late teens, when he began to slowly withdraw from social interactions and complain of difficulty concentrating. His hygiene deteriorated and his grades at school started to slip. Eventually he developed a paranoid delusion that the television had been rigged by a foreign government and was now sending him messages, trying to recruit him to join a conspiracy against the U.S. government. Because of this, he became very agitated when anyone in his family turned on the TV. Over the next few months, this fear generalized to all electronics and his family took to hiding their cell phones when in the room with him.

So how can we connect the typical schizophrenic symptoms to the Unlearned Core? In paranoia, a typical positive symptom of schizophrenia, we see over-activation of the FEAR and RAGE/Anger system. In the negative symptoms, we see suppression of the SEEKING system, similar to what occurs in depression. Negative symptoms also reflect suppression of the Social systems (decreased CARE/nurturance, PANIC/sadness and PLAY) as manifested in interpersonal indifference and withdrawal. However, neither the break with reality nor the cognitive impairment easily fit into this framework.

Therefore, it appears that these symptoms involve higher levels of the mind/brain associated with cognitive processing. Here I will speculate that these cognitive and perceptual deficits reflect the bottom-up influence of more fundamental pathology at the Unlearned Core.

The third reason to anchor the major mood and psychotic disorders in the Unlearned Core has to do with treatment response. Importantly, treatment response is one of the main ways that we distinguish disorders of the Unlearned Core from those located at higher levels. The first line treatments for disorders at this level involve medication and other physiological treatments (e.g., ECT), whereas disorders of higher levels of the mind/brain are primarily treated with psychotherapy. Relevant medications include antidepressants, mood stabilizers, and/or antipsychotics (Cf. Joska & Stein, 2008; Stroup et al., 2014). Treatment of major depression is more complicated due to the multiple types of depression. The more genetically-based major depressive disorder responds best to physiological treatments. While mild to moderate reactive depression also responds to medication, it responds equally well to various forms of psychotherapy or even physical exercise. Depression based in personality pathology responds well to psychotherapy but not as well to antidepressant medication (Limandri, 2018). Moreover, depressed mood and related behavioral problems in borderline patients are often treated with second generation antipsychotics (Martin-Blanco et al., 2017; Limandri, 2018).

Importantly, the main treatments for these disorders target specific neurotransmitter tracts, the cell bodies for which are all located in the deepest regions of the mind/brain, that is in the Unlearned Core. Most antidepressants work on the serotonin and/or norepinephrine tracts, whose cell bodies are located in the raphe nuclei and locus coeruleus, respectively, both of which are found in the brain stem. Antipsychotic medication has long targeted a tract of dopamine neurons known as the mesocorticolimbic dopamine system. The first-generation antipsychotics target these tracts directly while the second-generation antipsychotics alter them indirectly (Brisch et al., 2014). The cell bodies for these tracts are in the ventral tegmental area, which is in the midbrain (also in the Unlearned Core). Mood stabilizers are not linked as closely to any specific neurotransmitter tract and in general are much less understood, although there is evidence that they indirectly alter dopaminergic and glutamate transmission (Rapoport et al., 2009). Glutamate is an excitatory neurotransmitter found throughout the brain.

Additional support for anchoring these disorders in the Unlearned Core comes from a relatively recent brain imaging study looking at serotonin processing in the raphe nucleus, a region of the brain stem. The authors found that the amount of serotonin receptor binding in parts of the raphe nucleus offered a remarkably precise way to differentiate study participants with major depressive disorder from healthy volunteers (Pillai et al., 2018). Thus, there is considerable evidence to support anchoring the major mood and psychotic disorders in the Unlearned Core.

Temperament and the Unlearned Core

Now let us consider another critical aspect of human psychology that can be situated at the Unlearned Core. Specifically, I will ground the *temperament* component of personality here. Remember, "temperament" refers to the genetically transmitted elements of personality while "character" refers to the aspects of personality that have been learned (See Chapter 3). The notion that temperament is 1) dissociable from character and 2) more genetically based than character is far from proven and in some quarters may be quite controversial. Still, there is evidence to support this notion. I also propose that the distinction has real clinical utility.

Let us first consider the work of Ken Davis and Jaak Panksepp (2018). These researchers explored the relationship between Panksepp's core emotional systems[4] and human personality traits. Note, however, that as Panksepp holds the primary emotional systems to be largely genetic in origin, their analogues in personality should represent *temperament* rather than character. Indeed, Davis & Panksepp even used the term "temperament" when speaking of individual differences in these systems in non-human animals (Davis & Panksepp, 2018, p. 152).

First, Davis and Panksepp created a self-report questionnaire to measure traits related to the six core emotional systems in human beings. They termed this the Affective Neuroscience Personality Scales. The authors then correlated scores on this questionnaire to those from a measure of the 5-Factor Model of personality. The 5-Factor Model attributes most of the variation in human personality to the following five general traits: openness to experience, conscientiousness, extraversion, agreeableness, and neuroticism. As discussed in Chapter 3, these 5 traits have a strong genetic component and thus can be attributed more to temperament than to character. Hence to the extent Davis and Panksepp's questionnaire correlates with a measure of human temperament, the study supports the anchoring of temperament in the Unlearned Core.

The authors hypothesized that PLAY would correlate with Extraversion, SEEKING with Openness to Experience, CARE/Nurturance with Agreeableness, and RAGE/Anger, FEAR, and PANIC/Sadness with Neuroticism (termed Emotional Stability in their system). Their findings strongly supported these hypotheses, with correlations ranging from .46 to .75. Non-hypothesized correlations were much lower, averaging about .13. Thus, the temperament component of human personality appears to align closely with traits related to Panksepp's primary emotional systems.

Next, these authors addressed animal models to see if behavior associated with Pankepp's primary emotional systems could be genetically altered by *selective breeding*. Such findings would provide powerful evidence of the genetic basis of Panksepp's core emotional systems and, by extension, of human temperament. Studies of selective breeding provide very strong evidence for the genetic basis of behavior as they directly manipulate the animals' genetic make-up. In this light, the authors cited a famous study by a Russian geneticist named Dmitry Belyaev, who succeeded in domesticating foxes through selective breeding. As we all know, dogs are tremendously sociable with humans—tame, affectionate and easy to domesticate. Foxes are quite different. They are wild animals and do not make good pets. However, after selectively breeding the foxes most comfortable with human touch for only three generations, Belyaev succeeded in creating a domesticated fox. These foxes no longer showed fearful and aggressive responses to humans (reduced FEAR and RAGE). After a few dozen generations, the foxes spontaneously exhibited the kinds of affectionate behavior towards humans typically seen with dogs, such as tail wagging and face licking (increased PLAY and PANIC) (See Trut, 1999). Additionally, selective breeding of a very different species, three-spined stickleback fish, led to reduction of territorial aggression (RAGE), as measured by the fish biting and bumping against a glass tube containing an intruder placed into their territory (Bakker, 1994).

Taken together, these studies indicate that temperament is 1) highly correlated with Panksepp's primary emotional systems, 2) genetically based, and 3) cuts across many different species. As such, available research supports the grounding of the temperament component of personality in the Unlearned Core.

Additional support for the anchoring of temperament in the Unlearned Core comes from the brain imaging research of Fox, Kalin and colleagues (2015). The authors studied anxious temperament in humans and rhesus monkeys, who share many brain structures with humans. Anxious temperament (AT) refers to a personality trait that renders the individual prone to heightened anxiety reactions to potential threats. In children, AT is highly predictive of later development of anxiety disorders (Fox et al., 2015). The study of most interest here involves a sample of 592 young rhesus monkeys from a large multigenerational family pedigree. As such, the researchers could determine the degree of genetic relatedness among the monkeys in the sample. In a "genetic correlational approach," they used brain imaging techniques to identify brain regions where activity associated with AT has a strong genetic component. They measured AT in the monkeys by recording their behavioral freezing, suppression of "cooing" sounds, and levels of the stress hormone cortisol in response to a human presenting his or her face in profile to the monkey's cage for 30 minutes without making eye contact. This ambiguous threat has proven to reliably elicit the stress response in monkeys.

The authors found that the anxiety response activated a network of neurons cutting across all levels of the brain, ranging from the periaqueductal grey in the midbrain to the frontal cortex. This is an example of *vertical integration*, illustrating how our fundamental psychological processes integrate the entire history of our brain structure. However, the largest area where the AT-related brain activation was associated with genetic heritability was in the periaqueductal grey, a mid-brain region located in the Unlearned Core. Genetically-related activity was also found in other brain regions, such as the amygdala and hippocampus, but, based on the brain maps included in the article, such activity was dwarfed by that in the periaqueductal grey.

Treatment for Temperament

What does this all mean for clinical work? What are the implications for treatment? We do not generally treat temperament with medication as we do not tend to see different temperaments as pathological, but rather as the product of normal individual variation. Some people may *wish* that their temperaments were different. For example, introverted people may wish that they were more extraverted and people with low levels of conscientiousness may struggle with regard to time management, work performance, or financial behavior. In therapy, it can be beneficial to help people recognize and accept their basic temperament and then work to maximize adaptation to the environment given the realities of their personality. If temperament does manifest in pathology, then it can be treated a number of ways, with medication, or with self-regulation techniques utilizing other levels of the mind/brain. This will be discussed in greater detail in the next chapter.

LEVEL 3: PRE-CONCEPTUAL LEARNING

Now we will move up to the next level in the mind/brain, that of *Pre-conceptual Learning*. This level builds on top of the emotional systems of the Unlearned Core but modifies them with learning and memory. Although the nature of the emotional responses is genetically pre-programmed, the specific conditions in which they are elicited are determined by memories of prior experience. The Pre-conceptual level involves higher regions of the telencephalon, which is the newer part of the forebrain. Nonetheless, the Pre-conceptual level remains largely subcortical, that is below the cortex. (See Figure 5.1.) Relevant brain areas include the basal ganglia (central for motor learning), the amygdala (central for fear learning), and the nucleus accumbens (central for reward learning). Learning at this level is *Pre-conceptual* as it does not involve concepts, that is representations of objects or situations that can be thought about outside of the presence of the original object. Consequently, at this level, out of sight means out of mind. Emotional responses are very *cue-based*; they are activated when the cue is present but not when it is absent. We see this with a cat who shows intense fear when the vacuum cleaner is brought out of the closet but calms down pretty quickly after it is turned off and returned to the closet. Specific types of learning and memory found at this level include associative conditioning and motor learning. To some extent operant conditioning (learning from reward and punishment) occurs at this level too. Importantly, we are not seeing episodic memory at this level, that is conscious memory of lived events. That occurs at a higher level. Rather we are seeing pairing of particular emotional and behavioral responses to learned cues.

Pathology at the Pre-conceptual Level

It is at the Pre-conceptual level that we can locate anxiety disorders, such as phobias and panic disorder, as the amygdala plays an important role in fear conditioning. Addictive disorders can also be situated here as the nucleus accumbens has been implicated in both behavioral and chemical addictions. The nucleus accumbens is where the dopaminergic reward system hooks up with learned cues. In behavioral addictions such as gambling, kleptomania, or sexual addictions, relevant cues can elicit an overpowering urge to engage in the addictive behavior. In chemical addictions, ingestion of dopaminergically active drugs (e.g., cocaine, methamphetamine) alters the dopaminergic reward system, stimulating intense cravings in response to drug-related cues. Impulse control disorders may also be attributed to the Pre-conceptual level as they often reflect the failure to learn from punishment—a problem with operant conditioning (though the failure to *anticipate* punishment also involves higher cortical levels). Additionally, obsessive compulsive disorder (OCD) can be placed at this level as it is strongly linked to the basal ganglia. In this case the compulsion to perform motor programs, such as handwashing or ordering and arranging items, is elicited by relevant cues. Finally, early conditioning of the stress response through childhood trauma and neglect can train this system to be hyper-reactive to stressful cues. This can manifest in overcontrol of the stress response, under-control, or fluctuations between either extreme. Such behavior is fairly typical in individuals with severe trauma histories (Thomas, Gurvich and Kulkarni, 2019).

Finally, I will locate the emotional volatility of personality pathology at this level. By this, I am referring to the inappropriate outbursts of rage, excessively fearful reactions, sudden bouts of despair and other similar responses that are so typical of personality disorders. We will anchor these phenomena at the Pre-conceptual level (1) because of the centrality of Pre-conceptual brain regions in emotion research (e.g., amygdala, nucleus accumbens) and (2) because this kind of emotional volatility is always triggered by cues. Nevertheless, unlike the disorders listed above, such difficulties are not the primary pathology. Rather these problems may result *from* the personality disorder; they may be the consequences *of* it. For example, patients with borderline personality often respond to the cue of romantic conflict with sudden bouts of rage or suicidal despair because that particular cue has activated their abandonment schema. The threatened break-up is not just disturbing, it is experienced as almost life threatening. Therefore, while treatment of Pre-conceptual difficulties is often necessary with personality disordered patients—they have to learn to control their emotions and behavior—it will not be sufficient to change the maladaptive interpersonal representations fundamental to their pathology. For that, intervention at a higher level is necessary. This will be explored in greater depth in Chapter 6.

Treatment for Disorders at the Level of Pre-conceptual Learning

Treatment for mental disorders anchored in the Pre-conceptual level is level-specific. The primary interventions for disorders at this level target problems with conditioned learning. They largely aim to disconnect a problematic response from the triggering cue or forge a connection between a desired response and a new cue. For anxiety disorders, treatments such as gradual desensitization aim to extinguish associations between the fear response and the fear-arousing cue. Exposure and response prevention, which is used to treat OCD, works on a similar mechanism. For addictive behavior, treatment often involves controlling exposure to cues that elicit problematic responses, as when alcoholics are told to avoid bars and liquor stores. Problems of operant conditioning can be addressed with behavioral modification, as with a token economy. People are systematically rewarded for desired behavior. Hyper-reactivity to stress cues is managed by various kinds of skills training as exemplified by Dialectic Behavior Therapy (DBT). Skills training, via DBT and various forms of cognitive behavioral therapy (CBT), is also used for problems with impulse control and emotional regulation. People learn to inhibit or redirect their problematic, cue-induced behavior. As will be explored in the following chapter, these treatments utilize a range of interventions that involve different levels of the mind/brain.

LEVELS 4 AND 5: CONCEPTUAL LEARNING

The next general level of the mind/brain is called Conceptual Learning and is subdivided into the Basic and Verbal Conceptual levels. At this point we have moved to a much higher level of psychological complexity. At both the Pre-conceptual and Conceptual levels, emotional responses are modified by learning and memory. But while the Pre-conceptual level relies upon conditioned learning and cue-based responses, here we introduce the notion of *concepts*. Cue-based responses live entirely in the present. When the cues are not present the responses do not occur. Concepts, on the other hand transcend time and space. You can think about an idea regardless of whether or not the object of your thought is immediately present. You can also manipulate ideas in your mind. This means you can use your imagination to consider possible changes to an object or event. This allows for much greater flexibility in our responses to changing conditions in our environment.

With this advance in cognitive complexity, we move into the cortex, the uppermost, phylogenetically newest, and most elaborate section of our brain. (See Figure 5.1.) Thus, both the Basic and Verbal Conceptual levels of the mind/brain operate within cortical regions.

LEVEL 4: BASIC CONCEPTUAL LEVEL

The Basic Conceptual level is located in the *inner* or medial regions of the cortex as well as the limbic lobe, including the cingulate gyrus and hippocampal regions. I will speculate that, in some form, this system level dates back maybe 14 mya to the evolution of great apes, judging by their sophisticated social relations as well as the complex state of their medial cortical regions and limbic lobe.

The Basic Conceptual level mediates basic concepts of key emotional relationships, most fundamentally our primary attachment relationships. Relatedly, the hippocampus, part of the limbic lobe, is a central structure mediating episodic memory. *Thus, it is at the Basic Conceptual level that memories of formative attachment relationships coalesce into interpersonal representations.* As detailed in Chapter 3, experiences of emotionally powerful interpersonal relationships in childhood are consolidated and generalized in memory to form a schema or map of how self and other relate to one another. This notion aligns with the attachment theorists' concept of the internal working model of attachment, Daniel Stern's concept of Representations of Interactions that have been Generalized (RIGs), cognitive therapists' notion of self and interpersonal schemas, and the psychoanalytic notion of object representations. *As such, I propose the Basic Conceptual level to be the primary level subserving character pathology. While the temperament component of personality is located at the level of the Unlearned Core, the character component is located here.*

It is important to note, however, that the interpersonal representations anchored at this level do not require language and often operate outside of verbal capacities. People can learn to verbally describe their interpersonal representations but generally only with effort. Thus, the concepts at this level operate largely below conscious awareness and often outside the domain of language. In fact, it is frequently the work of psychotherapy to translate patients' interpersonal representations into a verbal narrative.

I will also speculate that we find the self-conscious emotions, such as guilt, shame, pride, and embarrassment (Lewis, 1997), at the Basic Conceptual level. The self-conscious emotions require a concept of self; one cannot feel shame if one has no concept of self to be ashamed of. Likewise, our self-conscious emotions are not present at birth. In fact, they do not make their appearance until after the first year, around the time that children can pass the mirror test, indicating emergence of a self-concept. Relatedly, I would put the emotions of guilt and moral disgust at the Basic Conceptual level. One needs a clear conception of social relations to feel moral emotions. Indeed, a 2015 review of brain imaging findings highlighted the involvement of the medial prefrontal, cingulate and insula cortices in the feelings of shame, guilt and embarrassment (Bastin, Harrison, Davey, Hally & Whittle, 2015). All of these brain regions are included here in the Basic Conceptual level. Thus, at the Basic Conceptual level, we not only see representations of self and other, we may also see the emergence of specific emotions that depend on the capacity for those representations.

Pathology at The Basic Conceptual Level

As already detailed, I will locate the core of personality pathology at this level. To be more precise, I will base the character component of personality pathology here, while the temperament component is anchored in the Unlearned Core. How does this work? The Basic Conceptual level is a central site for interpersonal representations, which form the basis for an individual's character. If we assume that character predominates over temperament in the etiology of personality pathology, then the Basic Conceptual level is the primary site for personality pathology in general. The evidence supporting this model is presented in Chapter 3 but let us briefly review it here. (1) A very robust literature connects personality pathology to maladaptive interpersonal representations. (2) An equally robust literature links personality pathology and maladaptive interpersonal representations in adulthood to adverse early environments, including multiple types of childhood trauma as well as poor attachment relations with caregivers. (3) Family studies show a high rate of environmental vs. genetic etiology for personality disorders, about twice that shown for bipolar disorder and schizophrenia. (4) Imaging studies show a central role for the medial neocortex and limbic lobe in psychological functions related to interpersonal representations, such as empathy, navigation of social power and intimacy, and self-related mentation. The medial frontal cortex has also been implicated in borderline personality disorder.

Treatment for Disorders at the Basic Conceptual Level

The primary treatment for personality disorders is psychotherapy (Caligor & Clarkin, 2010; Oldham, 2005). There are many types of psychotherapy for personality disorders, which we will explore in the next two chapters. Medication can also be helpful for personality disorders but it is adjunctive, not the primary treatment. This marks a critical distinction between personality disorders and the major mood and psychotic disorders. As noted above, the primary treatment for the major mood and psychotic disorders is medication, with psychotherapy providing supportive treatment. While certain personality and mood/psychotic disorders can present similar symptoms (for example, borderline personality disorder and bipolar disorder are often misdiagnosed for one another [Zimmerman et al., 2008; Ruggero et al., 2010]), effective interventions are level-specific. Once again, this underscores the importance of accurately identifying the primary level of our patients' psychopathology.

LEVEL 5: THE VERBAL CONCEPTUAL LEVEL

We now turn to the Verbal Conceptual level, the highest of the five levels of the human mind/brain. At this level, we encounter the extraordinary capabilities of language. It is here that emotions are elaborated with words. This system level is located on the *outer* part of the neocortex, the newest part of the human brain. This region mediates higher level cognition, including planning, abstraction, symbolic thought, and language. Reading, writing, and mathematical and spatial reasoning are also processed at this level. Specifically, Broca's area, in the posterior region of the left frontal cortex, is involved with speech production, and Wernicke's area, in the upper part of the left temporal cortex, is involved with language comprehension. This region is also important for semantic memory. Not surprisingly, this area is greatly impacted by education and culture (D.P. Eisenberg et al., 2005).

At the Verbal Conceptual Level, emotional experience is translated into words. Feelings are articulated into language, a shared symbolic system. We have already discussed the notion of concepts. Language goes several steps further. Language creates a *symbol* of the concept that can be communicated with others. For example, the word "rain" symbolizes small water droplets that fall from the sky. You don't need to be standing in the rain to know what the word means. And right now, as you read the word, you can *imagine* rain, what it sounds like and feels on your skin as it comes down. Thus, the word "rain" is not a private symbol, with meaning only to me, the author. It is a shared symbol with meaning to anyone who speaks enough English to understand the word. Moreover, this and the hundreds of thousands of other words in the English language (plus the millions of words in other languages) are combinatory. That means that they can be combined in an infinite number of sequences to create new meanings, all of which can be communicated to others.

It is at the Verbal Conceptual level where we introduce explicit notions of time and causation to our subjective experience. By labeling these concepts, we make them more amenable to mental manipulation. In other words, we make them easier to think about. We can consider events in the present moment in the context of the past and future. We can also analyze causation. What happened here? How did it happen and what caused it? These cognitive processes powerfully impact our emotional and behavioral responses. We can tell ourselves that bad moods always pass or control our urge to act aggressively by considering possible future consequences. We can also plan our actions to be more effective. Consider how we might respond emotionally to being physically pushed if we conclude it was an accident or if we determine that it was an intentionally aggressive act. In this way, we make meaning of our environment and our role within it and then modify our responses accordingly. Thus, the Verbal Conceptual Level is a critical part of human emotional experience. While we share the Unlearned Core and Pre-conceptual levels of experience with many other species, the Verbal Conceptual level is—to the best of our knowledge—uniquely human. This is not to say that other species do not have ways of processing time and causation, but, as far as we know, no other species can process them with the sophistication, flexibility and symbolic capacities of humans.

We know that the translation of emotion into words has a moderating effect. Certainly, the ability to identify and label emotional experience is a key part of emotion regulation. A fairly large literature within developmental psychology links children's language skills to their ability to regulate their emotions (c.f. Eisenberg, Sadovsky & Spinrad, 2005). It is believed that verbally labeling emotions helps children understand their emotional states. It helps them think about the causes and consequences of their emotions, and subsequently how best to manage them. Accordingly, this task of transforming unprocessed, unconscious or poorly understood emotional experience into ideas that can be expressed in words forms the cornerstone of many types of psychotherapy. For example, Mentalization Based Psychotherapy, developed by Peter Fonagy and colleagues, focuses on just this task.

On the other hand, cognition at the Verbal Conceptual level can also *intensify* emotional experience. When we think about something upsetting, consider all possible future problems, or ruminate about past regrets, this aggravates negative emotion. Likewise, if we look forward to an upcoming vacation or reminisce about good times with friends, this can bolster positive emotions. Further, mood and emotional states can bias our cognition to interpret our environment in a way that is consistent with our emotions. For example, people who are depressed describe the world in very negative and pessimistic terms. Thus, there is constant interaction between the Verbal Conceptual and lower levels of emotional processing.

Pathology at The Verbal Conceptual Level

What does psychopathology at the Verbal Conceptual level look like? Problems in high level cognitive processing, as found in learning disabilities, can be linked to this level (Ashkenazi, Black, Abrams, Hoeft, & Menon, 2013). Cognitive deficits due to dementing diseases, such as Alzheimer's, can be as well. There also seems to be pathology at this level in schizophrenia, as reflected in the significant cognitive deficits that are characteristic of patients with this disorder.

Most relevant for the treatment of personality disorders, pathology at the Verbal Conceptual level can compromise *coping skills*. These skills are also known variously as ego functions, executive functions, or even wisdom. We are not born with mature abilities in this realm and their development does not happen by itself. In every culture, such development requires appropriate education and a supportive environment. The bulk of this development occurs in childhood but also continues throughout the lifespan. When Verbal Conceptual development proceeds well, adults gain sufficient capacity to *analyze* their environment and their role within it to negotiate their world effectively. When development goes awry, coping skills are impaired. In such cases, people respond to situations impulsively and inappropriately. Emotional reactions may be disproportionate or poorly controlled. Deficient coping skills are found in most psychiatric disorders. Some deficits are due to adult-onset disease damaging the frontal lobe, which causes people to lose skills they once possessed. But in personality disorders, deficits in coping skills are due to problematic development; the individual never developed these skills in the first place.

Treatment at the Verbal Conceptual Level

Treatment for pathology at the Verbal Conceptual level depends on its etiology. Some disorders of executive functioning can be helped by cognitive remediation, for example after strokes. More severe disorders of executive function, as in advanced dementia, require outside supervision when patients can no longer care for themselves. In schizophrenia and other psychotic disorders, cognitive impairment is treated with antipsychotics, employing the bottom-up effects of interventions at a much lower level. When inadequate coping skills are due to stymied development, as we find with personality disorders, psychotherapy can be very helpful. In these cases, interventions at the Verbal Conceptual level can help patients learn to more effectively *reason out* the causes and consequences of their own and others' behavior. Patients can also learn to place events in a temporal context, to consider the past, present and possible future. In sum, we teach patients to regulate their emotions and behavior using thought; to think before they act. Thus, intervention at the Verbal Conceptual level can have enormous impact on behavioral control.

Nonetheless, as noted above, the Verbal and Basic Conceptual levels can operate somewhat independently of one another. As such, despite improved behavioral control, intellectual insight gained from verbal interventions does not necessarily translate into *felt change* in self and other representations. We frequently see this in psychotherapy when our patients complain that understanding their problems has done little to change the way they actually feel. While some intellectual insight is probably necessary, the structure of one's interpersonal representations will not change unless there is also change at lower levels. Our patients with personality pathology will only *feel* different, therefore, when there is reorganization at the Basic Conceptual level. Once again, this highlights the distinction between the different levels of the mind/brain.

We have now reviewed the 5 levels of this model of the mind/brain, including the brain regions involved, the psychological processes they mediate and the associated forms of psychopathology. Let us now consider two additional levels of the larger human system that have considerable relevance for clinical treatment, the Life Structure and Social Levels. While these levels cannot be placed with the mind/brain proper, they are emergent properties of these lower levels and both influence and are influenced by them.

LIFE STRUCTURE LEVEL

The Life Structure level sits between the psychological and the social levels. This concept is drawn from the work of Daniel Levenson (1979, 1997). In his 1979 book *Seasons of a Man's Life* and his later work *Seasons of a Woman's Life* (1997), Levenson defined the life structure as the totality of a person's life, including one's individual personality, relationships, work, and environmental setting. What is the life that you have created for yourself? What are the cumulative effects of the life that you have lived? This level is distinguished from the psychological levels in that it includes the actual environmental impact of one's actions as well as the resulting environmental conditions that, in turn, shape the individual's day to day life. Whereas the psychological levels address the person's modes of interacting with the environment, the life structure addresses the life within the environment that has been created over time. Psychological theory and research largely focus on the domains of the five psychological levels proper. Nonetheless, many of our patients come to us for help with problems in their life structure. This is particularly the case for patients with milder psychopathology, those whose ability to self-regulate and negotiate the environment is not notably compromised. Their complaints are the problems of life. How do I live a meaningful and satisfying life? What choices should I make? Should I leave my job?

THE SOCIAL LEVEL

The Social level has profound influence on the individual's psychological development and hence is highly relevant to psychotherapy. The social level refers to any kind of interpersonal pattern that involves more than one person. Although we bring our individual personality to all our interpersonal relationships, each relationship has a life of its own that transcends the individual traits of all participants. In this way, interpersonal relationships have emergent properties vis a vis their individual members. The whole is greater than the sum of its parts. These systems can be as small as a dyadic relationship, including friendships, marriages, parent-child relationships, or even co-worker relationships. Or they can be as large as a nation or a general culture.

When patients' complaints mainly concern interactions between themselves and another person close to them, such as a spouse, it is often advisable to intervene at that level, for example with couple's therapy. Sometimes the dysfunction is related to larger social systems, such as a work environment or a larger culture or subculture. In these cases, the therapy cannot directly intervene in the larger system, but consideration of the larger group dynamics can be helpful to the patient. Then therapy can focus upon strategies to help navigate such systems. Sometimes the social system can have a top-down influence on lower psychological levels, such as on self-esteem or mood. In these cases, we can help patients differentiate their sense of self (Basic Conceptual level) from the larger social dynamics over which they may have no control (Social level). Or we can help them manage their emotional reactions (Pre-conceptual level) given the social constraints they are facing.

DIFFERENTIAL DIAGNOSIS AND CLINICAL FORMULATION

So far in this chapter we have spoken about the different levels of the mind/brain and the distinct kinds of pathology that can be ascribed to each level. Now let us consider the method of differential diagnosis. This refers to the process by which we figure out what kind of pathology we are looking at. What level or levels of the mind/brain are involved? This is not always so easy to discern because similar symptoms can manifest from different types and levels of pathology.

To determine the appropriate diagnosis, we have to consider a range of factors, including the nature, timing and context of the symptoms. After identifying a pattern of related features, we can begin to make *causal* inferences. What is cause and what is effect? The notion of causation is a tricky one as it is very difficult to determine causation definitively. As taught in introductory statistics, correlation is not equal to causation. Nevertheless, we must try to do so in order to diagnose accurately and intervene effectively.

Importantly, when we see pathology at different levels of the mind/brain, we want to characterize the causal relationship between the different forms of pathology. In other words, we want to differentiate between primary and secondary pathology. The primary pathology is the original source of the dysfunction while the secondary pathology is caused by the primary one. For example, in a psychosis related to a medical condition, the medical condition is primary and the psychosis secondary. Further, these causal relations can be *top-down* or *bottom-up*. In top-down pathology, a dysfunction at a higher level of the mind/brain causes disturbance at a lower level. For example, personality disorders (Basic Conceptual level) cause top-down disruptions in cue-induced reactions (Pre-conceptual level), resulting in problems such as depression, suicidal behavior, and substance abuse. In bottom-up causation, primary pathology at a lower level causes secondary pathology at an upper level. In this way, a person with bipolar disorder (Unlearned Core level) can show bottom-up disruptions of emotion, cognition and behavior, manifesting in paranoid and grandiose ideation (Verbal Conceptual levels) as well as reckless and even violent behavior (Pre-conceptual levels).

When there is *comorbid* pathology, independent types of pathology can interact and influence each other. They may have a synergistic or mutually reinforcing effect on one another. Alternatively, additional vulnerabilities may not *cause* the pathology but can aggravate it. This additional complexity is more the rule than the exception in our real-world settings. In fact, the clinical presentation of most of our patients will stretch across multiple levels of the mind/brain and often into the Social levels.

Let us consider some case examples.

***Carlotta*:**

Carlotta is a 36-year-old woman with a recent diagnosis of liver cancer and a 20-year history of bipolar disorder that has been well controlled on lithium. Several hospitalizations in her teens, however, delayed her completion of college and at the time were a significant source of shame. Fortunately, Carlotta has had a successful career as a book editor, which has boosted her self-esteem. It has also provided gratifying work relationships and daily structure. She has had more difficulty in romantic relationships with men, however, in which she demonstrates emotional volatility, obsessional preoccupation with rejection, and even stalking behavior. Carlotta was raised in an intact, middle class family but had a conflictual relationship with her father, who died of cancer when she was in her early twenties. After her own diagnosis of cancer, she was told to stop her lithium in preparation for a medical procedure. She then became highly volatile and began to stalk a recent ex-boyfriend, calling him incessantly until he was forced to obtain an order of protection against her.

In Carlotta's case, we see the interaction of comorbid disorders at multiple levels. Sociologically, she has sufficient access to society's resources to develop a successful career (Social level). However, the social norms of marriage and family for middle class women also haunted her, contributing to her sense of shame and inadequacy due to her difficulty establishing a stable romantic relationship. At the Basic Conceptual level, her schemas of self and partners in romantic relationships are highly problematic, as she sees herself as unable to win the love of a man or even make an effect on him and the man as out of reach and uninterested. This causes top-down disruption in emotional responses, that is in cue-induced behavior (Pre-conceptual level). Such dysregulation is aggravated by her bipolar disorder (Unlearned Core), as manifest in manic irritability and impulsivity. Of course, the shock of her cancer diagnosis (at the sub-psychological, physiological level) has aggravated her pathology even more. Finally, development in her Verbal Conceptual level was stymied in adolescence about the time of her bipolar diagnosis and further stunted by the loss of her father in her twenties. She did not have the opportunity to develop a mature understanding of their problematic relationship before he died.

***Sammy*:**

Sammy is a 46-year-old man who came from a wealthy family. Throughout his life, Sammy experienced tremendous pressure to achieve, both directly from family members and indirectly via social comparisons with highly successful and affluent peers. Sammy had a fairly severe but undiagnosed learning disability, resulting in lifelong difficulty with focused attention and reading comprehension. He was able to hold a job obtained through family connections but never excelled. Less than optimal behavior at his work was often overlooked due to his employer's desire to avoid offending his family. When his wife started to advance in her career, he reacted impulsively, engaging in an affair with another woman who then introduced him to a self-help cult. Within a year he abandoned his family to devote himself to the cult. Several years later, he left the cult, finding it too restrictive. The affair had long ended. However, he soon found that he had little to return to. His wife had divorced him, his children held him at arm's length, and his parents and siblings were angry at him. At this point, he sought therapy for help with depression.

With Sammy we see how the socio-cultural context he was born into set very high expectations for his occupational functioning. When he could not live up to them, due to his undiagnosed learning disabilities (Verbal conceptual level), his self-esteem was deeply damaged (Basic Conceptual level). Moreover, his protected background (Social level) impeded his development of frustration tolerance (Pre-conceptual level), as he was never allowed to fail and learn from his failures. His wife's professional success triggered a crisis in self-esteem (Basic Conceptual level), which resulted in dysregulated behavior (Pre-conceptual level), which ultimately resulted in significant damage to his life structure. This in turn caused the depression, which brought him to treatment. Thus, in Sammy's case we see how difficulties at multiple levels interacted in complex ways.

***Filene*:**

Filene was a 76-year-old woman with a long history of schizoaffective disorder. When properly medicated she was quite organized and capable of holding a job. But when psychotic, she would wander across the country in a delusional state, behaving in bizarre and agitated ways. Filene came from a very different background than Carlotta or Sammy. She grew up poor in the American South, when segregation was the law of the land. Her parents were of different racial backgrounds, her mother white and her father South Asian. Her parents divorced early and her father died soon after. When she was 4 years old, her mother remarried to a white man. Not wanting to be hindered by a biracial child, she put her daughter in a convent and promptly abandoned her. Filene recalled how at

> Christmas all the other children would be picked up by their families and taken home for the holidays, but that no one came for her. When she was in her mid-teens, her paternal uncle arrived to claim her and take her home but she did not adapt well to this new arrangement. She said he was too strict and she rebelled and eventually ran away. It is also possible that she could not tolerate the attachment due to fear of abandonment. By middle age, she was chronically mentally ill. She had a fixed delusion that every night 50 Mexicans invaded her motel room to rape her. She stated that she knew this was true as she put a Kleenex between her legs when she went to sleep and every morning it was wrinkled and mushy, proving that her rapists had been at work. She would even nail up boards on the windows to protect herself. After one of her many hospitalizations, she settled down in outpatient treatment, adhering to her medication regimen and engaging in psychotherapy with a social worker. She attended a day treatment program and had a small job, in which she took great pride. While her delusions quickly cleared up on medication, she maintained the belief the rapes had actually occurred in the past. Sadly, when the therapist became pregnant and resigned from the clinic, Filene abruptly quit treatment. She was last seen leaving her supervised residence with two large suitcases in hand.

Filene's primary pathology is schizoaffective disorder (Unlearned Core) but her tragic childhood of abandonment and rejection left her with deeply damaged interpersonal representations (Basic Conceptual level). Her rejection sensitivity, impulsivity, and disturbed capacity for attachment suggest a comorbid diagnosis of borderline personality disorder. This pathology aggravates the psychosis by undermining her ability to tolerate disruptions in her therapeutic relationships and thus to sustain her treatment. It is also tempting to interpret her delusions as reflective of her own personal history. Might the 50 Mexicans reflect the paternal relatives finally coming to get her? Might there be a wish to be *wanted* mixed in with her professed fear of rapists? We also see how the socio-cultural context is crucial to her story. Raised in a time of intense racism, her mother abandoned her rather than be stigmatized by a biracial child.

In conclusion, we have now reviewed a model of the hierarchical structure of the human mind/brain and located different clinical phenomena on the different levels of this model. At this point, we can turn to issues of treatment. In the next chapter we will review many of the major forms of psychotherapy and address the specific levels of the mind/brain that they target.

NOTES

1. However, there is evidence of epigenetic changes in regions of the Unlearned Core, specifically, the raphe nuclei and locus coeruleus in the brain stem. This has

been found in psychiatric conditions, such as Alzheimers disease (Iatrou et al., 2017). Epigenetic changes allow for environmental events to temporarily change gene expression without actually changing the structure of the gene.

2. Panksepp uses the capitalized terms (e.g., LUST, PANIC) to refer to the primary emotional systems that are found across mammalian species. He adds qualifiers (e.g., PANIC/Sadness) when applying these concepts to human psychology. I will follow the same convention here.

3. These four emotional systems align with the "four Fs" commonly cited in evolutionary biology. These stand for fighting, fleeing, feeding and fornicating. A cruder term is sometimes substituted for the fourth F.

4. They addressed only 6 of the 7 primary emotional systems as they excluded LUST from consideration, deeming it more of a physiological drive than a personality dimension.

Chapter Six

The Different Parts of the Elephant

In the last chapter, we discussed Emergent System Theory's hierarchical model of the mind/brain. We reviewed the psychological characteristics of each level and their associated psychological disorders. Now we are going to apply this model to a broad range of psychotherapeutic modalities available to today's psychotherapist, with particular attention to the treatment of personality pathology. Let's look back to the parable about the blind men and the elephant mentioned at the beginning of this book. If you recall, the parable describes a group of blind men who discover an elephant. Each grabs a different part of the elephant and declares the whole of the elephant to be exactly like the part that they have encountered. One man takes hold of the tail and asserts that the elephant is very much like a rope, another clasps the trunk and states that the elephant is very much like a snake. In their focus on the separate parts of the elephant, therefore, they miss the larger whole. They miss the forest for the trees.

In this chapter I will present a model of the whole elephant, an attempt to synthesize the many different forms of psychotherapy into a coherent whole. *My premise here is that the different schools of psychotherapy address different levels of the mind/brain.* For example, some treatments focus on psychological functions at the Verbal Conceptual level, others on the Basic Conceptual and still others on the Pre-conceptual. Of course, most therapies address more than one level—few are restricted to only one. But most *prioritize* one level of the mind/brain over the others. And it is this that gives it its distinct character. Therefore, in order to give focus to the therapy, each school restricts its range to one or perhaps two levels of the entire mind/brain. This is probably necessary for practical purposes and there is nothing inherently wrong with it. The problem lies in the discounting of other modalities that address different levels of the mind/brain or in thinking that any one modality can cover all mental phenomena. From this vantage point, no one treatment is a panacea.

In the rest of the chapter, we will review some of the most commonly practiced modes of psychotherapy and classify them according to the mind/brain level where we find their primary focus. (See Table 6.1 for an overview of this classification scheme.) We will address both the level of the *primary target* and the level of the *primary entry point* for treatment. The primary target refers to the predominant type of pathology the treatment aims to ameliorate. In some cases, there may be secondary targets as well. The primary entry point refers to the main level of intervention, which in turn determines the means by which the treatment is conducted. Sometimes the primary target and entry point are found at the same level and sometimes at different levels. For example, in couples therapy the primary target and entry point are both found at the social level. Both the problem targeted and method of treatment used involve the relationship between two people. In contrast, in Alcoholics Anonymous, the primary target is addiction, anchored at the Pre-conceptual level, while the primary entry point is at the level of the group, i.e., at the social level.

Now, in order to match the different types of psychotherapy with their respective level(s), we will take a walk down the mind/brain hierarchy, stopping at each level and considering the treatments we may find there. While in the last chapter we walked from the bottom floor up to the top, in this chapter we will reverse the process, starting at the top and walking down. We will do this because most of the treatments relevant to personality pathology are found on the upper levels of the hierarchy.

Of note, I will not address the relative efficacy of the different treatments or the literature either supporting or critiquing each approach. Each mode of therapy included in this chapter is well known in the mental health field and has robust support for its clinical efficacy. My goal here is to provide an integrated model rather than to critique any one therapy.

It is also worth considering the multi-level impact of the different types of treatments. While this chapter focuses upon the primary levels of the mind/brain that are targeted in each therapy, we should also keep in mind that most treatments, when successful, have far reaching multi-level effects. For example, effective treatment of severe alcoholism (at the Pre-conceptual level) can improve job performance, elevate self-esteem and strengthen mood and anger-management, reflecting benefits on the Life Structure, Basic Conceptual and Pre-conceptual levels, respectively. Nonetheless, here we will focus on the level where we find the *primary* targets and entry points for each treatment described, as it is this that gives each treatment much of its distinctive qualities. This is what separates the elephant's trunk from its tail.

Table 6.1. Psychotherapy Targets and Entry Points According to System Level

System Level	*Type of Therapy*	*Primary Target Level*	*Primary Entry-point Level*
Social	Group Therapy	Social, Pre-conceptual	Social
	Family and Couples Therapy	Social	Social
Life Structure	Acceptance and Commitment Therapy (ACT)	Life structure	Verbal conceptual
	Motivational Interviewing (MI)	Pre-conceptual	Life structure
	Supportive Therapy	Life structure	Life structure
Verbal Conceptual	Cognitive Therapy	Verbal conceptual	Verbal conceptual
Basic Conceptual	Psychodynamic Therapy	Basic conceptual	Basic conceptual
	Mentalization-Based Therapy	Basic conceptual	Basic conceptual
	Schema-Based Therapy	Basic conceptual	Basic conceptual, Verbal conceptual, Pre-conceptual
	Humanistic Therapies	Basic conceptual, Life structure	Basic conceptual
	Psychedelic Therapy	Basic conceptual	Basic conceptual, Unlearned core
Pre-conceptual	Behavior Therapy	Pre-conceptual	Pre-conceptual
	Dialectical Behavior Therapy	Pre-conceptual	Verbal conceptual, Unlearned core, Sub-psychological
Unlearned Core	Psychiatric Medication	Unlearned core	Unlearned core
	Mindfulness Meditation	Unlearned core	Unlearned core
	Relaxation Techniques	Unlearned core	Sub-psychological

THE SOCIAL LEVEL

We will start with the Social Level. This level does not actually belong to the mind/brain per se; rather it lies above it in the larger hierarchy. Nonetheless, it has a strong impact on the psychological levels such that social issues permeate the psychotherapy of personality disordered patients. At this level we are looking at the patterns of interactions between individual people. In keeping with the holistic approach of Emergent Systems Theory, there are properties of the social group that cannot be reduced to the personalities of the individual group members. Groups have their own personalities, so to speak, that can persist even when the group members change. For example, groups can be cohesive, fractured, polarized, insular and/or porous in relation to outsiders. Groups also have norms, values, and rules. Further they are judged in terms of social value both by group members and those outside the group. Importantly, belonging to a devalued group can cause significant psychological distress to group members. We will discuss the properties of the Social level in more detail in Chapter 9, but for now we can address some of the therapies that operate at this level.

Group Therapy

This is a common mode of therapy that offers significant benefits not found in individual modalities. Human beings are profoundly social animals and our group-oriented nature has a powerful impact on our mental life. Therefore treatments aimed directly at the Social level offer unique advantages over treatments that only engage lower levels within the individual mind/brain. There are many types of groups, including process-oriented, task-oriented, and support groups for specific issues (Vinogradov & Yalom, 1989). One of the prime goals of groups is to provide a sense of belonging to people who may feel alienated, either due to generalized social isolation or to their grappling with particular challenges, such as alcoholism, weight loss, bereavement, or illness in a family member. The sense of belonging to a community is extremely important to mental health and acts as a buffer for many types of mental and physical stresses (Fulginiti et al., 2020). Another important function of groups is to establish group norms. This is a powerful means of motivating change as people are compellingly drawn to follow the norms of a group that they both value and identify with (Cohen, 2016). This is a key ingredient behind the success of Alcoholics Anonymous and other 12-step groups. Dialectical Behavior Therapy (DBT) also makes use of groups to teach self-regulatory skills. Further, group members can provide encouragement for change and offer useful advice and information about shared goals.

Finally, group membership provides an identity to its members. Think of all the people you have known who suddenly show a surge of self-confidence, visible even in their body posture, when they claim membership in a group they value. The young man who was lost and aimless may stand straighter once he becomes a U.S. Marine. Many people get that same sense of self-worth by belonging to a church, a community organization, or a profession. More specifically, many of our patients feel stigmatized by their psychiatric difficulties. Joining a supportive group of people with similar conditions can offer a potent corrective to such stigma. Thus, group therapy is an excellent resource for people who feel socially alienated, need help in changing stubbornly problematic behaviors, or want to feel connected to others in similar circumstances.

Primary Targets and Entry Points

The primary *targets* of group therapy can vary. Often, they fall at the level of the social group, as with socially isolated or anxious people or those who feel stigmatized by membership in a socially devalued group. But therapy groups can also target the Pre-conceptual level, as with the many 12-step programs and DBT, which address impulsive, cue-based behavior. In contrast, the primary *entry point* for group therapy is the same across all groups. Interventions occur at the Social level.

Family and Couples Therapy

Many patients in individual therapy complain of problems in family or romantic/intimate relationships. Indeed, this is one of the most common reasons patients seek out therapy (Göstas, Wiberg, Engström & Kjellin, 2012). Frequently, it is sufficient to focus on patients' individual difficulties, either in how they repeat similar patterns across different relationships or in their coping with current circumstances. At other times, however, when the problem does not lie entirely in the patient's control, it is more helpful to intervene at the level of the social group, i.e., the family or couple.

When we intervene this way, we are addressing the social group as a coherent whole, as a unit in itself. Like other groups, families have properties of the whole that are not reducible to their individual members. Families have boundaries between in-groups and out-groups, between individual members and between generations. These boundaries can be overly porous, as when intrusive parents try to control adult children's life choices, or overly rigid, as when parents fail to inform their adult children of a terminal illness. Families range in terms of cohesion, from enmeshed to distant. Families also have different styles of managing emotion and communication.

An important concept in both family and couples therapy is the notion of vicious cycles, a destructive type of feedback loop. Joe may behave in a particular way which elicits a problematic response from Sarah which in turn aggravates the original behavior in Joe which then further aggravates Sarah's response. Before long the interactions escalate into a highly contentious cycle. This can be found in the withdraw/chase cycle, such that one partner withdraws emotionally and the second becomes increasingly intrusive in order to wrest a response from the other, who in turn withdraws further. This can also be found in a control and defy cycle, where one partner feels overly controlled and becomes increasingly resistant to any request from the partner, who in turn becomes increasingly aggressive and demanding. Such concepts have been elucidated in a number of schools of family therapy such as the structural family therapy of Salvador Minuchin, the strategic family therapy of Virginia Satir, and the experiential family therapy of Carl Whitaker and Virginia Satir (For a classic review, see Guerin, 1976).

Primary Targets and Entry Points

All family and couples therapies target the Social level, specifically that of the family or couple relationships. The intention is to change the patterns of interaction that are causing distress within the relationships. The primary entry point for this mode of treatment is also the same; all such therapies intervene at the Social level.

THE LIFE STRUCTURE LEVEL

We will now move down one level to Life Structure. This lies below the Social level and above the purely psychological levels. The life structure refers to the totality of the lives people have developed over time. This includes their occupational history, financial condition, marital or romantic circumstances, and larger family relations, as well as their guiding values, morals, and/or religious tenets. How have people lived their lives and how do they want to do so? While this level lies above the 5 psychological levels of the mind/brain proper, it has direct impact upon them and conversely, is greatly impacted by them. Almost all modes of individual psychotherapy hope to make an impact on this level, to ultimately improve the patient's life satisfaction. A few therapeutic modalities make the life structure their primary focus of treatment.

Acceptance and Commitment Therapy (ACT)

Acceptance and Commitment Therapy (ACT) is a relatively new therapy that has become quite popular in recent years (Hayes, 2015; Hayes, Follette & Linehan, 2004). While it is not specifically designed for personality disordered patients, it is used with disorders which frequently co-occur with personality pathology, such as anxiety, depression, alcohol abuse, and even physical pain. ACT comes out of the behavioral tradition and in fact is known as part of the "third wave" of cognitive behavioral therapy; the first wave being behaviorism, the second cognitive treatment, and the third integration of cognitive, behavioral and experiential approaches (Hayes et al., 2004). Steven Hayes, the founder of ACT, lists cognitive behavioral therapy and Eastern meditational traditions as his primary influences. Additionally, Relational Frame Theory, ACT's underlying conceptual framework, is reminiscent of post-modern philosophical theories which propose our view of reality to rest on a network of linguistic symbols (D'Angelo, 2020).

In somewhat of a departure from other CBT approaches, however, the fundamental aim of ACT is to help patients remove barriers to a meaningful and vital life rather than to reduce symptoms. As such, we will locate ACT at the level of the life structure. Although ACT also focuses upon thought patterns associated with the Verbal Conceptual level, we will nevertheless place ACT at the Life Structure level because ACT's primary goal is to enhance life satisfaction. In this way, the cognitive interventions serve as a means towards a larger purpose. Indeed, as Hayes states in his 2015 book:

> This book is not about solving your problems in a traditional way so much as it is about changing the direction of your life, so that your life is more about what you value. (Hayes, 2015, p. 16)

Hayes believes that the primary barrier standing between patients and a fully realized life is the tendency towards *experiential avoidance*, the use of various mental strategies to avoid pain. But because pain is ultimately inescapable, attempts to avoid it create more suffering than the pain itself. Over time, experiential avoidance causes a narrowing and depletion of the person's life, which in turn magnifies the very suffering the person was trying to avoid. For example, a person afraid of panic attacks can become so agoraphobic that they sacrifice all engagement with the outside world. Hayes describes these avoidant maneuvers as "an adorable tiger kitten" that turns into an "uncontrollable, savage beast" (Hayes, 2015, p. 36).

ACT makes a distinction between pain and suffering. Pain is natural and unavoidable. We feel pain when we are physically ill, suffer a loss, or when we have any serious stressor. However, pain is generally time-limited. Suffering, however, is more long-term. It reflects ongoing pain, the extension of pain over time. (Hayes, 2015). It is the basic premise of ACT that we turn pain into suffering when we try to avoid the inevitable experience of pain.

Why and how do we do this? ACT conceptualizes psychopathology in profoundly linguistic terms. As humans, we are verbal creatures. We see the world in terms of the abstract symbols called words. Language both describes and evaluates situations; we can judge events as good or bad. Language also allows us to move out of the here and now and into the future and the past. Thus, with our temporal, verbal mind, we not only feel pain in the present when actually encountering something painful, like non-human animals do, but we also suffer from *anticipating* pain in the future and *recalling* pain from the past.

Relatedly, we tend to confuse our thoughts with actual reality. In this case, there is inadequate separation between the subjective products of the mind and external, objective reality. This is called *cognitive fusion* and is seen by Hayes as the basis of experiential avoidance. I feel unattractive so I am unattractive; I believe I am not likeable so you must not like me. Inevitably, such thinking leads to avoidant life choices, hence greatly constricting life.

How does ACT treat this? First, the patient has to commit to being *willing*, which means being open to the full range of human emotions, to relinquish experiential avoidance. This allows patients to move towards *acceptance*, that is the acceptance of the entirety of who they are as people and of their felt experience, including pain. But in order to arrive at full acceptance, patients have to first recognize their maladaptive thoughts *as* thoughts and to cognitively defuse them. For this, ACT introduces *mindfulness meditation techniques*. In Hayes' words "Mindfulness is the defused, nonattached, accepting, nonjudgmental, deliberate awareness of experiential events as they happen in the moment" (Hayes, 2015, p. 98). By mindfully observing their thoughts, they defuse the cognition. They step outside of it and in so doing, the maladaptive thought loses its power. While there are many ways to practice mindfulness, ACT utilizes multiple written exercises as well as visualization techniques. One of the more conventional mindfulness practices asks patients to mindfully observe their sensations, emotions, memories, bodily impulses and thoughts. In a less conventional meditation exercise, patients are instructed to visualize their disturbing thoughts as an object in front of them. They are then asked to characterize the object in terms of its physical properties and then to imagine physically moving the object to the side and finally to take it back inside of themselves.

Once these skills have been mastered, it is time for patients to make changes to their lives. They are now asked to commit to making life changes in line with their *values*. Here, the concept of values appears to be less about ethics and morality than what is personally important to the patient. What do patients really value in their life? Written exercises are provided to help with this task. Once a patient's values are identified, the patient is helped to set goals, both short-term and long-term. For example, if family life is important, then a short-term goal could be to spend 3 hours a week with one's children on the weekend. A long-term goal would be to find a job that allowed for better work-life balance. Importantly, the goals are not seen as ends in themselves but rather as guide posts along a life path, to help patients proceed through life in line with their expressed values. Note that anxiety-provoking goals can be reached incrementally, in small steps that are less anxiety producing.

Primary Target and Entry Point

I propose that the primary target of ACT lies at the Life Structure level. Even though ACT gives considerable attention to mindfulness techniques and maladaptive thoughts, the clearly stated aim of this treatment is to open up life experience, to help people move towards a vital and fully embraced life. Indeed, the title of Hayes' 2015 book is "Get Out of Your Head and into Your Life."

Although the primary target of ACT lies at the Life Structure level, the primary *entry point* for this treatment lies at the Verbal Conceptual Level. In ACT, the basis of maladaptive behavior is attributed to the inherent properties of language. Relational Frame Theory, the underlying conceptual framework, is a theory of language. Indeed, a significant proportion of ACT is devoted to helping the patient cognitively defuse, that is to identify their thoughts as thoughts and not as objective reality. At first glance, mindfulness meditation may not appear to belong to the Verbal Conceptual level. Indeed, as we will see, in other treatment modalities meditative techniques will be situated at a lower level of the mind/brain. But in ACT, these methods have become highly verbal and cognitive, often involving written exercises. Once again, the intention is to shift patients' relationship to their thoughts.

ACT does acknowledge phenomena at lower levels of the mind/brain, including those at the Basic and Pre-conceptual levels. More specifically, the concepts of experiential avoidance and incremental goal setting are based on associative conditioning and gradual desensitization, both Pre-conceptual forms of learning. ACT also addresses patients' self-concept (Basic Conceptual level), noting that one of the greatest barriers to relinquishing one's problematic thoughts is attachment to a fixed self-concept, to a fixed identity. If I am not my thoughts, who am I? ACT also distinguishes between the experience of self as an observing agent vs. a static, objectified entity (the "I" vs. the "me"). But to my mind, neither the nature of the self-concept nor its origins are explored in detail. ACT also acknowledges the importance of childhood memories in forming the cognitive matrix underlying experiential avoidance but, as with self-concept, this is not explored in detail. In ACT, therefore, the overwhelming focus of interventions involves language and cognition.

Motivational Interviewing

Motivational Interviewing (MI) is a very targeted, time-limited treatment designed to enhance motivation to change in people struggling with addiction (Miller, 2009; Miller & Rollnick, 1991; Miller, Zweben, DiClemente, Rychtarik, 1992; Lewis, Larson, & Korcuska, 2017). I have included it in this chapter as it is widely used in the treatment of addictions, which are frequently comorbid with personality disorders. Additionally, the basic principles of MI are widely applicable to any self-destructive behavior pattern that is resistant to change. Certainly, such patterns are a hallmark of personality pathology. MI is placed at the Life Structure level because its primary mode of action is to help patients reflect upon the stark discrepancy between their life goals and values and their current life of addiction.

MI was started by William Miller in the early 1980s. He was influenced both by the behaviorist tradition and by Carl Rogers' client-centered school of psychotherapy. Miller's background in behaviorism led to a focus on specific behavioral change as is relevant to substance abuse disorders. The Rogerian tradition, however, is evident in MI's insistence on a collaborative, empathic, non-judgmental, and non-argumentative mode of engaging with patients. In his early training experiences, Miller was disturbed by the confrontational and authoritarian approach that he observed in the treatment of patients with substance abuse. Patients with addiction were perceived as manipulative, resistant and deceptive. Treatment was confrontational and directive. Miller found, however, that when he engaged patients in a non-directive and respectful way, without judgment or argument, his patients were far more open with him and far more honest.

He also reconceptualized these patients' "resistance" as ambivalence about change. Patients both do and do not want to change, to give up their dependence on mind-altering substances. With colleagues such as Steve Rollnick, he developed the notion that the therapists' goal is to facilitate patients' resolution of their ambivalence to change. Nonetheless, such motivation must ultimately come from the patient and not the therapist. If a therapist becomes too invested in one side of a patient's ambivalence (i.e., sobriety), this will only strengthen the pull of the other side (i.e., addiction), and the patient will become that much more entrenched in their opposition to change. The therapist must place both sides of their patients' ambivalence squarely in their own lap.

Thus, it is the goal of the therapist to elucidate the full extent of their patients' ambivalence. When frequently relapsing patients emphasize their motivation to change, the therapist can question what might be attractive about their addiction. When patients insist on no interest in change, the therapist can explore any behavior that indicates otherwise. But the therapist is not without a desired outcome; the aim of MI is to enhance motivation to change. More specifically, by use of techniques such as skillful questioning and active listening, the therapist elicits patients' life goals and values and ultimately helps them to see *discrepancies* between their personal goals and their current life. Additionally, individuals with addictions are often quite demoralized about their ability to change as they have generally failed in their efforts many times before. Therapists therefore highlight positive steps that have been taken, what has been accomplished rather than what has not. For example, if a patient manages to stay sober for a week, this is emphasized rather than the fact that he or she relapsed soon after. In this way, therapists reinforce self-efficacy and self-agency.

Once the patient can voice motivation to change in a believable, authentic, and elaborated way, rather than in a pat, compliant and superficial way, it is time to set goals for change. MI uses the acronym of SMART goals, which are specific, measurable, achievable, relevant and time bound. These guidelines help set the patient up for success rather than failure. Overly broad and vague goals and those without a set time limit are less likely to succeed.

Although MI is a short intervention, generally delivered in a matter of days or even hours, it has been shown to be highly effective when used in conjunction with more intensive substance abuse treatments (Miller, 2009). As such, it serves to prime the patient's motivation to fully engage with substance abuse treatment.

Primary Target and Entry Point

In MI, the primary target for treatment is ultimately the cessation of substance abuse; therefore, we can situate MI's treatment *target* at the Pre-conceptual level. However, the primary *entry point* falls at the life structure level. It is through the heightening of discrepancy between the person's values and life goals on one hand and their current life of addiction on the other that the treatment strengthens motivation for change. It is only with some resolution of their ambivalence towards change that patients can mobilize themselves to fight the inordinately strong pull of their addiction. Nonetheless, the actual behavioral change is not achieved in MI; rather, that occurs in specific substance abuse programs.

Supportive Therapy

Supportive therapy can also be placed at the level of the Life Structure. In this treatment, the therapist serves as a caring figure who offers useful, practical guidance in negotiating the challenges of daily life. The goal is less to resolve specific symptoms or change underlying personality structure than to support stable functioning within the parameters of the patient's life. While this type of therapy is most typically used with lower functioning, psychiatrically impaired patients, it is also relevant for patients with personality pathology. For one, it is likely that most therapists, regardless of orientation, incorporate supportive techniques to some degree. Even the highest functioning patients can benefit from emotional support and guidance at times. While an excessively supportive approach might undermine patients' independence and contribute to the avoidance of difficult truths, it is a rare person who does not need a helping hand now and then. This is particularly true with personality disordered patients, whose emotional instability can periodically undermine their reasoning and judgment.

Although supportive techniques date back as far as Sigmund Freud (who even gave money to one of his patients!) (Wolf-Man, 1971), this approach has traditionally received little recognition as a valid treatment in and of itself. Since the early 2000s, however, Arnold Winston and colleagues have examined the benefits and characteristic features of supportive therapy (Winston, Rosenthal, & Pinsker, 2011; Winston, Rosenthal & Roberts, 2019). As hospital-based psychiatrists, the authors were well aware that severely ill psychiatric patients had distinct therapeutic needs.

To clarify the parameters of supportive therapy, the authors contrasted this type of therapy with traditional psychoanalytic methods. Psychoanalytic techniques focus on uncovering intense, unconscious emotion in order to facilitate greater self-awareness and insight. Directive interventions, that is suggestions on what to do, are seen as not only unnecessary but actually harmful in that they interfere with the self-discovery process. Likewise, therapists maintain a "neutral" stance and disclose very little personal information so as not to impinge upon the patients' self-exploration.

In contrast, supportive methods do not assume that patients are capable of regulating their emotions or of negotiating daily life on their own. The goal of supportive therapy therefore is to help patients maintain stable functioning in their environment and to live as satisfying and meaningful a life as possible. Self-awareness is less important. Consequently, supportive therapists do not challenge patients' defenses or seek to elicit strong emotions. These therapists focus on conscious (rather than unconscious) experience and provide direct advice where needed. "Have you thought about buying an appointment book? That might help you get to your job on time." They aim to support intact daily functioning, boost self-esteem, and maintain emotional stability. Supportive therapists also relate to their patients differently; they are warm and "real" rather than "neutral." Instead of withholding all personal information, they may disclose minor aspects of their life in order to put their patients at ease and normalize their experience. "Yes, I have also felt nervous when attending a party where I don't know people. I think that's quite common."

Primary Target and Entry Point

The life structure level provides both the primary target and the primary entry point for supportive therapy. When patients are having a difficult time negotiating their lives, either due to cognitive limitations, acute situational stress, or emotional difficulties, therapists provide additional support, in effect coaching the patient to engage with their lives in the most adaptive way possible. While this is rarely the sole form of psychotherapy with personality disordered patients, it is an important part of the therapeutic toolkit as, despite normal intelligence, these patients often experience significant challenges navigating interpersonal or occupational situations and making appropriate decisions. Nonetheless, overreliance on such techniques with personality disordered patients can ultimately impede their growth towards mature independence. As the old saying goes: Give a man a fish and you feed him for a day. Teach a man to fish and you feed him for a lifetime.

THE VERBAL CONCEPTUAL LEVEL

Now we move into the 5 levels of the mind/brain proper. The Verbal Conceptual Level is the highest of the mind/brain levels. It includes the most recently evolved segments of the brain, the outer portions of the neocortex. The psychological functions associated with this level include language, complex cognition, abstract thought, and high-level executive functions, such as planning, consideration of future consequences, and generation of alternative courses of action. This is, in essence, the seat of our intellect and is central for regulating goal-oriented behavior. It is also important for monitoring and controlling emotion but it does not generate emotion per se. In this way, the Verbal Conceptual level is the seat of "cold cognition" as opposed to "hot cognition," which is more directly involved with emotion.

Cognitive Therapy

Cognitive Therapy was born of the cognitive revolution in the 1960s in which the anti-mentalist tradition of behaviorism gave way to a recognition of the mental processes that mediate between stimulus and response. Throughout the first half of the 20th century, behaviorists had regarded the subjective processes of the human mind as a "black box" inserted between external stimulus and behavioral response, something impossible to observe and thus irrelevant to scientific psychology. During this period, psychoanalysis ruled the consulting room and behaviorism ruled the laboratory. But, over time, it became impossible to ignore the mind. Even rats running mazes showed signs of cognitive processes. Hence the study of cognition became scientifically respectable (Hunt, 2007). With that development, cognitive and behavioral approaches began to make inroads into the clinical world, a territory that psychoanalysis had long dominated.

Albert Ellis and Aaron T. Beck are considered the fathers of cognitive therapy. In this chapter we will focus on the Beckian tradition as that is arguably more influential today. Cognitive therapy is now subsumed under the umbrella family of therapies called cognitive behavioral therapy (CBT), which integrates basic behavioral principals of change with cognitive approaches. A large number of different types of CBT have been developed to deal with a great range of behavioral problems, such as insomnia, eating disorders, and substance abuse (J.S. Beck, 2011). Here, however, we will focus on cognitive therapy per se as it is most pertinent to the Verbal Conceptual Level. Its focus is almost entirely on the conscious beliefs that drive patients' emotional and behavioral responses. Behavioral treatments will be addressed at the Pre-conceptual level.

Like almost all psychiatrists in mid-20th century America, Aaron Beck was trained in psychoanalysis. He was taught to attend to patients' unconscious beliefs and that depression reflected suppressed hostility. But when listening to his depressed patients, he found instead that they generated quite explicit and conscious beliefs related to low self-esteem, pessimism, and helplessness. Over time he became interested in an alternative approach to his patients' depression, one that focused more on the here and now rather than childhood, that addressed conscious maladaptive thoughts rather than unconscious beliefs, and that utilized a more directive and goal-oriented approach than was found in the classical psychoanalysis of the time. Throughout the 1960s and 1970s, he developed a new therapeutic approach to depression that focused upon these conscious and distorted beliefs. The underlying assumption was that the content of a person's beliefs shapes emotional experience. This is a very old concept, dating all the way back to ancient Greece. In fact, both Beck and Albert Ellis credit the Stoic philosopher Epictetus with this core idea.

As explicated by his daughter Judith Beck in her classic textbook on cognitive behavior therapy (J.S. Beck, 2011), the focus of cognitive therapy is on identifying and restructuring patients' maladaptive thoughts. Beckian therapy specifically focuses upon what is called "*automatic thoughts*," spontaneously generated cognitions that occur in response to a stimulus. Such thoughts are emotionally fraught, often quite distorted, and lead to maladaptive emotional and behavioral responses. To use an example noted earlier, if a young woman sends a text to her boyfriend and does not receive a response within the hour, she might have the automatic thought of "He must not like me anymore. I think he's met someone else." Obviously, this would cause distress and might lead to impulsive action on the woman's part.

Automatic thoughts are linked to underlying *core beliefs* about the self and the world, otherwise known as schemas. Core beliefs originate from past experience, often in childhood, and give people a view of who they are and how they fit into the world. Automatic thoughts, which reflect our interpretation of the day-to-day situations we encounter, are shaped by our core beliefs. For example, if we see ourselves as helpless, we would be prone to automatic thoughts such as "I can't do this. It will never work." As such, automatic thoughts serve to confirm a person's core beliefs; they bias our reactions to events to be consistent with them. This is a general property of human cognition, but it becomes a serious problem if the core beliefs are rigidly maladaptive.

Beck also addressed the specific information processing biases, known as *cognitive distortions*, that ensure our automatic thoughts remain consistent with our core beliefs. In depressed people this can include exaggerating the negative aspects of a situation, minimizing its positive aspects, or overgeneralizing from a conclusion. David Burns, an early popularizer of Beck's work (Burns, 1999), elaborated on this notion. He created a list of cognitive distortions, such as all or nothing thinking (e.g., something is either all good or all bad, with no middle ground), disqualifying the positive, jumping to conclusions, emotional reasoning (i.e., reasoning from emotions instead of facts) and mind reading.

Cognitive therapy is highly structured but also collaborative. Together therapists and patients use written exercises to track and identify automatic thoughts and cognitive distortions. A thought record is commonly used for this purpose. Patients are asked to keep a log of situations that were troubling to them during the day. This information is recorded in a table, with each incident entered on a separate row. The first column describes the challenging situation or incident, the second the automatic thought generated in response to it, and the third the resulting emotional response along with a rating of its intensity (often 0–100). The fourth column lists an alternative, more adaptive thought, and the fifth the outcome, with a new emotional intensity rating.

In order to identify the core belief underlying the automatic thoughts, exercises such as the downward arrow can be used. This involves repeated questioning of the automatic thought until the core belief is elicited. What does it *mean* that this would happen? What is so bad about it? Once identified, the core beliefs can be challenged by techniques such as testing the evidence. What evidence do you have that you are unlovable? What evidence do you have *against* that belief? The automatic thoughts can also be challenged by testing the evidence, specifically, with behavioral experiments. For example, to test the accuracy of the automatic thought "I can't go to that party, because I will have a terrible time," the patient can be asked to attend the party as a behavioral experiment. Homework assignments like these are central to cognitive therapy as well as many different types of CBT.

Note, while ACT and cognitive therapy both focus upon maladaptive cognitions as drivers of psychopathology, they differ in their proposed goals with regard to maladaptive thoughts. Whereas cognitive therapy aims to restructure the thoughts, replacing maladaptive with adaptive thoughts, ACT aims to change the person's *relationship* to the thoughts, assuming that maladaptive thoughts are unavoidable products of the verbal mind. Likewise, over time CBT has incorporated other aspects of treatment, such as mindfulness meditation, and has elaborated its theoretical framework. In 2014 Aaron Beck published a conceptual paper on the Generic Cognitive Model, expanding his focus to incorporate the role of emotions, genetics, attentional biases, etc. (A.T. Beck & Haigh, 2014). Nonetheless, the primary focus on cognition as a driver of psychological distress remains.

Primary Target and Entry Point

Both the primary target and entry point of Beckian cognitive therapy lie at the Verbal Conceptual level. Although this treatment aims to reduce depression and anxiety and improve overall life adjustment, the emphasis is clearly on cognitive processes. It is assumed that shifts in cognitive evaluations will result in improved emotional functioning. While cognitive therapy has been adapted to treat a range of psychological disorders, including personality disorders, the strongest evidence of efficacy is for depression and anxiety (J. S. Beck, 2011). Hence personality disorders that are characterized by depression and anxiety, particularly Cluster C disorders, would be well suited for this approach. Additionally, to the extent that patients with other personality disorders are also highly ruminative and ideational, they could benefit from the explicit focus on maladaptive cognitions.

There are likely to be beneficial top-down and bottom-up effects of cognitive therapy. Reduced depression and anxiety reflect top-down improvement at the Pre-conceptual levels. Likewise, reduction of depressive ruminations can reduce behavioral inhibition which would have salutary bottom-up effects on the Life Structure and Social levels. It is the contention of this book, however, that although Beckian therapy incorporates self and interpersonal schemas in its conceptual framework, this therapy does not extensively address the dysfunctional interpersonal representations that underly personality disorders. Thus, there is unlikely to be significant top-down change at the Basic Conceptual level. Hence the ability to transform personality disordered patients' fundamental experience of self and relationships is likely to be limited. Indeed, schema therapy was developed to address just this gap in the cognitive behavioral tradition (Young, Klosko & Weishaar, 2003). Schema therapy will be addressed in the section on the Basic Conceptual level.

THE BASIC CONCEPTUAL LEVEL

We will now move one level down to the Basic Conceptual level. This is the home of interpersonal representations, emotional cognition ("hot" vs. "cold" cognition; Stein, 2021), and episodic memory. It involves the interior, medial parts of the cortex as well as the limbic lobe. From the vantage point of Emergent Systems Theory, the Basic Conceptual level is the seat of the mental structures underlying personality pathology. In effect, this is the primary residence of personality pathology. A number of well-established psychotherapy modalities focus upon this level. Accordingly, these therapies typically aim to treat personality pathology per se rather than common comorbid conditions, such as alcohol abuse, anxiety disorders or depression. All of the therapies in this section, therefore, are placed at the Basic Conceptual Level because they primarily target patients' maladaptive interpersonal representations, often in the context of significant personality pathology.

Psychodynamic Therapy

The oldest and best known of these therapeutic modalities is psychodynamic psychotherapy, a descendant of Freudian psychoanalysis. More specifically, I am referring to the offshoots of object relations theory and other psychoanalytic schools that focus primarily upon patients' interpersonal representations. Such psychoanalytic schools include British object relations, interpersonal psychology/psychoanalysis, self-psychology, and, most recently, the relational school. The more orthodox Freudian approach, typically known as "classical" psychoanalysis, focuses more on the "instinctual drives" (specifically sex and aggression) and defenses used against them. For simplicity's sake, we will use the term psychodynamic approaches to refer to the psychoanalytic schools that concern themselves with interpersonal representations.

As reviewed in Chapter 3, interpersonal representations are concepts of self and other that guide affect, cognition, and behavior in relevant situations. They derive from lived experience of actual interpersonal relationships, primarily those in childhood. Although fairly malleable in childhood, by adulthood they are conservative and difficult to change. Considerable evidence points to dysfunctional interpersonal representations as the primary contributor to general personality pathology. Hence treatments that focus upon personality pathology tend to emphasize interpersonal representations.

While several treatment approaches address analogous concepts (e.g., core beliefs in Beckian cognitive therapy), psychodynamic therapy has a number of characteristics that distinguish it from other modalities. This is most clear when comparing it with treatments in the behavioral tradition. The behavioral school came out of American academia. It is based on empirical research and understands knowledge to reflect measurable information about observable behavior. Behavior is coded into quantifiable variables and the efficacy of treatment is tested mathematically, with statistics. In contrast, the psychoanalytic tradition is an import from Europe. It has a scholarly tradition. Intellectual discourse focuses upon *theory*, which develops from careful reflection upon one's predecessors' ideas. Of course, actual events matter and psychoanalytic theorists are almost all clinicians themselves. Their theoretical work is informed by their own clinical experience. But until recently, clinical phenomena were not studied with empirical research. Instead, psychoanalytic writers carefully reflected upon their clinical experiences in the context of analytic theory. As such, knowledge in this tradition is seen as an internally coherent and trenchant system of ideas. In short, while the academic behaviorists seek out *facts*, the analysts seek out *ideas*.

Now why is this important to the actual performance of psychotherapy? Because these different worldviews lead to different emphases in the actual treatments. Therapists in the behavioral tradition tend to be goal-oriented, directive and very structured, frequently offering homework in the form of charts and tables. They focus upon measurable behavioral change. Therapists in the psychoanalytic tradition tend to be process-oriented, non-directive, and largely unstructured. Sessions involve open-ended conversations, in which patients speak about whatever is on their mind. Therapists listen attentively, ask clarifying questions, and offer interpretations of patients' motivations and behavioral patterns. Most of all, psychodynamic therapists focus on the process of *reflection*, seeing the achievement of an internally coherent and complete narrative of one's own life as curative in itself. They aim to help their patients develop a maturely organized, nuanced and internally consistent understanding about who they are in the social world. In effect, they are helping their patients create a better "theory" about themselves.

Importantly, this type of treatment is not a mere intellectual exercise. All psychoanalytic schools have long noted how dry, intellectualized insight does not bring about change. Rather insight has to be deeply felt. The patients must engage with their deepest emotions and only in the process of doing so, learn to understand their own experiences from a healthier perspective. It is this combination of direct feeling and greater insight that leads to reorganization of the patient's interpersonal representations; it is through this process that true transformation takes place. The patient can fully experience her or himself as different—freer and yet more secure, more grounded. Likewise, the world becomes a different place to such patients, more open and inviting, with more possibilities and fewer threats. Importantly, unlike the other approaches discussed so far, psychodynamic treatment does not specifically aim to change behavior, affect, or cognition. It does not aim to resolve symptoms. Rather it aims to rework the underlying mental structures that lead to problems in all these other areas. In this view, psychodynamic therapists attempt to treat the cause and not the symptoms. The assumption is that change in interpersonal representations will naturally lead (i.e., in a top-down manner) to resolution of the other problems.

There are two other features that distinguish the psychodynamic approach, the developmental perspective and an emphasis on the therapeutic relationship. From its inception, psychoanalysis has looked at psychological function through a developmental lens. The assumption was that we best understand our patients' present psychological structure by considering how it developed over time. The developmental history of patients' interpersonal representations is reflected in both content and form. The *content* of interpersonal representations is a function of episodic memory, as discussed in Chapter 3. Memories of (largely) childhood relationships are consolidated into a template of self and other in the social world. For example, a young man, having grown up with a highly authoritarian and controlling father, may see himself as incompetent and dependent on others' direction. He may also reflexively rebel against such guidance, perceiving it as intrusive and humiliating, but do so recklessly and ineffectively, thus reinforcing his self-view as incompetent. As such, the psychodynamic therapist aims to a) uncover the content of the patient's interpersonal representations, b) identify its roots in childhood experience, and c) trace its manifestation in adult life.

The *form* of interpersonal representations reflects the structure of patients' mental processes and not just the content. Psychodynamic writers such as Sidney Blatt (Blatt, Brenneis, Schimek & Glick, 1976) and Irene Fast (Fast, 1985) have developed sophisticated ways of talking about the formal organization of patients' interpersonal representations from a developmental perspective. Poorly organized interpersonal representations are seen as inadequately developed, as immature and regressed. Such views of self and other lack complexity; they are crude and simplistic. As a result, there is a tendency towards overwhelming affect and an inability to step outside of the immediate emotional state to reflect upon cause and effect. To the patient, these emotional states are experienced as outside of time. They exist in an eternal present; nothing has come before, and nothing will come after. This includes both positive and negative experience, involving states of "oceanic bliss" as well as "annihilation anxiety" (Hurvich, 1989). Consequently, by paying attention to subtle fluctuations in the *organization* of patients' ways of speaking about self and others, psychodynamic therapists can identify problematic areas of personality functioning and then foster the development of more maturely organized world views. For example, consider a young woman, who, at the start of treatment, described her ex-husband in simplistically negative and egocentric terms ("He was a selfish shithead. He hated me!"). One year later, she showed a more objective and nuanced perspective, better able to understand cause and effect ("He really had a horrible childhood. I guess if no one ever cared for what he felt, it's not surprising he couldn't care about what I felt."). This more sophisticated understanding allowed her to negotiate contact with her ex-husband more effectively, with far less antagonism.

Another distinguishing characteristic of the psychodynamic approach is the emphasis on the therapeutic relationship. Although other therapeutic modalities address the relationship between patient and therapist, they do so mainly as a background condition for effective treatment, not as a central element of the therapy. For example, Dialectical Behavior Therapy (DBT) discusses the problem of therapy-interfering behavior (Linehan, 2015). Beckian cognitive therapy promotes a collaborative relationship between patient and therapist (J.S. Beck, 2011). Additionally, psychotherapy research supports the role of the therapeutic alliance and therapeutic empathy for treatment efficacy (Muran et al., 2009). Psychodynamic therapy, however, places the therapeutic relationship at the forefront of the treatment, as embodied in the concepts of *transference* and *countertransference*.

These two concepts have a long history in psychoanalysis (See Harris, 2012 for a review). It was Freud himself who first realized that the patient's emotional reaction to the analyst may be less of a response to the real person and more a projection, or "transfer," of the patient's internal desires and conflicts. That is not to say that all aspects of the patient's feelings toward the analyst are transference. There is, of course, a reality-based relationship as well. But within the psychoanalytic tradition, emotionally intense, disproportionate, and often quite distorted reactions to the therapist are understood as transference. In this way, transference offers a unique opportunity to bring the patient's core interpersonal representations directly into view.

The therapist's version of transference is called countertransference. This refers to the therapist's intense and often disproportionate emotional response to the patient. Countertransference can arise as a direct reaction to the patient's transference or to the therapist's own personal psychology. Distinguishing the two sources is often difficult. Originally, countertransference was seen as a hindrance to the therapeutic work, a messy impingement on the patient's personal space, best kept tightly under wraps. But with time, the informative value of countertransference was increasingly recognized.

Many therapists will tell you that they often have strong emotional reactions to their patients. When these feelings are acknowledged and reflected upon carefully, they can be enormously instructive. For example, therapists can feel bored when their patients are emotionally detached, sleepy when their patients are desperately trying to shut out emotional pain, depleted and draggy when their patients are depressed, and irritated when their patients are unconsciously passive-aggressive. I once supervised a student who dreamed that her patient on the psychiatric inpatient unit would go home and commit suicide. The next day he did just that.

More than once I have found myself fighting tears when patients relay very sad stories while remaining emotionally detached themselves. If I call their attention to this phenomenon, they quite often start to cry. I then feel immediately relieved of the emotional intensity. It is as if I have handed them back their own emotions. Thus, countertransference is a complex and powerful phenomenon, and we ignore it at our peril.

The object relations theorist Melanie Klein introduced the term *projective identification* to the psychoanalytic lexicon (Britton, 2012). This occurs when patients unconsciously elicit a psychological state in the therapist that either parallels or complements their own emotional state. This most frequently occurs in the treatment of patients with severe personality pathology and can be quite uncomfortable for the therapist. The more recent relational school of psychoanalysis focuses upon similar phenomena, but uses the term *enactments* (Harris, 2012). This refers to a co-creation by both patient and therapist of an emotionally fraught interaction which ultimately reveals important information about the patient's interpersonal representations.

Let us consider an example. A middle-aged woman told her therapist that she was very upset after the previous session when the therapist suggested that she had prioritized her new boyfriend over her daughter's need for time and attention. The patient had been distraught for several hours. The therapist realized that he had felt judgmental of the patient during the prior session and had probably communicated these feelings unintentionally. While he did not immediately disclose this insight to the patient, he used it to inform his understanding of the incident and to guide further investigation. Eventually, the conversation addressed the patient's fear and shame about behaving like her mother, who had frequently prioritized her own interests over the patient's needs. Because the patient felt so judgmental of her own mother's behavior, she could not allow herself to recognize that she had replicated some of her patterns. In response, the therapist fell into an enactment in which he also became judgmental, triggering a catastrophic sense of guilt on the part of the patient.

Now, perhaps this sounds like hocus-pocus, like some sort of a magical telepathy. But if we think about the neuroanatomy of emotional responses, we can see that much of emotional processing is done subcortically, certainly below the Verbal Conceptual level, and likely beneath consciousness (See Chapter 2). If we think about it this way, it is not surprising that emotion can be communicated subliminally, from one amygdala to another, so to speak. Additionally, as shown in the work of Beatrice Beebe (See Chapter 3), careful analyses of mother-infant interactions show split second sequences of mutual influence. This occurs so quickly that it is not always evident to the naked eye. In sum, human beings are master communicators and much of our communication is not conscious.

The task of the therapy, therefore, is for both patient and therapist to recognize enactments as such and to collaboratively untangle it in the interest of a greater understanding of the patient's internal world, that is their matrix of interpersonal representations. Importantly, the relational school believes in a two-person rather than a one-person psychology (Aron, 2012; Harris, 2012). They do not assume that the therapist is a neutral bystander and that all difficulty in the therapeutic relationship stems from the patient's pathology. Nonetheless, the focus of the therapy is on the patient's psychology and not the therapist's and therapists are very careful in what they disclose to patients of their own subjective experience.

Primary Targets and Entry Points

In psychodynamic therapy, the primary target and entry point both lie at the Basic Conceptual level. More than any other modality of psychotherapy, psychodynamic therapy focuses on self and other representations and sees development in this realm as sufficient to ensure improvement in other areas. Hence, psychodynamic therapy presumes powerful top-down effects on the Pre-conceptual level, resulting in improved affect regulation and impulse control. Importantly, psychodynamic treatments do not *directly* address problems stemming from the Pre-conceptual level, such as panic disorder, addiction, impulsive aggression, or self-injurious behavior, common comorbid conditions in patients with severe personality pathology. For patients with significant difficulties in these areas, therefore, alternative modalities may be needed. Such approaches will be addressed below in the Pre-conceptual section.

Additionally, not all patients are capable of the self-reflection necessary for psychodynamic work and certainly not at all times. In order to benefit from psychodynamic interpretations, patients must be capable of distinguishing between their own subjective processes and external reality; they must be able to think about their own thoughts, a process known as meta-cognition. Psychodynamic therapists recognize this and emphasize careful and tactful timing of their interpretations in order to be most effective. Other therapeutic modalities also address this challenge. For example, ACT uses the notion of cognitive fusion while Mentalization Based Therapy uses the notion of non-mentalizing states (see below) to describe problems with meta-cognition. Nonetheless, all three modalities assume meta-cognitive limitations are temporary and surmountable with treatment. In contrast, supportive therapy is designed for patients who are not able to make this mental leap, often because of cognitive or psychiatric limitations. By focusing on the concrete, here-and-now and avoiding discussion of unconscious material, supportive therapy skirts the need for meta-cognition. This is the primary reason that psychodynamic and supportive therapy are seen to reside on opposing ends of a therapeutic spectrum (Winston et al., 2019).

In recent decades, empirical research has made inroads into the psychoanalytic world, resulting in numerous studies of psychodynamic treatment (Fonagy, 2015) and several evidence-based treatments, such as Mentalization-Based Therapy (Bateman & Fonagy, 2019), Transference-Based Therapy (Clarkin, Caine, Lenzweger & Levy, 2018), Interpersonal Psychotherapy (Weissman et al., 2000) and Brief Relational Therapy (Muran et al., 2009). In the next section, we will discuss mentalization-based therapy (MBT) as one of the best supported of these psychodynamically-informed treatments.

Mentalization-Based Therapy

MBT is an evidence-based therapy developed by Peter Fonagy and Anthony Bateman that was originally designed to treat borderline personality disorder (BPD) (Bateman, Unruh & Fonagy, 2019). Fonagy, a psychoanalyst trained at the Anna Freud Centre in London, has also been strongly influenced by attachment theory. Bateman was trained in Interpersonal Psychotherapy, an evidence-based therapy for depression (c.f. Weismman et al., 2000). Over the past 20 years, MBT has been elaborated and adapted to many other disorders, including eating disorders, antisocial personality disorders, substance abuse, and depression (Bateman & Fonagy, 2019). Although MBT was originally intended to blend individual and group modalities, it is now used in either modality alone or in combination (Bateman, Kongersleve & Hansen, 2019).

MBT clearly comes out of the psychodynamic tradition and there are many similarities. But it differs in important ways. For one, it is more structured than psychodynamic treatment, with clear guidelines. It also has a wealth of concepts and terms that are unique to MBT, although many of the concepts overlap with psychodynamic notions. Most importantly, MBT has a more specific focus. MBT is single-mindedly concentrated upon patients' capacity to *mentalize*. This refers to the ability to thoughtfully, flexibly, and coherently reflect upon mental states, one's own and others. Such mental states include people's thoughts, emotions, motivations, and unique perspectives. When people mentalize they also consider causation and the person's historical context. Why does someone react the way he or she does in a given situation?

The concept of mentalization is very similar to the psychodynamic notions of introspection and psychological mindedness. It also overlaps with the meta-cognitive capacities addressed above. Importantly, while psychodynamic approaches consider such abilities to be a necessary *precondition* for insight-oriented therapy, MBT makes it the *end goal* of the therapy. MBT sees the failure of mentalization, particularly in the context of emotionally important attachment relationships, as the primary deficit underlying borderline personality disorder. Thus, the aim of MBT is to enhance patients' mentalization abilities, with the assumption that other problems characteristic of BPD, such as impulsivity, suicidality, mood dysregulation, and interpersonal instability, will improve as a result.

Mentalization incorporates 4 dimensions: controlled vs. automatic, self vs. other, internal vs. external, and cognitive vs. affective mentalizing (Fonagy & Bateman, 2019). The ability to flexibly shift along these dimensions is seen as necessary to mental health. Controlled mentalizing is deliberate, thoughtful, and cognitive, in contrast to automatic mentalizing, which is quick, intuitive and automatic. It is the difference between analysis and intuition. Self vs. other mentalizing refers to the effort to mentalize the internal state of either the self or the other. Healthy people can balance attunement towards one's own mental state with that of the other person but patients with BPD often emphasize one at the expense of the other. Internal mentalizing refers to the capacity to integrate what is known about other people and their circumstances to infer their internal state. In contrast, external mentalizing is more concrete; the other person's mental state is inferred from external cues, such as facial expression or body posture. Cognitive mentalizing refers to the ability to identify, label, and think about mental states in oneself and others. Affective mentalizing refers to the ability to *feel* these mental states. The former is an intellectual understanding, the latter experiential. A balance between the two is optimal. BPD patients tend to overemphasize automatic, external, and affective mentalizing, contributing to the emotional volatility that they are known for. Such patients are hyper-reactive to external clues about other people's mental states, quickly become emotionally aroused, and then jump to conclusions without checking their intuitions against actual evidence.

In addition, MBT identifies 3 non-mentalizing modes, in which people fail to reflect upon either their own or others' mental states. In psychic equivalence, people do not differentiate between their own internal state and the outside world; external reality is defined by their subjective experience. I fear that you are angry so therefore you are angry. In the teleological stance, one's internal state is solely defined by external behavior. If you do not hug me, you do not care about me. The pretend mode is often more subtle. The person appears to engage in mentalization, analyzing the internal states of either the self or other, but the internal mental world, while recognized, does not feel truly real. This includes a sort of intellectualized mentalization, characterized by emotional disconnect. Two other modes of disturbed mentalizing include hypermentalizing, in which the person is overly attuned to others' internal states and over-attributes extreme mental states to others, and pseudomentalizing, a more intentionally superficial intellectualization, lacking authentic engagement with one's own or others' subjective experience, and often used in self-serving ways. Finally, relational mentalizing is used to address the patient's understanding of interactions within the therapeutic relationship.

During therapy sessions, the therapist promotes mentalizing of both self and others. Patients are invited to talk about whatever is on their mind. Through skillful questioning, carefully timed interpretations, and targeted reflections, the therapist draws attention to non-mentalizing modes and promotes flexibility among mentalizing dimensions. For example, let's say that the patient gets "stuck" in the psychic equivalence mode, insisting that the therapist finds him boring. At this point, the patient is not able to differentiate his own insecurities from the therapist's actual experience. This calls for a focus on relational mentalizing. Here, the therapist might shift the focus along the self vs. other dimension, away from the other and onto the self. In other words, the therapist turns the discussion away from what the therapist *might be* feeling onto what the patient *is* feeling. This, in turn, leads to exploration of the patient's fear that no one will ever care enough to consistently pay attention to his feelings.

Primary Target and Entry Point

Both the primary target and entry point of MBT lie at the Basic Conceptual level. Like traditional psychodynamic therapy, the main focus of Mentalization Based Therapy is on patients' interpersonal representations, how patients understand themselves in relation to others. As with psychodynamic therapy, it is assumed that problems at the Pre-conceptual level (e.g., emotional volatility, impulsivity) will resolve with improvements at the Basic Conceptual level in a top-down manner. Nonetheless, there is a subtle difference between the two approaches to interpersonal representations. In psychodynamic therapy, a person's system of interpersonal representations is treated like a *noun*, as a fairly static entity, whereas in MBT it functions as a *verb*. In MBT it is the moment-by-moment ways of making sense of self and other's subjective processes that is key. The *process* of mentalizing is emphasized rather than the product. This is probably a more accurate reflection of how the mind/brain functions. The brain does not store interpersonal representations like photos in a photo album. Interpersonal representations are not things per se, rather they are consistent modes of reacting. They are repeated patterns of neuronal firing.

Schema Therapy

Let us now consider another type of therapy that targets interpersonal representations, but from a cognitive behavioral rather than psychodynamic vantage point. Schema Therapy is the brainchild of Jeff Young, who was initially trained in Beckian cognitive therapy (Young, Klosko & Weishaar, 2003). Although this treatment comes out of the cognitive-behavioral tradition, it incorporates ideas from psychodynamic and attachment theory as well as Gestalt therapy. We will locate it at the Basic Conceptual level as it primarily targets interpersonal representations, known in this modality as *early maladaptive schemas* (EMS). As in the psychodynamic tradition, schema therapy considers these representations, or schemas, to form the foundation of personality pathology. Nonetheless, there are important differences between this approach to character pathology and those of the psychodynamic tradition. As noted above, the psychodynamic tradition emphasizes a relatively unstructured, open-ended exploration of mental life, providing great theoretical depth and richness but less in the way of precision and clarity. Consistent with other cognitive behavioral treatments, schema therapy emphasizes precise, measurable concepts; structured goal-oriented interventions; and measurable behavioral change.

Schemas are defined as mental structures, based in memory, that depict a specific class of events and incorporate sensory, motor, emotional and cognitive components. Schemas serve to guide our responses in relevant situations, functioning as a kind of mental map. While schemas are a fundamental cognitive structure and operate in many psychological domains, personality pathology derives from those schemas based on problematic early childhood relationships with significant attachment figures. These are known as early maladaptive schemas (EMSs). While people develop schemas of other relationships encountered in later life, it is the EMS that have the most powerful and pervasive emotional effect.

Schema therapy posits a finite number of EMS, captured empirically in the Young Schema Questionnaire (Louis, Wood, Lockwood, Ho, & Ferguson, 2018). The most recent version of this questionnaire was published in 2005 and proposes 18 EMSs, such as abandonment/instability, enmeshment/undeveloped self, and defectiveness/shame (from Schematherapy.com, retrieved 8/30/2019). Young proposes that EMSs develop as a result of the frustration of core developmental needs. In his 2003 book on schema therapy (Young et al., 2003), five such needs are listed: 1) secure attachment to others; 2) autonomy, competence, and sense of identity; 3) freedom to express valid needs and emotions; 4) spontaneity and play; and 5) realistic limits and self-control. Caregiver failure to meet any of these needs often leads to specific maladaptive schemas. For example, frustration of a child's autonomy needs can result in a helplessness schema; frustration of a child's need for secure attachment can result in an emotional deprivation or defectiveness/shame schema; and frustration of the child's needs for healthy limits may lead to a schema of entitlement/grandiosity.

Additionally, Young makes a distinction between the schema itself and people's characteristic strategies for managing it, their *coping modes*. These are defensive maneuvers designed to reduce the negative emotions associated with activating the EMS. Young proposes three basic coping modes, *compensation*, *avoidance,* and *surrender*. These correspond to fight, flight, and freeze reactions, which are basic responses to threat found across the animal kingdom. In compensation mode, the person tries to counteract the EMS, for example, using a grandiose stance to compensate for an underlying schema of inadequacy. In avoidance, the person avoids any situation that might trigger the EMS, for example, avoiding intimate relationships so as not to trigger an abandonment/instability schema. In surrender, the person gives in to the EMS, making choices that are consistent with the EMS. For example, a person with a subjugation schema may choose dominating or even abusive partners.

Importantly, EMS are not always salient in the person's day to day functioning. They are activated by cues that are evocative of the original experiences that underlie the EMS. When any type of schema is activated, a psychological response termed the *schema mode* is triggered. When an EMS is activated, a *dysfunctional* schema mode is triggered. People enter an altered psychological state in which their experience of the present moment is dominated by the EMS and thereby awash in negative emotion. The more painful the EMS, the more all-encompassing the dysfunctional schema mode and the less integrated with the rest of the personality. It is in these circumstances that personality pathology is most evident and symptomatic behavior is most likely to occur. For example, a person with a dependence/

incompetence or failure to achieve schema may function well at a job until unfairly criticized by a supervisor, at which point the person becomes highly distressed, convinced that she is failing at her job, and suddenly unable to manage challenges that previously caused no problem.

According to Young and colleagues, there are 4 main types of schema modes, the Child, Maladaptive Coping, Dysfunctional Parent, and Healthy Adult modes (Young et al., 2003). In a Child mode (i.e., Vulnerable, Angry, Impulsive/undisciplined, or Happy), people are identifying with their childhood role in the schema. In the Dysfunctional Parent modes (i.e., Punitive/critical or Demanding), they are identifying with the role their parents played. Ultimately, schema therapy aims to weaken the Maladaptive Coping mode and strengthen the Healthy Adult mode.

As important as the original source of the maladaptive schemas are the mechanisms that *perpetuate* them. What are the specific processes that keep them going, that keep the past so active in the present? Schema therapy posits two main processes in this regard, cognitive distortions and a discomfort with change. As described above in the section on cognitive therapy, cognitive distortions reflect biases in attention, memory and reasoning which serve to process information in a way that confirms one's core beliefs. Contradictory information is disregarded or explained away (Oh, he only likes me because I help him with his workload. I did well on that test because it was easy. Anyone could have done it). Additionally, despite the high cost they incur, people are generally reluctant to part with their maladaptive schemas as they provide a wholly familiar lens with which to view the world. They also serve to define the person's identity. Remember, schemas are a fundamental property of cognition and serve a critical purpose in our adaptation to the environment; they are, in effect, our GPS. EMS are problematic because they provide *dysfunctional* maps of the world; they are *bad* schemas. Nonetheless, they are the only maps our patients have known. To take away patients' EMS is to rob them of their entire orientation to the world as well as their identity. Hence to avoid eliciting significant resistance to change in the patient, therapy has to move slowly without expecting too much change too soon.

The purpose of therapy is to *heal* the EMS, to help the person truly overcome their maladaptive schemas and interrupt the cycle of self-perpetuation. It is not expected that maladaptive schemas will entirely disappear; they will still be activated on occasion. Nevertheless, the person will gain greater understanding of and control over them and thereby reduce their negative impact.

Schema therapy has two general phases, assessment and schema change. The first is achieved through multiple modalities, to provide a comprehensive understanding of the patient's early schemas and related psychological structures. The patient is educated in the schema therapy model in this phase, using the results of structured assessments as well as assigned readings. This may take several weeks or even months. By the end of the assessment phase, the therapist and patient have collaboratively achieved a comprehensive formulation encapsulating the patient's characteristic EMS, coping mechanisms, and schema modes.

Assessment modalities include structured questionnaires, such as the Life History Assessment Forms and the Young Schema Questionnaire (See Young et al., 2003) as well as intensive, open-ended interviews. The patients' interactions with the therapist also provide information about maladaptive schemas, for example, overly dependent or demanding behavior might reflect dependence/incompetence or entitlement/grandiosity schemas. Interestingly, Young recognizes that schema identification cannot solely rely on patients' verbal reports of their own schemas, in effect acknowledging that interventions at the Verbal Conceptual level will be insufficient to elicit underlying schemas. Maladaptive schemas are often unconscious and elude intellectualized insight. Therefore, an imagery task is employed, in which patients are guided through a visualization focused on memories of painful interactions with parents during childhood. This elicits much more experience-near and deeply felt emotions. It can also yield results that contradict the questionnaires.

Once the maladaptive schemas have been identified, the schema change phase begins. The first step involves cognitive strategies. In this phase, the therapist helps patients develop an intellectual understanding of their schemas and how they work. Several structured exercises support this endeavor, including listing the evidence for and against the schemas, creating schema flashcards as reminders, and arguing the costs and benefits of the schemas and related coping styles. This greater awareness is used to "combat" the schema whenever it is triggered. Young uses strikingly militaristic language in this regard; therapy involves "doing battle" with the schemas, it is "like waging war" (See Young et al., 2003, pp. 53 and 32). He also uses the term *empathic confrontation* to describe the therapeutic stance used during cognitive challenges. Therapists must empathize with the patients' experience of the schema, acknowledging the reasons that the schemas appear so true to the patient and how they may have been useful in the past. But therapists must also challenge the schema's accuracy and highlight the dysfunction it causes in the present.

Importantly, and in a significant departure from much of the cognitive behavioral tradition, schema therapy recognizes the limitations of purely intellectual understanding. As in the psychodynamic tradition, insight must be paired with genuine emotional experience in order for true change to occur. Therefore, schema therapy utilizes a number of exercises to elicit schema-related emotions. Many of these exercises, known as experiential strategies, are borrowed from Gestalt therapy. Imagery is a common technique, often focused on early childhood memories, and particularly useful when strong emotion is already activated but the source of it is not understood. Asking a patient in the throes of strong emotion to close his or her eyes and describe any images that come to mind is a powerful means of eliciting schema-related material. Imaginary dialogues are also used. These take place with people who originally caused the schemas, generally parents, and anyone who reinforces them in adulthood. The aim of these dialogues is to help the patient directly experience and process schema-related emotions, particularly anger and grief, in order to create more distance from the schemas, to make them *ego dystonic*. In this way the therapy "battles" the schemas emotionally as well as intellectually.

Finally, schema therapy focuses upon behavioral change, which is seen as necessary for a successful outcome. For personality disordered patients, however, behavioral change cannot occur until patients have gained some mastery over maladaptive schemas. Ultimately, people must replace their schema-driven behavior with healthier goal-oriented behavior that allows them to fulfill the core needs that were frustrated in childhood (e.g., attachment, autonomy, identity). The technique used for such change is called *behavioral pattern-breaking* and focuses upon behavior related to the three schema coping modes of avoidance, surrender, and compensation. For example, a young man with schemas of failure and unrelenting standards may struggle with procrastination as an avoidance coping mode. Procrastination then becomes the behavior to be changed.

Together patient and therapist make a list of target behaviors matched with healthy alternative behaviors. This phase of treatment utilizes many of the techniques mentioned above, such as imagery for identification of problematic behavior and cost-benefit analyses to address ambivalence about behavioral change. Additional methods from traditional behavior therapy, such as gradual desensitization to overcome phobic avoidance and functional analyses to illuminate the sequence of events leading to problematic behavior, are also employed to support behavioral change.

Primary Target and Entry Point

Both the primary target and entry point of schema therapy lies at the Basic Conceptual level as the explicit focus of this treatment is on maladaptive interpersonal representations. However, when employing the cognitive and experiential strategies, this treatment also uses entry points at the Verbal Conceptual and the Pre-conceptual levels, respectively.

The emphasis on the Basic Conceptual level ties schema therapy to treatments in the psychodynamic tradition. In fact, of all the CBT approaches, schema therapy has the most in common with psychodynamic approaches. Nonetheless, schema therapy differs in fundamental ways from the psychodynamic tradition. In contrast to psychodynamic therapy, schema therapy focuses solely upon the *content* of interpersonal representations and not on the *form*. There is no attention to the organizational quality of the schemas, to their level of integration and differentiation, although this is addressed to some extent with regard to schema modes. In this way, schema therapy has less of a developmental approach despite the focus upon the schemas' childhood roots. In contrast to Mentalization-Based Therapy (MBT), maladaptive schemas are perceived as a noun rather than a verb. While MBT emphasizes the *process* of mentalizing or of representing relationships on a moment-by-moment basis, schema therapy treats representations as a fixed entity that is either quiescent or triggered. This might account for the emphasis on "battling" the schemas. In psychodynamic approaches, personality change occurs through a process of growth and development that the therapy fosters and facilitates. In schema therapy, the maladaptive schemas and associated behaviors must be removed (or vanquished) and then replaced with healthier responses. Change is directive and controlled rather than emergent and facilitated. The distinctions between these two approaches to change will be further explored in Chapter 8.

Humanistic Therapies

The last family of talk therapies that we will consider at the Basic Conceptual level includes the humanistic therapies. These are a group of therapies that developed in the mid-1900s and were very popular throughout the 20th century. Indeed, they remain influential today, particularly through their impact on newer forms of psychotherapy. Humanistic therapies were seen at the time to be the third force in psychology, as they provided an alternative to psychoanalysis and behaviorism, the reigning schools for most of the 20th century. Humanistic treatments all focus on the development of the patient's sense of self and aim to foster a freer, more purposeful, and joyful way of being in the world. There is less focus on resolving psychopathology and more on positive self-development. While there is acknowledgment of how childhood experiences have thwarted healthy self-development, therapeutic interventions primarily aim to unlock and foster the unfolding of the person's innate potential (See Hunt, 2007; King, Viney & Woody, 2009). Because of their emphasis on the self-concept, humanistic therapies are located here at the Basic Conceptual level; however, they can also be seen to straddle the

Life Structure level given their focus on values, attitudes towards life and full engagement with life as lived. Specific treatments to consider include Carl Rogers' Client Centered Therapy and Fritz Perls' Gestalt therapy. Abraham Maslow's concepts of self-transcendence and self-actualization, although not integrated into a treatment per se, have also been influential concepts that derive from this tradition.

The humanistic approaches often protested against the mechanistic reductionism found in science, which they felt had negatively impacted the view of human psychology promoted in both behaviorism and psychoanalysis. They argued that human beings are multifaceted, intentional, and growth-oriented beings, not passive objects acted upon by abstract forces. Importantly, humanist psychologists were holistic in their approach to human psychology; to understand another person, one must consider the totality of their subjective experience within the world in which they live.

Abraham Maslow was an academic psychologist and never functioned as a clinician. Although he did not develop a specific form of psychotherapy, he introduced concepts that have had considerable influence on the development of other treatments. His best-known concepts are the *hierarchy of needs, self-actualization, and self-transcendence* (Maslow, 1968, 1971). In contrast to the emphasis on a single motivation prevalent at the time, Maslow proposed that human beings are motivated by multiple goals which can be organized hierarchically in terms of priority. The most pressing needs pertain to basic physical survival, including hunger, thirst, warmth, and physical health. Once these are met, the need for safety becomes more salient and tolerance for risk declines. After safety is achieved, the need for belonging becomes more pressing and people look to commune and connect with others. After the need for belonging comes the need for self-esteem, for a sense of mastery, competence, and social recognition as such. The final need is for *self-actualization*. This is a state of being in which people have fully actualized their own potential. They have become all that they can be. This does not imply a single-minded, self-absorbed focus on personal gratification, but rather an unfolding of self-awareness, wisdom, courage, and creative development. Paradoxically, it allows for much stronger connection to others through greater wisdom and through acceptance of the challenges and beauties of life. In his later work, Maslow added another layer to the hierarchy of needs, self-transcendence, which refers to a state of consciousness that expands beyond the narrow limits of the individual self, such that one feels absorbed into the larger totality of reality. Maslow refers to these blissful states as peak experiences. While similar to spiritual experiences, self-transcendence is not restricted to any specific religion nor tied to any religious dogma.

Carl Rogers' client centered therapy, later termed person-centered therapy, is highly consistent with Maslow's ideas (Hunt, 2007; King et al., 2009). This treatment has also been quite influential over the years, for example in the development of Motivational Interviewing. Rogers had an optimistic view of human nature and believed that human beings have a natural drive towards growth. The role of therapy is to foster such development, particularly for those whose self-development has been thrown off track through parental failures of empathy. Rogers made a distinction between unconditional positive regard and conditional love. Children who feel unconditionally loved are free to self-actualize, to grow into their full selves. Children whose parents communicate to them that their love is conditional on the child's fulfillment of certain demands become stunted in self-development. The parts of themselves that were not acknowledged or permitted become suppressed or distorted. Therapy therefore aims to heal these developmental failures through empathic responses and unconditional positive regard during discussion of the patient's life challenges. While Rogers has been criticized for being uncritically supportive and for not challenging patients' pathological behavior, decades of research have shown the importance of therapeutic empathy in treatment outcome. Indeed, the incorporation of Rogerian techniques into Motivational Interviewing shows that it is fully possible to empathically accept the person while still addressing his or her problematic behavior.

Gestalt therapy was developed in the mid-20th century by Fritz Perls along with his wife Laura Perls, Paul Goodman, and Ralph Hefferline (Perls, Hefferline, & Goodman, 1951). Over the ensuing decades, Gestalt therapy has been elaborated by many other practitioners and theorists (See Brownell, 2010). Gestalt therapy was highly influenced by the philosophical school of phenomenology (along with many other psychological and philosophical schools). In phenomenology, subjective experience is explored directly without the interference of preconceptions. What are you actually feeling or perceiving in this moment rather than what you think you should or might be feeling? Gestalt therapy is also very contextual; the individual is always understood holistically, particularly in the context of the interpersonal world. The ultimate goal of this therapy is to facilitate the emergence of a more open, authentic, and aware self-experience in dialogue with the therapist. While the childhood roots of self-disturbances are addressed, the focus is more on the present way of being than on the past. The empty chair technique is a well-known component of Gestalt therapy. By engaging in a role play with an empty chair, the client tries out new ways of engaging with split-off parts of the self or with significant others, expressing feelings and thoughts which might previously have felt threatening or otherwise uncomfortable. This technique is what many people associate with Gestalt therapy and has been incorporated into newer treatments, such as schema therapy.

Primary Target and Entry Point

As noted above, this family of treatments has been ascribed to the Basic Conceptual level because of its focus on the sense of self and, in several treatments, on the childhood roots of emotional suffering. However, it clearly reaches into the Life Structure level as well, given the emphasis on purpose and meaning in life as well as on personal values and philosophy.

Psychedelic Therapy

We will close this section with a very different type of treatment, namely psychedelic therapy. Psychedelic therapy diverges from traditional talk therapy in that it requires ingestion of psychoactive agents, such as psilocybin (from "magic" mushrooms), mescaline (from peyote cactus), DMT (N,N-dimethyltryptamine, from ayahuasca), MDMA (*3,4-methylenedioxy-methamphetamine)*, or LSD (lysergic acid diethylamide). The first 3 agents are extracted from plants while the last two were synthesized in laboratories. LSD, psilocybin, mescaline, and DMT are considered "classic psychedelics" as they share similar mechanisms of action, while MDMA operates somewhat differently (Doss et al., 2020; Pollan, 2018). Although most psychedelic therapy is still technically illegal, FDA approval for specific forms of psychotherapy with certain clinical populations will likely be granted in the relatively near future and multiple clinical trials are now underway. I include psychedelic therapy in this chapter as it has garnered a good deal of attention in recent years and raises intriguing questions about the interaction between different levels of the mind/brain in the psychotherapeutic process.

Psychedelic therapy with a variety of agents has shown efficacy in the treatment of multiple conditions, including depression, anxiety, addiction, posttraumatic stress disorder, and death anxiety in terminally ill patients (Doss et al., 2020; Johnson, Hendricks, Barrett & Griffiths, 2019; Pollan, 2018). Treatment effects have been attributed to patients experiencing a greater sense of unity with the larger world (Johnson et al., 2019; Pollan, 2018) as well as greater psychological flexibility (Carhart-Harris, 2019; Carhart-Harris et al., 2014; Davis, Barrett & Griffiths, 2019), suggesting that the treatment disrupts entrenched emotional patterns and replaces them with a more flexible outlook. Additionally, the intensification of emotional experience allows people to access and reflect upon feelings that may have otherwise been suppressed or avoided.

According to Michael Pollan, in his book on the "new science" of psychedelics (Pollan, 2018), there are two types of psychedelic experiences (known colloquially as trips) dependent on the dosage. At a low dose, people can have "aesthetic trips," in which both perception and emotions are intensified and perceptions infused with emotion. Colors may appear remarkably beautiful and music profoundly moving. People may feel great sadness, love, or other emotions but reality testing is intact and perceptions are not grossly distorted. Trips at higher doses, however, are more hallucinogenic, with perception distorted to the point to defy the laws of space and time. People may experience themselves as melting, giving birth, or looking over a great precipice into death itself. A number of psychedelic researchers and writers speak of "ego death," in which the boundary between self and non-self dissolves and people experience themselves to be a seamless part of a larger, cosmic consciousness.

This notion is often interpreted as spiritual, as if psychedelics occasion a mystical experience. In fact, psychedelics have been used for millennia across premodern societies to commune with the supernatural world. Journeys to the spirit world and back again have been used as rites of passage or as shamanistic opportunities to gain special knowledge or aid in healing. Moreover, both waves of scientific psychedelic research—the first from the late 50s to the early 70s and the current one starting in the late 1990s—were driven by proponents of some type of mystical experience (Barrett, Johnson & Griffiths, 2015; Johnson et al., 2019; Pollan, 2018). It was believed that psychedelics potentiated a true spiritual experience with life changing and profoundly healing effects. In fact, the Mystical Experience Questionnaire (MEQ30; Barrett et al., 2015) was designed for psychedelic research. It measures the intensity of a specific psychological state characterized by feelings of blissful serenity, a profound sense of communion with the entire world, transcendence of time and space, and ineffability, the sense that the experience cannot be conveyed in words. While there is clear evidence that many people do experience such a state during psychedelic trips, there is considerable debate as to whether such states are purely psychological phenomena or reflect encounters with a genuinely numinous, transcendent reality (Pollan, 2018).

One fact that is well recognized and entirely germane to this debate is the centrality of "set and setting" in the psychedelic experience (Pollan, 2018; Horgan, 2017). Psychedelic experiences are profoundly suggestible. Set refers to the mindset of the individual engaging in the psychedelic experience, the state of mind at the time of the trip, as well as the expectations of the experience and the beliefs, values and memories that might influence psychological reactions to the drug. Setting refers to the context of the trip, including the physical setting, the instructions given before and during the trip, and the behavior of the people with whom the individual interacts throughout the trip. As the journalist John Horgan states, "The same compound can evoke psychotic paranoia, psychological insight, or blissful communion, depending on whether it is consumed as a party drug in a nightclub, a medicine in a psychiatrist's office, or a sacrament in a tepee" (Horgan, 2017). Thus, when people are told that they are likely to have a spiritual experience during a trip, they are conditioned to do just that. Nonetheless, there is no question that many people have profound emotional experiences during psychedelic trips which can have long lasting, transformative effects on their sense of self in the world (Carhart-Harris et al., 2014; Johnson et al., 2019; Pollan, 2018).

Given the chemical source of these transformative experiences, it is inevitable that researchers would investigate the neurobiological substrates of psychedelic intoxication. So, what does neuroscience have to say? Results have been largely consistent. While multiple brain chemicals are activated by different psychedelics, the primary neurotransmitter appears to be serotonin. More precisely, classic psychedelics are serotonin agonists at 5-HT_{2A} receptor sites. What this means is that psychedelic molecules that closely mimic serotonin (i.e., 5-HT) land on specific serotonergic receptor sites and activate their neuronal firing (Doss et al., 2020; Pollan, 2018). Importantly, 5-HT_{2A} receptors are densely concentrated across the cortex and specifically cluster in the Default Mode Network (DMN) (Carhartt-Harris, 2019; Carhart-Harris et al., 2014; Pollan, 2018), a network of medial cortical structures linked to self-related mental processes. As discussed in Chapter 5, we have located the DMN at the Basic Conceptual level.

There is also a burgeoning neuroimaging literature on the effects of psychedelics. Robin Carhart-Harris was one of the first researchers to use brain imaging techniques to investigate psychedelics. His work produced two important findings that have been replicated in later studies (Carhart-Harris, 2019; Carhart-Harris et al., 2014). The earliest studies showed a dampening of activity in the DMN, which corresponded to the intensity of psychedelic experiences. Later studies revealed a reduction in the coherence of neuronal firing in these networks, such that brain activity was less organized. In fact, across the brain, neuronal activity was less coordinated *within* distinct neuronal networks but more integrated *across* networks that normally do not talk to each other much. Carhart-Harris referred to this as an increase in *entropy*, reflecting a break down in normal structure allowing for newer types of organization to emerge. In other words, the regular structures of consciousness were shaken up in ways that allowed for creative, new psychological connections to arise. For people stuck in a mental rut, this provided new possibilities. Additionally, the DMN is strongly connected to lower level, emotional regions of the brain; by loosening up the DMN, the lower emotional systems are similarly unchained, precipitating the intense emotional experience typical of psychedelics.

Primary Target and Entry Point

Both the primary target and entry point of psychedelic therapy can be placed at the Basic Conceptual level of the mind/brain. The major effect of psychedelic therapy is to change the person's experience of self in the world. When successful, psychedelic trips facilitate the emergence of a freer, more open and serene sense of self. This appears to be accomplished through the loosening up of mental maps at the Basic Conceptual level. Chemicals that mimic the neurotransmitter serotonin land on receptor sites in the DMN, a network of brain regions included in the Basic Conceptual level, which causes relevant brain circuitry to both disintegrate and dedifferentiate. What was coordinated becomes uncoordinated and what was separate starts to overlap. The resulting subjective experiences are new and disorienting but ultimately allow for a fresh organization of mental maps. Importantly, such *reorganization* is not automatic. Sometimes chaos just causes chaos. For that reason, all psychedelic treatments are highly structured, with careful monitoring of set and setting plus a discussion of insights gained after the trip is complete (Carhart-Harris et al., 2014).

It is worth questioning why psychedelics are placed at the Basic Conceptual level whereas other psychiatric medications are placed much lower, at the level of the Unlearned Core (See Chapter 7). Although all these drugs work on neurotransmitters such as serotonin, traditional psychiatric medications serve to correct dysfunction in neuronal tracts whose cell bodies lie in the Unlearned Core. Psychedelics, on the other hand, cause dysfunction (temporarily) rather than correcting it and go directly to the Basic Conceptual level. They do not impact pathology at the Unlearned Core nearly to the same extent; in fact, they are more likely to exacerbate such pathology rather than cure it. Hence, most clinicians would be highly reluctant to treat a psychotic or manic person with psychedelics.

This completes our survey of the types of treatments aimed at the upper levels of the mind/brain (and the levels immediately above the mind/brain proper). In the next chapter, we will continue our journey down to the remaining levels.

Chapter Seven

The Bottom of the Elephant

THE PRE-CONCEPTUAL LEVEL

In this chapter we complete the journey we started in the previous chapter. Here we will explore treatments targeting problems at the lower levels of the mind/brain, at the lower floors of the building, so to speak. Or to refer back to the parable of the blind men and the elephant, we will check out the lower parts of the elephant. To start with, let us step down to the Pre-conceptual level of the mind/brain. In doing so, we are leaving the parts of the mind/brain that process *ideas*. This means we have moved out of the *conceptual* realm where events can be kept in mind separate from their actual occurrence in time or space. Instead, we have arrived at a realm where our psychological reactions are bound to the present, to the here and now. This does not mean that our Pre-conceptual reactions are disconnected from learning and memory, but rather that they are dependent on simpler and evolutionarily older forms of learning and memory which do not involve concepts. That is why this level is called *Pre*-conceptual. Likewise, this realm of the mind/brain is not unique to humans. Rather, it is a place we share with all mammals and many non-mammalian animals as well.

At the Pre-conceptual level, learning and memory are *cue-induced*. That is, they are dependent on cues that trigger memories of past events and give emotional significance to present circumstances. Such types of memory include habit learning, associative conditioning, and operant conditioning. At this level, our emotions are far more central than cognition to the way we process information and have far more impact on our behavior. The Pre-conceptual level of the mind/brain accords with Jaak Panksepp's secondary emotional systems (See Chapters 2 and 5). It is in this region that the core, unlearned emotional systems—Panksepp's primary emotional systems—are first linked to simple learning and memory. Relevant brain regions are subcortical, that is they lie beneath the cortex, and include the amygdala, nucleus accumbens, and other areas of the basal ganglia.

We frequently see Pre-conceptual learning in our pets; our dogs get excited at the sight of the leash, knowing that the leash signals a walk outside. Likewise, our cats get terrified at the sight of the vacuum cleaner (or at least mine did), knowing that it signals a loud, threatening noise. Human pathology at this level involves maladaptive cue-based emotional responses, such as emotional volatility, anxiety attacks, suicidal urges, and rage reactions. Impulsive and compulsive behaviors, such as substance abuse, impulsive aggression, binge eating and even obsessive compulsive disorder, also fall at this level. Of note, while patients with personality pathology frequently struggle with these types of problematic responses, Pre-conceptual pathology is neither necessary nor specific to personality pathology. Many people *without* personality pathology can have Pre-conceptual difficulties while people *with* personality pathology may not. Likewise, as proposed throughout this book, the Pre-conceptual level is not the primary locus of personality pathology. Nonetheless, it is frequently impacted by it in a *top-down manner*. As such, interventions at this level can be enormously helpful in curtailing pathological behavior and responses, that is in reducing symptoms, but they will not change the core disturbance in interpersonal representations.

Behavior Therapy

We will start with behavior therapy, as it both preceded and arguably provides the foundation for all other Pre-conceptual treatments. Unlike psychoanalysis, which originated as a clinical discipline, behavior therapy came out of a purely academic tradition. The clinical applications followed the academic research by several decades (See Hunt, 2007; King et al., 2009 for a history). Behavior therapy is based on the academic school of behaviorism, which identifies two basic types of learning, *associative conditioning* (also known as classical or Pavlovian conditioning) and *operant conditioning*. Both forms of learning cut across many animal species. As such, we see again how psychological processes at the Pre-conceptual level predate the evolution of human beings.

Associative Conditioning

Associative conditioning dates back to the work of Ivan Pavlov from the turn of the 20th century. Pavlov was actually studying the digestive processes of dogs and stumbled upon his famous discovery by accident. He noticed that the dogs learned to salivate not only in the presence of food, but eventually at the sight or sound of any cue indicating the food was coming.

He elaborated on this observation with additional experiments, eventually defining the terms of associative conditioning. An unconditioned (or unlearned) response is an inborn, biologically-based reflexive response linked to the unconditioned (or unlearned) stimulus, such as fear in response to threat or pleasure in response to tasty food. When the unconditioned stimulus is paired with a neutral stimulus, then the animal learns to associate the two stimuli. For example, imagine if a cat gets a shock every time it steps into a cage. The cage will become paired with the shock. Ultimately, the cat will come to fear the cage as much as it fears the shock. The fear response to the cage is termed the conditioned response.[1] Additionally, Pavlov investigated the process of *extinction*, how conditioned responses can be unlearned. He found that if the conditioned stimulus is repeated enough times *without* the unconditioned stimulus, for example if the animal is put in the cage without a shock, the conditioned response will be extinguished. The animal will lose its fear of the cage. In short order, this form of learning was studied in numerous different species (often with little concern for the animal's suffering) by many different researchers, soon becoming a dominant psychological paradigm.

However, it was not until the 1950s that the principles of associative conditioning were applied to clinical work with humans (c.f. Hunt, 2007). Joseph Wolpe was a general practitioner in South Africa who became intrigued with Pavlov's work, particularly the issue of extinction. After studying the extinction of conditioned fear in animals, he sought to apply the principles to his human patients. His methods formed the basis of *systematic desensitization*, the primary technique for treating anxiety disorders today. The aim of the treatment is to extinguish the pairing between conditioned stimulus and conditioned response. The way to do this is to gradually expose the patient to the conditioned stimulus. When the negative event (unconditioned stimulus) does not occur, the connection between the conditioned stimulus and conditioned response will degrade. At the same time, a new pairing can be created between the conditioned stimulus and a positive unconditioned stimulus, creating a new, positive conditioned response.

What does this look like in practice? Let's say George has a phobia of heights. First George must create a hierarchy of anxiety provoking situations, say from standing on a 1st floor balcony all the way to standing on an 8th floor balcony and looking over the side. Next George will be taught relaxation techniques, such as progressive muscle relaxation or deep breathing. Then, once the relaxation techniques are mastered, George is asked to go to a shopping mall with an indoor atrium. First, he must go the first-floor balcony and look over. There he practices his relaxation techniques until he can tolerate being on the balcony without anxiety. In this way, the first floor balcony is decoupled from fear and instead paired with the pleasant feeling of relaxation. This process is repeated until George reaches the top floor. It is important that the exposure to the feared stimuli be introduced gradually because if the process occurs too quickly, then the phobic anxiety reaction will be traumatizing in and of itself. The link between unconditioned stimulus and unconditioned response will only be strengthened.

This simple process has been applied to many other clinical conditions. In fact, some form of systematic desensitization is used in the treatment of all anxiety disorders, such as social anxiety disorder, panic disorder and agoraphobia (e.g., Barlow, Craske, Cerney, & Klosko, 1989). It is also used in the treatment of posttraumatic stress disorder (PTSD) (Foa & Rothbaum, 1998). Likewise, exposure and response therapy is used to treat obsessive-compulsive disorder, such that patients are asked to engage in obsessive worry (e.g., fear of contamination), then to engage in the exact behavior that they fear (touching the garbage can) but are then prevented from the compulsive behavior that would typically alleviate the anxiety caused by the obsession (e.g., hand washing) (Foa, Yadin, Lichner, 2012). In the 1960s, Masters and Johnson applied similar techniques to sex therapy, as sexual function is dependent on a state of relaxation and can be compromised by anxiety (Hunt, 2007).

Operant Conditioning

In the 1950s, B. F. Skinner introduced the concept of *operant conditioning*, expanding upon the much earlier work of Edward Lee Thorndike with his puzzle boxes (King et al., 2009). While Pavlovian conditioning concerned automatic reflexive responses (such as salivation or the fight/flight response), operant conditioning addressed intentional, goal-directed behavior. The animal's motivation to repeat a specific behavior will depend on the consequences of that behavior, otherwise known as its reinforcement. There are three main types of reinforcement. Positive reinforcement (or reward) increases the likelihood of the behavior being repeated. If an animal receives a tasty pellet every time it presses a bar, it will continue to press the bar. Negative reinforcement also increases the likelihood of the behavior but does so by removing aversive stimuli. Pressing a bar might stop a loud, noxious noise. Punishment reduces the likelihood of the behavior. The animal might receive an electric shock after pressing the bar. The process of extinction is also a factor in operant conditioning. When the reinforcement stops following the behavior, the conditioned behavior will be extinguished. Therefore, to reduce the frequency of an objectionable behavior, one can remove the rewarding consequences.

While Skinner's original research was conducted on various non-human species, operant conditioning is equally impactful on human behavior. For example, we go to work, in large part, because we get paid to do so (positive reinforcement). If the pay stopped, most of us would stop going to work (extinction). We shower to remove dirt and embarrassing body odor (negative reinforcement). Also, we restrain ourselves from committing crimes because we do not want to go to jail (punishment). Thus, operant conditioning is a pervasive influence on human motivation.

Skinner also investigated different schedules of reinforcement. An important finding was that *intermittent reinforcement* makes a behavior more resistant to extinction. This is evident in many aspects of human behavior, such as addiction and child rearing. For example, gambling works by intermittent reinforcement. If you only win every so often and you don't know when the win will occur, you are much less likely to stop gambling when you start to lose. Likewise, when a child throws a temper tantrum to get a new toy, the child is using negative reinforcement on the parents, stopping the tantrum when the toy is obtained. This trains the parents to give in to temper tantrums. However, if the parents want to extinguish this behavior, they will need to stop rewarding it by no longer giving into the child's demands. At first the child will continue to throw tantrums, likely escalating when first frustrated. If the parents hold their ground, the child will eventually give up and the parents will have succeeded in stopping the temper tantrums. However, many parents will eventually give in. In the short run it is easier for them. In the long run, however, this is highly problematic as the intermittent reinforcement only teaches the child to continue the tantrum long enough for the parents to give in.

Skinner was a bit of a Utopian and envisioned using operant conditioning in many aspects of social planning, such as child rearing, education, and the workplace, pointing towards what others considered an objectionable and unrealistic goal of a tightly controlled society (King et al., 2009; Skinner, 1948). Nonetheless, these ideas build on our common-sense notions of rewards and punishments, which are thoroughly integrated into most social systems, such as government, education, and the criminal justice system, and have been throughout human history. What Skinner contributed was a systematic analysis of how they work. Skinner also emphasized positive reinforcement over punishment as he felt that the latter had too many negative consequences and did not offer an alternative behavior.

It is important to note, however, that operant conditioning does not translate so easily into psychotherapy. It works best in hierarchical social systems in which the person controlling the reinforcement contingencies (e.g., the parent or the manager) is distinct from and has more power than the person performing the behavior (e.g., the child or the employee). This poses considerable challenges in individual psychotherapy, where the patient enters into a voluntary therapeutic relationship. It is not the therapist's job to control the reinforcement contingencies as that would deprive the patient of the autonomy and personal responsibility necessary for psychotherapy to work. It would also put the therapist in a highly authoritarian role, which raises ethical dilemmas (American Psychological Association, 2017; Beauchamp & Childress, 2001). Further it would be problematic to put patients in charge of their own reinforcement contingencies as they would then both be performing the behavior they need to stop and in charge of stopping it. The fox would be in the henhouse, so to speak.

Nonetheless, what *is* helpful in psychotherapy is a collaborative investigation into the subtle reinforcements that perpetuate unwanted behavior. Such chain analyses of problematic behavior and symptoms (also known as functional analyses) can help the patient understand on a step-by-step basis what function various behaviors serve and how they might be reinforced or punished. This allows patients to try alternative behaviors that yield more desirable results. Chain analysis is particularly useful for people with impulse control problems, those who repeat problematic behavior and do not know why. In fact, it is a key component of Dialectical Behavior Therapy, a therapy aimed at reducing impulsivity and affective over-reactivity in patient with borderline personality disorder. (See below.) Chain analysis can also help parents figure out how to set effective limits with their children and how their current actions may be reinforcing the very behavior they are trying to stop.

Primary Target and Entry Point

Behavior therapy both targets pathology anchored at the Pre-conceptual level and uses the Pre-conceptual level as its primary entry point. Thus, it is a qualitatively distinct type of therapy compared to those aimed at the Conceptual levels of the mind/brain or at the Life Structure or Socio-cultural levels (e.g., psychodynamic, schema-focused or group therapy, respectively). Both associative and operant conditioning are found in many non-human species, supporting the ancient evolutionary role of Pre-conceptual learning. This further underscores the difference between treatments aimed at the Pre-conceptual level and those aimed above it, at the phylogenetically newer levels of the human mind/brain. In effect, therefore, the different types of therapy are targeting different points in our evolutionary history!

Dialectical Behavior Therapy (DBT)

Dialectical Behavior Therapy (DBT) is a widely used treatment designed for patients with borderline personality disorder (BPD) who engage in frequent suicidal and/or self-injurious behavior, such as cutting their wrists and arms (Linehan, 1993, 2015, 2020; Linehan et al., 2006). Although DBT originally targeted a fairly narrow clinical problem, like many successful treatment modalities, it has expanded to treat a wider array of clinical conditions, such as alcoholism, depression, and eating disorders (Linehan, 2015).

DBT is the brainchild of Marcia Linehan, who recently revealed she had suffered from profound suicidal crises of her own when she was young (Linehan, 2020). Linehan developed DBT, therefore, with the unique insight of someone who has successfully overcome the very behaviors DBT treats. DBT is considered one of the third-wave treatments in the cognitive behavioral tradition. Likewise, Linehan was originally trained in the behaviorist approach. DBT also borrows from Eastern meditation practices, however, and mindfulness is a key part of the treatment. The dialectical nature of DBT refers to the balance struck between the need to accept and validate patients' emotional experience and the simultaneous need to challenge patients' maladaptive behavior and promote the need for change.

Like other CBT treatments, DBT is highly structured, using hand-outs, diary cards, work sheets and other written exercises. In its full form, there are four components to DBT: individual therapy, group therapy, a therapist consultation team (for therapists to support one another in this frequently stressful work), and phone coaching. The latter requires the therapist to be available by phone to reinforce patients' use of their DBT skills in everyday life, especially during crises. As DBT has become more popular, however, many clinical settings provide only the individual and group components.

The main purpose of individual therapy is to collaboratively conduct chain analyses of incidents of cutting, suicidal gestures or other forms of behavioral dyscontrol. Each problematic behavior is broken down into a sequence of component steps, including contributing thoughts, emotions and behaviors. Particular attention is paid to choice-points, where the patient could have instituted a different response or practiced DBT skills (Linehan, 2015). Patients are asked to fill out diary cards as homework, so they can learn to perform their own chain analyses to be discussed in session.

The four modules of DBT skills are taught in group therapy. DBT skills help the patient manage thoughts and emotions that are triggered by various stressors in the environment and to replace maladaptive behavioral responses with more effective ones. The four modules include Mindfulness, Distress Tolerance, Emotion Regulation, and Interpersonal Effectiveness. The skills learned in group therapy are then reinforced in individual therapy and phone coaching.

Mindfulness is defined as "the act of consciously focusing the mind in the present moment without judgment and without attachment to the moment" (Linehan, 2015, p. 151). The ultimate function of this practice is to calm the mind in order to achieve a state of mental clarity. This is a critically important skill for people prone to intense emotional reactivity and consequent impulsivity. Linehan refers to such a state as "wise mind," in which people can be in touch with their emotional experience but still maintain rational thought and objectivity. It is in wise mind that people are most likely to exercise good judgment and make effective decisions. Numerous mindfulness practices are introduced in this module, including mindful breathing, mindful observation of sensations, thoughts, and emotions, and mindful movement. Multiple handouts are provided that describe different exercises. Interestingly, DBT makes a distinction between mindfulness and meditation, the latter described as mindfulness practiced while either sitting or standing still. As such, meditation is seen as a subset of mindfulness practice.

The module on Distress Tolerance can be seen as an outgrowth of the one on Mindfulness. Painful distress is an inevitable and inescapable aspect of life and the capacity to tolerate such discomfort is necessary for optimal functioning. Likewise, emotional distress is often the trigger for suicidal, self-injurious and other destructive behavior in patients with BPD. These symptoms serve as maladaptive coping mechanisms to help patients escape feeling bad. The aim of this module, therefore, is to teach patients how to acknowledge, accept and manage emotional distress. The concept of "radical acceptance" is paramount and refers to a calm acceptance that an unpleasant reality exists and cannot be denied. Strategies utilize sensory, behavioral, and cognitive techniques. Acronyms for many strategies are spelled out in handouts. For example, the TIP hand-out lists sensory techniques to immediately reduce autonomic arousal: Tip the temperature of your face with cold water, Intense exercise, Paced breathing, and Paired muscle relaxation. The STOP hand-out addresses reactions to emotional crises: Stop, Take a step back, Observe and Proceed mindfully. Finally, the ACCEPT hand-out lists distracting techniques: Distracting with Activities, with Contributing (to others), with Comparisons (with worse situations), with different Emotions, with Pushing away (painful thoughts and situations), with other Thoughts, and with other Sensations.

The module on Emotion Regulation is related to that of Distress Tolerance. BPD patients are characterized by intense and poorly controlled emotions which precipitate destructive behavior. This module helps patients learn to recognize, label and effectively cope with negative emotion using cognitive and behavioral techniques. Importantly, the aim of the module is not to eradicate or suppress negative emotions but to help patients manage them better. The concept of Emotion Mind is emphasized here, referring to a state of mind, common to patients with BPD, in which intense emotions overwhelm rational thought. A good part of this module involves teaching the function and mechanics of emotion—what emotions do and how they work. The assumption is that people who understand how their emotional reactions work are better able to anticipate emotional responses to events and respond effectively. Strategies for changing unpleasant and disproportionate emotions include checking the facts (making sure the interpretation of the situation is grounded in facts), opposite action (performing the opposite action from the maladaptive behavioral urge) and problem solving. DBT also emphasizes the need for repetition, that the new skills will not be effective without considerable practice. With sufficient practice, however, they will become automatic, a function of habit.

The final module is termed Interpersonal Effectiveness. BPD patients are highly sensitive to interpersonal interactions and their emotional dysregulation is typically precipitated by real or perceived interpersonal ruptures. Further, their disruptive behavior is highly damaging to their relationships. The core aims of this module are to teach patients how to "obtain [interpersonal] objectives while retaining relationships and self-respect" (Linehan, 2015, p. 231). Additional skills for building healthy relationships and ending destructive ones are also covered. Hand-outs with acronyms are emphasized in this module as well. The acronym DEAR MAN addresses assertiveness in relationships: Describe, Express, Assert, Reinforce, stay Mindful, Appear confident, and Negotiate. Strategies for maintaining relationships during conflict are encapsulated in the acronym GIVE: be Gentle, act Interested, Validate, use an Easy manner. Strategies for maintaining self-respect during conflict are captured in the FAST acronym: be Fair, no Apologies (do not over-apologize), Stick to values (maintain your integrity), and be Truthful.

Primary Target and Entry Points

The primary treatment targets for DBT lie at the Pre-conceptual level. Cue induced behaviors, such as cutting, burning, and suicidal gestures, are the primary targets though general emotional hyper-reactivity and impulsivity are also covered. As discussed in Chapter 5, we have allocated these psychological phenomena to the Pre-conceptual level, where hard-wired emotional and behavioral responses are triggered by learned cues. DBT uses multiple entry points to ameliorate these problematic responses, however. The most common interventions are cognitive, such that patients are taught to control their impulsive emotional and behavioral responses with reason. Thus, the primary entry point falls on the Verbal Conceptual level. But many core DBT interventions operate on a lower level as well. Mindfulness, as will be discussed below, engages with the Unlearned Core. The overall state of consciousness is altered and general hyperarousal calmed in order for verbal reasoning to be possible. Additionally, *sub-psychological* levels of organization are also recruited. The TIP skills are purely physical—tip your face with cold water, engage in intense exercise, and employ progressive muscle relaxation. Thus, DBT recruits multiple levels of the mind-brain to treat Preconceptual dysfunction. DBT also addresses difficulties in the social level with the interpersonal effectiveness module. DBT does not, however, address the Basic Conceptual level. Nowhere in the treatment does DBT deeply engage with patients' core views of self and other; rather DBT's focus is on the downstream or top-down results of pathology at the Basic Conceptual level.

THE UNLEARNED CORE

We now take one more step down to the lowest of the 5 levels of the mind/brain, the Unlearned Core. This level involves the oldest and lowest regions of the brain, including the hindbrain (specifically the brainstem), the midbrain, and the oldest parts of the forebrain (the diencephalon and ventral telencephalon). In short, this is the realm of animal instinct, of unlearned, inborn emotional reactions to preset stimuli. It is only at the higher levels that learning and memory come into play. More specifically, we ground Jaak Panksepp's seven primary emotional systems at this level: FEAR, LUST, RAGE, SEEKING, PANIC, CARE and PLAY.

Medication

The most common mental health intervention at the level of the Unlearned Core is not a form of psychotherapy. Rather I am referring to the vast armamentarium of psychiatric medications available today. As explored in Chapter 5, these medications provide the first line treatment for mood and psychotic disorders and other mental conditions anchored in the Unlearned Core. As discussed previously, these disorders are more heavily genetic than environmental in etiology; they reflect disturbances across Panksepp's seven primary emotional systems and are mediated by multiple neurotransmitter systems whose cell bodies lie in brain regions of the Unlearned Core (i.e., the midbrain and brain stem). Specifically, disorders such as schizophrenia, bipolar disorder, and the genetic form of major depression are treated by antipsychotics, mood stabilizers and antidepressants, respectively. The drugs serve to normalize the function of neurotransmitter tracts whose cell bodies lie in the Unlearned Core. It is important to note, however, that these drug classes are not precisely labeled and many medications are used with more than one kind of disorder.

Medication is also used with patients with personality disorders to help them manage depressive, anxious and impulsive symptoms as well as affective volatility. Nonetheless, pharmacotherapy is generally seen as an adjunctive treatment for personality disorder, with psychotherapy serving as the first line treatment (Caligor & Clarkin, 2010; Oldham, 2005).

Mindfulness Meditation

Mindfulness meditation has garnered considerable attention over the past several decades and is now incorporated into multiple forms of psychotherapy. Here, we will not distinguish between the two very similar constructs of mindfulness and meditation, though others have done so previously (See Linehan, 2015; Newberg & Iversen, 2003). In general, meditational practices have shown broad and dramatic benefits for mental and physical wellbeing, including reduced stress, better impulse control, and even improved immune function (Cohen, 2016; Kabat-Zinn, 2013; Linehan, 2015). For a fairly simple intervention, it certainly packs a punch.

So far, we have mentioned mindfulness practice in the context of other forms of psychotherapy assigned to higher levels of the mind/brain, specifically, ACT, located at the Life Structure level, and DBT, located at the Pre-conceptual level. In both cases, mindfulness practice is integrated into a broader treatment. If we look at mindfulness meditation practices in isolation, however, we can see that they are best placed at the level of the Unlearned Core. Why is that?

As above, many definitions of mindfulness involve controlled, directed attention and cultivation of a passive, receptive state of mind that suspends judgment. Jon Kabat-Zinn, the originator of mindfulness-based stress reduction, defines mindfulness practice as "paying attention in a particular way: on purpose, in the present moment, and non-judgmentally" (Kabat-Zinn, 2013). Marcia Linehan defines it as "the act of consciously focusing the mind in the present moment without judgment and without attachment to the moment" (Linehan, 2015, p. 151). Hayes, the founder of ACT, defines it as "the defused, nonattached, accepting, nonjudgmental, deliberate awareness of experiential events as they happen in the moment" (Hayes, 2015, p. 98). In contrast, Buddhist or Hindu meditation techniques focus upon a particular word, image or object or aim to empty the mind of any content (Newberg & Iversen, 2003). Many of these practices include a focus on the breath.

Despite minor differences across practices, all aim to achieve an altered state of consciousness characterized by feelings of serenity and mental clarity. *I will argue that this process fundamentally recruits the Unlearned Core and that the salutary effects on other aspects of psychology reflect bottom-up effects on higher levels of the mind/brain.*

Let's look at what neuroscience has to say about meditation and mindfulness. Much of the neuroimaging data suggest a wide range of brain regions are involved, particularly the medial cortical regions such as the ventromedial and dorsomedial frontal cortex and the insula (Hatchard et al., 2017). Note that these brain regions are part of the Basic Conceptual level, where we have anchored interpersonal representations. This supports the notion that mindfulness practice impacts the representation of self in relation to others. Nonetheless, most imaging studies over-emphasize cortical regions as they are larger and easier to capture with imaging technology than are deeper brain structures (c.f. Carhart-Harris et al., 2014; Newberg & Iversen, 2003). Thus, I would argue that imaging studies do not tell the whole story.

Here are my arguments for placing the mindfulness meditation practices at the level of the Unlearned Core:

1. These practices rely on physiological techniques such as deep breathing, which are mediated by the brain stem, part of the Unlearned Core (Newberg & Iversen, 2003).
2. Fundamentally, mindfulness techniques serve to modify states of alertness and arousal. Such variation is found across animal species, suggesting it arose early in evolution, and therefore will be processed in the oldest parts of the brain. Indeed, these states are subserved by the brain stem and other regions of the Unlearned Core (specifically, the reticular activating system).
3. All mindfulness practices rely on a general inhibition of behavioral responses. As such, they require a form of *stillness*. Even when performed during some form of action, they require a degree of emotional detachment and slowing of responsiveness, as in mindful eating or mindful walking (Kabat-Zinn, 2013; Linehan, 2015; Newberg & Iversen, 2003). This necessitates a quieting of Panksepp's seven primary emotional systems, which are anchored in the Unlearned Core.
4. Mindfulness practices are particularly effective at reducing anxiety and stress (Kabat-Zinn, 2011, 2013), implicating Panksepp's FEAR system. The fear response is associated with norepinephrine activation in the locus coeruleus, also in the Unlearned Core (White & Depue, 1999). Fur-

> ther, the fear response is dependent on the hypothalamic-pituitary-adrenal axis (HPA), an evolutionarily ancient stress response system reaching from the Unlearned Core down into the body outside the brain (Newberg & Iversen, 2003).

There are, of course, higher cortical processes involved with mindfulness, including language, cognition, and visual imagery. But all forms of psychotherapy address complex cognitive and emotional processes. What distinguishes mindfulness from every other psychotherapy is the emphasis on the more fundamental processes of breathing, motor stillness, physiological arousal and the quality of alertness. Through modifying these basic physiological processes, mindfulness creates an altered state of consciousness that somehow and somewhat miraculously allows for bottom-up reorganization at higher levels of the mind/brain.

Indeed, Newberg & Iversen (2003) present a model of meditation which incorporates vast brain circuitry ranging from the prefrontal cortex (Verbal Conceptual Level) to the limbic system (Pre-conceptual Level) down to the midbrain and brain stem (Unlearned Core) and even into the peripheral autonomic nervous system (i.e., at a sub-psychological level, in the body outside the brain). For example, they suggest that a general increase in the inhibitory neurotransmitter GABA in the thalamus serves to deactivate the parietal cortex, where our representation of body in space is integrated. This is an example of the *bottom-up effect* of processes at the Unlearned Core onto the higher, cortical levels of the mind/brain. In this way, lower-level brain activity influences our higher-level perception of our physical self. Going in the opposite direction, reduced secretion of norepinephrine from the locus coeruleus in the brainstem inhibits the HPA axis and dampens the body's stress response. Here we see a top-down effect of the Unlearned Core onto sub-psychological levels of the human body.

Primary Target and Entry Point

In sum, I suggest the primary *target* of mindfulness meditation practices to lie at the Unlearned Core. A problematic state of consciousness inhibits optimal cognitive and emotional functioning. In other words, agitation at a lower level of the mind/brain prevents healthy functioning at a higher level. When the brain's foundation is out of order, it is hard for all of the higher levels to function properly. Remember our metaphor of the multi-story office building? Here the building foundation is rickety, so the higher floors are not stable. They sway in the wind.

The primary entry point for mindfulness meditation practices also lies at the Unlearned Core as these techniques are primarily noncognitive and nonverbal. Breathing, stillness, and shifts in attention are not high-level cognitive processes but rather fundamental psychophysiological processes that underlie all higher-level cognitive processes. They live in the basement, not the penthouse. Nonetheless, higher level processes are also involved in mindfulness meditation practices. We need verbal understanding and directed, intentional behavior (Verbal Conceptual level) to engage in meditation at all. But that is the case for any type of psychotherapy—in fact, any complex, intentional behavior. Likewise, I'd argue that this only accounts for a small piece of the action.

As noted above, mindfulness practice can have dramatic bottom-up effects on both Basic Conceptual and Verbal Conceptual levels of the mind/brain as it creates shifts in our understanding of our self in the world. Perhaps it is why mindfulness has been so central to DBT, a treatment for personality disordered patients. Still, it is unlikely that mindfulness practices alone are sufficient to create the type of change in interpersonal representations necessary to fully treat patients with personality pathology. Rather mindfulness techniques create the *precondition* for work at more conceptual levels of the self.

Interestingly, this has long been understood within the psychodynamic tradition. While meditation techniques per se have not been employed, Freud spoke of the necessity of an even hovering attention in the analyst and Wilfred Bion spoke of the need for the analyst to enter every therapeutic session without memory or desire (Britton, 2012). Likewise, the patient requires an "observing ego" in order to benefit from psychoanalytic investigation. Thus, a mental state similar to mindfulness was seen as a necessary precondition for the therapeutic work. The role of this state of mind to therapeutic work will be addressed further in the next chapter.

A note now about the relationship of meditative techniques to psychedelic therapy. I would stipulate that the ultimate mechanisms of action of these two forms of treatment are similar. They both serve to shake up the Basic Conceptual level, allowing new forms of organization to emerge. In this way people can find new ways of experiencing themselves in their world. However, I have placed meditation on the level of Unlearned Core, as explained above, while I have placed psychedelic therapy at the Basic Conceptual level. This is because meditation accesses the Basic Conceptual level through a *bottom-up process*, whereas psychedelic therapy *directly* accesses the Basic Conceptual level through targeting $5HT\text{-}2_{1A}$ receptor sites in the Default Mode Network (Pollan, 2018; Carhart-Harris et al., 2014).

Relaxation Therapy

Relaxation therapy includes a variety of techniques that serve to calm the autonomic nervous system and create a relaxed mental state. The autonomic nervous system (ANS), a network of nerves reaching throughout the body, is controlled by the hypothalamus, a brain region in the Unlearned Core. There are two components to the ANS, the sympathetic and the parasympathetic nervous systems. The sympathetic nervous system prepares the body for action, for example by making the heart pump faster and by sending blood to the gross muscle groups and away from the extremities. The parasympathetic nervous system steps on the brakes. It helps the body rest and recuperate. Relaxation techniques activate the parasympathetic and quiet the sympathetic nervous system. These techniques by and large do not rely on ideas or concepts but rather address the core physiological elements of emotional tension and stress. For that reason, they are placed at the level of the Unlearned Core.

Common relaxation techniques include deep breathing, progressive muscle relaxation, yoga stretches, and visualization of peaceful scenes. For an excellent guide to these relaxation techniques, see Edmund Bourne's *The Anxiety & Phobia Workbook* (Bourne, 2010). Deep breathing entails long, slow, and deep breaths, which fill up the entire lungs. In contrast to rapid, shallow breaths from the upper chest, which occur in states of tension and during physical exertion, deep breathing promotes a state of relaxation. In progressive muscle relaxation, people sequentially tense and release isolated muscle groups, starting at the feet and working up to the head. The felt contrast between the muscle tension and release promotes a calm, serene state. Yoga involves a series of slow, deliberate stretches, in which people move their bodies into specific poses and hold them for a period of time. Yoga originated as a Hindu form of moving meditation. Over the past few decades, it has become increasingly popular in the Western world, where it sometimes loses its ties to meditative practices. Nonetheless, when used as a slow, meditative practice rather than as a weight loss technique, it has potent relaxation capacities. Visualization is the least physical of the techniques mentioned here. This involves visualization of a peaceful scene, such as a beach, forest, or babbling brook. Generally, there is a script to follow describing the scene and drawing attention to the sensory elements, such as the feeling of warm wind on one's cheek, the sound of the waves, or the smell of the grass.

These easily taught techniques are useful tools for anyone who struggles with anxiety and tension, doubtless a large portion of the population. Patients with personality pathology, in particular, have difficulty regulating their emotional reactivity and are often prone to anxiety and stress. Hence relaxation techniques are useful additions to the therapeutic toolkit for these patients. Of course, as noted previously, this will not address the core problems with interpersonal representations underlying personality pathology, but can alleviate the top-down difficulties such problems cause.

Primary Target and Entry Point

The primary target for these relaxation techniques lies at the Unlearned Core. The point is to reduce anxiety and create a calm, restful state, in other words to quiet Panksepp's FEAR system, a feature of the Unlearned Core. The primary entry point for deep breathing, yoga, and progressive muscle relaxation is entirely physical, however, involving sub-psychological levels of organization. In turn, these physical interventions have a *bottom-up impact* on the Unlearned Core, which, as the lowest of the 5 levels of the mind/brain is most closely tied to the rest of the body. In contrast, visualization of peaceful scenes employs verbal and sensory imagination, recruiting perceptual and language centers in the outer cortex and therefore anchored at the Verbal Conceptual level. In this case, there is a *top-down effect* on the Unlearned Core.

CASE EXAMPLES

We have now completed our walk down through the different levels of the mind/brain, considering which types of therapy can be assigned to each one. Now let us consider some case examples and think about which treatments would be most effective for each patient. Specifically, we will look back to three of the patients presented in earlier chapters. Martin and Sarah were presented in Chapter 4 and Filene in Chapter 5. Let us start with Filene.

> ***Filene*:**
> Filene is a 76-year-old woman with a long history of schizoaffective disorder. When properly medicated she is quite organized and capable of holding a job. But when psychotic, she wanders across the country in a delusional state, behaving in bizarre and agitated ways. She also has a tragic history of early loss and rejection. Her parents were of different racial backgrounds, her mother white and her father South Asian. Filene was born in the American South in the 1940s, when racial segregation was the law of the land. Her parents divorced early and her father died soon after. When she was 4 years old, her mother remarried to a white man. Not wanting to be hindered by a biracial child, she put her daughter in a convent and promptly abandoned her. Tragically, Filene grew up to lead an extremely chaotic life. She had difficulty sustaining relationships and abandoned her own children when they were the same age she had been at the time of her own parental abandonment.

Although Filene's primary pathology is schizoaffective disorder (Unlearned Core), her painful childhood experiences of rejection and abandonment left her with deeply damaged interpersonal representations (Basic Conceptual level). She struggles with rejection sensitivity, impulsivity, and a disturbed capacity for attachment, consistent with a comorbid diagnosis of borderline personality disorder. This pathology aggravates the psychosis by undermining her ability to tolerate disruptions in her therapeutic relationships and thus to sustain her treatment. Because her primary pathology lies at the level of the Unlearned Core, however, psychiatric medication is the primary form of treatment. Indeed, her psychosis resolves quickly with antipsychotic medication. Nonetheless, her considerable personality pathology also requires clinical attention as it has repeatedly interfered with her sustaining psychiatric treatment. Thus, some form of psychotherapy is indicated. However, Filene has significant cognitive limitations due to her psychotic disorder. Moreover, her ability to tolerate emotional stimulation is limited and fairly minimal emotional arousal can precipitate psychotic decompensation. Therefore, supportive therapy is the most appropriate form of psychotherapy. However, given her difficulty tolerating loss and separation, she is likely to stop her medication and decompensate if the therapist has to leave. We saw that in the history given in Chapter 5. To guard against this, some exploratory work will be necessary, at least to help her recognize, anticipate and plan for difficulties with separations. This work can be fairly concrete and behaviorally-oriented, keeping exploration of her past traumas at a superficial level. Additionally, as noted, she has an extreme history of acting out behavior (Pre-conceptual level), although when medicated this is less of a problem. If these behaviors occur even when medicated, DBT would be indicated. Finally, given her long history of dysfunction, she has not been able to create a viable life structure on her own (Life Structure level). In this case a structured day program to help develop job skills and to provide structure for her day would also be indicated.

***Martin*:**

Martin provides an example of a patient with much milder psychological difficulties. Still, his dysregulated behavior causes him distress and interferes with his functioning. Martin is a 62-year-old married man with three grown children. He owns a successful contracting business which he built up himself over three decades. He has a solid marriage and his adult children are doing well. However, he has considerable difficulty managing his finances. He has a particularly hard time putting together his invoices and procrastinates for months before billing his clients. This leads to considerable stress about unpaid bills and to frequent arguments with his wife. Sometimes he loses money as he has not adequately documented the work he has done. As explored in Chapter 4, this quite circumscribed difficulty reflects unconscious guilt about success and about taking from others, related to his having received greater love and attention from his parents than his younger brother did.

Overall, Martin is a high functioning man who is capable of logical reasoning with adequate emotion regulation and behavioral control. However, he lacks insight into the psychological reasons behind his financial procrastination, generally failing even to recognize it as a product of his own choices rather than external circumstances. Accordingly, he does not understand that this behavior is motivated by unconscious thoughts and feelings related to childhood familial dynamics. Given the circumscribed nature of his difficulties and their relation to his interpersonal representations, any of the psychotherapy modalities aimed at the Basic Conceptual level, such as psychodynamic, mentalization or schema focused therapy, would seem reasonable choices. Even cognitive therapy, with a focus on helping him identify his automatic thoughts and their relationship to his core beliefs would be helpful. Which one to use, therefore, might be more a function of personality style than pathology. By personality, Martin is a practical and rather concrete man; he is not given to introspection or psychological mindedness. Although intelligent, he is more of a doer than a thinker. As such, he might be more responsive to cognitive therapy as it is more explicitly linked to his conscious thoughts and less focused on a complex matrix of unconscious schemas.

***Sarah*:**

Sarah provides an example of a patient with severe borderline personality disorder. She is a 27 year old female whose parents divorced when she was 6 years old. Although her father was reasonably stable, her mother was far from that. She had bipolar disorder coupled with polysubstance abuse and was highly erratic and often abusive. While Sarah was able to obtain a college education and to maintain a meaningful job, she was far from stable herself. She was extremely dependent on her boyfriends and consistently made very poor choices, turning to emotionally and physically abusive men who also abused drugs. Men who treated her well disquieted her as she assumed she didn't deserve them. One night after a particularly long and intense fight, in which her boyfriend berated her mercilessly, she took off for a casino in a nearby state, where she gambled, drank and smoked cigarettes until the next morning. She was sick in her hotel room, vomiting repeatedly, and returned home thousands of dollars in debt. Such episodes occurred every few months.

Sarah is clearly struggling with a severe personality disorder. Despite her genetic loading for bipolar disorder, there is no evidence of a mood disorder independent of her personality disorder. In contrast to Martin whose difficulties are fairly mild, Sarah's pathology manifests in severely disturbed, addictive, and impulsive behavior. Such seriously problematic behaviors require interventions aimed at the Pre-conceptual level. For that reason, DBT and a treatment for alcohol abuse (which might include Alcoholics Anonymous) are recommended. Her significant emotional dysregulation might also be helped by relaxation and mindfulness techniques and possibly by psychiatric medication. Only after her addictive/impulsive behaviors are under control would more depth-oriented treatment, aimed at interpersonal representations, be indicated. Either psychodynamic, schema-focused or mentalization-based treatment should be appropriate at that point. Mentalization based therapy might be particularly helpful as Sarah can be very introspective and mentalize her own and others' internal states quite well when in a calm state. When activated, however, she can easily regress into disturbed mentalization.

But now we can ask, how can the typical therapist make use of these case examples? It's all very easy to match patients to specific treatments in the abstract but this may not be realistic in the real world. No one will become an expert in all treatments available. Do we refer our patients out when they could benefit from a treatment that we do not practice? In some cases, yes, as when the fit between patient and therapist is truly poor and there is considerable distance between the therapist's typical mode of practicing and the patient's needs. This is especially the case for high-risk patients, such as those who are acutely violent, suicidal, or actively abusing substances. In other cases, we can refer our patients for adjunct therapy while still continuing to treat them. For example, patients can be referred out for conjoint medication, substance abuse treatment, behavior therapy, or DBT skills groups. But frequently, it only takes a minor modification of our own technique to adjust to the patient's needs. This is when education about the different therapy modalities is most helpful. By expanding our knowledge about different modalities, we pack more tools into our therapeutic toolkit, allowing us greater flexibility in treating our patients. What this book has aimed to accomplish, therefore, is to provide a coherent theoretical framework to guide the selection of the most applicable techniques.

In the next chapter we will look at two different modes of information processing and how that influences the process of change in psychotherapy. For this we will turn back to our discussion of Emergent Systems Theory in Chapter 1. Specifically, we will consider the role of emergent processes in psychotherapy, the mysterious and even miraculous ways that change sometimes unfolds in treatment.

NOTE

1. Actually, Pavlov used the terms "reflexes," but modern behavior theory refers to "responses" (King et al., 2009).

Chapter Eight

The Accountant and the Artist

In this chapter, we are going to look at the kinds of information processing that therapists engage in when performing therapy. Previously, we have addressed the *patients'* processing modes, the nature of their pathology and of the kinds of treatments necessary to help them, but here we will turn our attention to how the therapist makes sense of the clinical material. I propose that there are two general modes of information processing at the conceptual level and that different kinds of therapy can be categorized according to which mode they prioritize.

Why is this important? Because there is a tendency for clinicians to misunderstand the aims, values and perspectives of treatments that operate differently from the ones they are familiar with. In this way, proponents of different treatments can talk past each other, dismissing the other approaches out of hand, without fully understanding them. By identifying this distinction in general information processing, I hope to mitigate that impasse, and help clinicians think about what kinds of treatments work best both for themselves and for different patients.

So far, in chapters 5 through 7, we have addressed the mind/brain as a *vertical* structure. We have considered the different levels of the mind/brain where we can anchor common mental disorders and their associated treatments. We have walked from the basement of this structure up to the top floor and back again. However, when psychotherapists are performing their work, they are operating at the upper levels of their *own* mental processing, at the level of thoughts and ideas. Although any complex brain process recruits the whole brain, conducting psychotherapy is a high-level, cognitive process that requires intense cortical activity. In other words, the therapeutic processing modes all take place at the Conceptual levels of the therapist's mind/brain, levels 4 and 5. Likewise, to the extent patients are active participants in their own treatments, therapy engages their own Conceptual levels as well.

Therefore, as our discussion is largely confined to one or two levels, this chapter addresses *horizontal* alignment, from left to right. In fact, these two distinct processing modes are to a large extent anchored in the left and right cortex, as will be discussed below. We will now visit these two processing modes in more detail. But, to return to our metaphor of the multi-storied building, instead of walking from the top of the building to the bottom, we are going to walk across the upper floors, from the left to the right side of the building.

ANALYTIC INFORMATION PROCESSING MODE

We will now consider the *analytic mode,* which rents offices on the left side of the building. Analytic reasoning tends towards highly logical, precise, and rule-based ways of making sense of the world. We can think of this processing mode as top-down. In other words, knowledge is based on an understanding of the parts that make up the larger whole. Complexity is reduced to simplicity. The dopamine model of schizophrenia is a good example. We investigate the psychiatric disorder of schizophrenia by studying the action of dopamine molecules in the brain. This type of knowledge is *reductive*. Knowledge is based on reducing the whole to its constituent parts. Moreover, the parts tend to be seen atomistically; they are considered in isolation rather than in relationship to the other parts of the system. When causal relationships between parts are addressed, they are typically considered sequentially, not simultaneously. A leads to B, which leads to C. This kind of reasoning process relies on *deductive* as opposed to inductive logic. This means that a) one reasons from the general to the particular and b) from general premises to logically necessary conclusions. If the general premise is valid, then the conclusion must be true. An example of deductive logic (adapted from ancient Greek studies of logic) may go like this: All men are mortal. Socrates is a man. Therefore, Socrates is mortal (See D'Angelo, 2020). This kind of information processing lends itself to the creation of and reliance upon algorithms, fixed rules for action. Likewise, the analytic mode is well suited for quantification, for translating verbal statements into numbers. In turn, the analytic mode is highly useful for generating precise, detail-oriented rules to guide behavior when circumstances are well understood. It is good for determining course of action. However, it is slow and laborious and does not do as well in complex, uncertain conditions when a quick reaction is necessary. The analytic mode is the dominant kind of reasoning in fields like computer programming, engineering, and accounting. It is not as dominant in creative endeavors or those which rely upon emotional communication.

Synthetic Information Processing Mode

The synthetic mode of processing has its offices on the right side of the building. This processing mode can be thought of as bottom-up. Parts are synthesized into a coherent whole. Complexity *emerges* from simplicity. While analytic processing is slow and meticulous, synthetic processing is quick and intuitive. It is less precise than analytic processing, yielding a sense of the gestalt, an overall truth, rather than a detailed analysis of component parts. It is ultimately about the recognition of patterns.

With synthetic processing, it is the relationships among parts that is studied, rather than the parts in isolation. Moreover, the interactions among parts are highly complex; they are reciprocal and simultaneous rather than sequential. A, B, C, D and E all interact with one another, constantly being modified in the process. Think of a crowd in motion. Rather than detailing the precise movements of all participants, it is easier to characterize the whole. The crowd is restive, enthusiastic, or tense. It is likely to disperse or ready to explode.

Synthetic knowledge comes through insight, in a somewhat unpredictable and even unexplainable way. Because the whole is *emergent* from the parts, synthetic reasoning arrives at something new, an emergent insight whose origins cannot be pinned down or entirely predicted. Consequently, synthetic knowledge can be fostered and facilitated but it cannot be controlled. The stance of the person engaging in the synthetic mode is passive and receptive rather than taking an active, directive, or controlling approach.

Likewise, synthetic reasoning tends toward *inductive* rather than deductive logic, which means a) that one reasons from the specific to the general and b) that the resulting insights cannot be certain; many possible insights can be gleaned from the same information. Because the outcome is neither certain nor predictable, the synthetic mode does not yield reliable algorithms to guide clinical behavior. Neither does it easily lend itself to quantification. Therefore, synthetic insights cannot be captured or taught in specific, precise and reproducible rules. As such, synthetic reasoning does not provide rules for action in the same way that analytic reasoning does. Nonetheless, it is flexible, adaptable and can provide a good read of a complex situation fairly quickly. (See Table 8.1 for a comparison of analytic and synthetic reasoning.)

Table 8.1. Analytic vs. Synthetic Information Processing Modes

	Analytic	*Synthetic*
Direction of Causation	Top-down	Bottom-Up
Part to Whole Relationship	Emphasis on parts, reductionistic	Emphasis on whole, holistic
Precision	Highly precise, detailed	More impressionistic, Gestalt
Speed of Processing	Slow, meticulous	Quick, intuitive
Part to Part Relationship	Atomistic, consider parts in isolation	Systemic, parts defined and construed as inter-related
Part to Part Interactions	Emphasis on sequential influence	Simultaneous, reciprocal interaction
Type of Reasoning	Deductive: General to particular; start with proposition, which if valid, results in necessary outcome. All people are mortal; Socrates is a person, therefore Socrates is mortal.	Inductive: Parts to whole, pattern recognition. Never provable; any future example could be different. Every person I have ever known is mortal, therefore all men are probably mortal.
Relationship to Logic	Careful logical analysis, deductive logic	Inductive logic, pattern recognition, intuitive leap
Relationship to Emotion	Cold cognition, unemotional	Hot cognition, inherently emotional
Rules	Algorithmic, identification of stable rules, rule-driven	General guidelines, outcomes probabilistic, less certain
Quantification	Lends itself to quantification	Less focused on quantification
Stability of mental structures	Static, mental structures defined as stable entities	Dynamic, system in constant flux
Stance of Therapist	Active, directive	Passive, receptive
Control of Therapist	Controlling	Passive, receptive
Brain Regions Involved	Left cortical hemisphere	Right cortical hemisphere
Characteristic Tasks	Engineering, mathematics, computer Programming	Creativity, artistic endeavors

The *synthetic mode* of information processing is predominant across the many artistic practices, such as creative writing, visual arts, dance and music. It is also well suited for making sense of emotions, for empathic and socio-emotional understanding.

Let us now consider some examples of the synthetic mode as described by two writers of fiction. These passages illustrate how important this mode of thought is in the creative process and, I will argue, in the therapeutic process as well.

Ursula Le Guin is an award-winning writer of fantasy and science fiction. This is how she describes the process of finding story ideas. Note the passive, receptive stance of the author.

> For a fiction writer, a storyteller, the world is full of stories, and when a story is there, it's there, and you just reach up and pick it.
>
> Then you have to be able to let it tell itself.
>
> First you have to be able to wait. To wait in silence. Wait in silence and listen. Listen for the tune, the vision, the story. Not grabbing, not pushing, just waiting, listening, being ready for it when it comes. This is an act of trust. Trust in yourself, trust in the world. The artist says, the world will give me what I need and I will be able to use it rightly. (Le Guin, 2004, p. 262)

Here Le Guin describes the process of creating fictional characters. Note the unpredictable outcome of the process.

> Whether they invent the people they write about or borrow them from people they know, fiction writers generally agree that once these people become characters in a story they have a life of their own, sometimes to the extent of escaping from the writer's control and doing and saying things quite unexpected to the author of their being. (Le Guin, 2004, p. 235)

Amy Tan is another well-known novelist. She describes the writing process in similar terms. Frequently, writing for her is laborious, hampered by self-consciousness, but occasionally she experiences flights of inspiration. In this passage, she uses a metaphor of upward movement in her description of powerful but unpredictable moments of intuition.

> Spontaneous epiphanies always leave me convinced once again that there is no greater meaning to my life than what happens when I write. It gives me awareness so sharp it punctures old layers of thought so that I can ascend—that's what it feels like, a weightless rising to a view high enough to survey the moments of the past that led to this one. Too soon, that feeling dissipates, and I am hanging

> on to contrails as I come back down to a normal state of mind—the one that requires me to write in the more laborious, conscious, pre-planned way, all the while hoping I will soon have another intuitive run in which the pieces join, lose their seams, and become whole. (Tan, 2017)

Clinical Relevance of the Analytic vs. Synthetic Distinction

Importantly, these distinctions in information processing style are not new to the field of psychology. Psychoanalytic writers such as David Shapiro contrasted obsessive-compulsive and hysterical cognitive styles (Shapiro, 1965), which are largely analogous to analytic and synthetic processing modes, respectively. Likewise, attachment theory distinguishes between Dismissing and Preoccupied attachment styles (Main, Cassidy & Kaplan, 1985), which also overemphasize analytic and synthetic processing, respectively. An excessive bias towards either analytic or synthetic processing may also underlie certain psychiatric disorders. Individuals with autism spectrum disorders characteristically view the world with highly logical, rule-based, and detail-oriented cognition with deficits in intuitive, socio-emotional understanding (Baron-Cohen, Wheelwright, Robinson, & Woodbury-Smith, 2005). Indeed, Frith and colleagues have long proposed a "weak coherence" model of autism, in which this particular cognitive style is attributed to a local, detail-oriented mode of processing that disregards or fails to recognize the overall gestalt. These individuals miss the forest for the trees (Happé & Frith, 2006). Although their symptom profile is quite different, patients with body dysmorphic disorder (BDD) exhibit a similar dominance of analytic processing. BDD patients experience great distress over perceived physical flaws. Sometimes this reflects exaggerations of minor physical imperfections but at other times there are wholly delusional misperceptions. This disorder can be extremely serious, even leading to suicide attempts. Research shows that a similar detail-oriented, local bias underlies the perceptual distortions of BDD (Feusner, Yaryura-Tobias & Saxsena, 2008). BDD patients also miss the forest for the trees. You can try this yourself. Stare at your face in the mirror. Fixate on your nose. Before long, it might look out of proportion to the rest of your face. You might become overly concerned with a mole or a small asymmetry. In so doing you have lost sight of the gestalt of your face, becoming overly focused on a facial part.

In contrast, individuals with Attention Deficit Disorder may privilege synthetic over analytic processing modes. In comparison with autistic subjects, they have been shown to lack the excessive focus on details and parts found in the autistic counterparts (Happé & Frith, 2006). In fact, they typically have considerable difficulty attending to details but often have excellent interpersonal intuition (Honos-Webb, 2008) and score higher on tests of creative problem solving and real-world success in creative tasks (White and Shaw, 2011). As such, they miss the trees but catch the forest.

Typically, we think of the scientific method as based on the analytic mode of information processing. However, both analytic and synthetic modes are necessary for science to progress. Hypotheses are generated via synthetic modes and tested via the analytic mode. Think of the legend of Isaac Newton being hit by an apple as he sat under a tree. This led to a sudden insight about the force of gravity. However, the theory required testing through rigorous empirical observation and mathematical analysis before it could be considered scientifically valid. Actually, this is also true in art; inspiration comes from the synthetic mode but editing and revising takes place in the analytic mode (See Ellamil, Dobson, Beeman & Christoff, 2012 and Mayseless, Iran & Shamay-Tsoory, 2015 for similar concepts). Furthermore, this is equally the case in psychotherapy. We must both generate and test hypotheses about our patients' psychological world. Nonetheless, as we will discuss below, the different types of psychotherapy vary in terms of the degree they emphasize either mode.

NEUROBIOLOGICAL SUBSTRATES

Let us now consider the neuroscience behind this distinction. To what extent does the science support location of the analytic mode on the left side of the brain and the synthetic mode on the right? Early neuropsychologists, who based their observations on brain damaged patients, noted an important distinction between the psychological impact of brain damage on either side of the brain. Language was strongly impacted by left hemisphere damage while visuo-spatial functions by the right. Emotional processing also appeared to privilege the right hemisphere. This distinction had mass appeal and was picked up in the popular press, generally to the point of gross oversimplification. In response, scientists came to pooh-pooh the left brain vs. right brain distinction, stating that the brain worked as a complex and interconnected system.

Indeed, in recent years, there has been a push towards "myth busting," stating that the left brain-right brain distinction is in fact myth (e.g., Blacker, 2016). Indeed, a number of brain imaging studies have investigated tasks typically attributed to the right brain, specifically creative tasks, and found bilateral activation (i.e., both sided) with no right brain preference. For example, in an fMRI study by Ellamil et al. (2012), subjects were asked to design book covers while instructed to alternate between generation of novel ideas and evaluation of the utility of these ideas, two different components of creativity. Comparison of the brain regions involved in each task revealed bilateral activation of multiple brain regions. Similar findings were found in an imaging study in which participants were asked to find novel uses for common objects (Mayseless et al., 2015). In other words, both right and left hemispheres were involved in creative tasks. On the other hand, Gansler et al., (2011) found a correlation between right parietal gray matter volume and performance on a visual creativity test. They posited this may be due to the critical role of the right parietal role in global attention.

In general, however, these studies may not be the best means to address the question of *lateralized* modes of information processing, that is tasks that differ across hemispheres. For one they are looking at too blunt a distinction. Creative thinking is extremely complex and involves multiple component processes including executive functions, sensory-motor functions, memory and language (Abraham, Beudt, Ott, & von Cramon, 2012). It is very difficult to isolate the specific processes that might distinguish the two hemispheres, particularly in brain imaging studies that pick up all brain activity at any given moment. Instead, it seems we find more consistent support for the distinction between right vs. left hemisphere processing modes in clinical studies, those investigating individuals with neurological or psychiatric disorders (c.f. Gurin and Bloom, 2017; Sacks, 1985).

Thus, I will argue that we must not throw the baby out with the bathwater. In his 2009 book, Iain McGilchrist revisited the left brain/right brain distinction and produced a sophisticated synthesis of many decades of prior research (McGilchrist, 2009). Reviewing multiple types of neuropsychological studies, including data from brain imaging research, stroke patients, split brain patients (whose hemispheres are either temporarily or permanently cut off from communicating with each other), and electroencephalographic (EEG) studies of brain waves, he concluded that there is indeed a significant distinction between the ways that the left and right cortical hemispheres process information, and that these modes work together to make sense of the world in which we live. We will spend some time on McGilchrist's findings as they provide dramatic support for the distinction between analytic and synthetic modes of information processing. Of note, other reviews of the scientific literature reported many of the same findings (Gansler et al., 2011; Gurin & Blum, 2017; Schore, 2003).

Firstly, there are, on average, biological differences between the two cortical hemispheres. The right hemisphere (RH) is larger, develops earlier than the left hemisphere (LH) (see Schore, 2003) and has far more connections with the rest of the brain, particularly with the limbic system and other subcortical areas. In contrast, neurons in the left hemisphere are largely connected with one another; they play in their own front yard. Further, the neurotransmitter profiles differ across hemispheres—in neurological terms, they are lateralized. Dopamine is predominant in the LH, whereas norepinephrine is more common in the right. Dopamine mediates expectations, anticipating future experience based on representations of past experience. This includes expectations of rewarding experience, as evident in its central role in the reward circuitry. Norepinephrine is associated with novelty, with detecting the unexpected.

McGilchrist proposes that the hemispheres vary according to *overall style of processing*, such that the differences in specific psychological functions are subsumed under more general processing differences. He states that the LH processes isolated parts while the RH synthesizes the parts into a global, coherent whole. In the LH, parts are seen in isolation, atomistically, while in the RH, parts are seen in context, in relation with each other. Further the LH sees the world as static and unchanging, operating according to stable rules, while the RH perceives the world as ever-changing, a dynamic flow, which, like a river, maintains its identity in the face of constant flux. This has implications for the processing of time; McGilchrist states that the RH is much better at estimating time duration than the LH, which processes time as a sequence of isolated moments.

As above, these general processing differences manifest across different psychological functions. Take attention, for example. In the LH, attention is narrow, highly focused, and rigid. In the RH, attention is global and diffuse, holistic. We see this in a neurological condition called hemi-neglect, in which, following damage to the RH, patients fail to attend to the left side of their visual field. As the hemispheres work contralaterally, that is each hemisphere processes information on the opposite side of the body, RH lesions lead to left-sided neglect. If asked to draw a picture of a flower, a patient with left hemineglect will only draw the right side of the picture, entirely neglecting the other half. Of note, patients with LH lesions rarely exhibit hemineglect.

McGilchrist also includes drawings of flowers from several patients who have had each hemisphere temporarily inactivated by a medical procedure (p. 78). Patients with RH inactivation are entirely dependent on their LH. These patients draw tight little pictures in the middle of the page. The drawings attend only to parts, such as circular petals around a circular center. They are cramped and mechanical. In contrast, when the LH is inactivated and the RH dominant, the drawings are much stronger. The drawings are larger, take up the page with grace and include the petals, center, stem and leaves. In short, they depict a convincing whole. Moreover, they are dramatically more lifelike and aesthetically pleasing. Interestingly, the drawings done under normal conditions are less impressive than when the LH is inactivated. These drawings fall in between the RH and LH drawings in terms of their aesthetic and lifelike quality.

We see analogous distinctions with language. Although we typically think of language as a LH activity, the picture is actually more complicated. The LH mediates vocabulary and the rules of grammar. When the LH is significantly damaged, receptive and/or expressive language is deeply compromised. However, according to McGilchrist, in the LH, words have a 1:1 relationship with meaning; they are signs rather than symbols in the full sense of the word. In contrast, the RH is sensitive to multiplicity of meaning in words and symbols; it is also sensitive to context. As such, it is dominant in the appreciation of metaphor, poetry, irony and humor.

We see analogous distinctions with regard to the brain's representation of the body. The LH understands the body in terms of isolated parts; it is the RH that grasps the whole, the gestalt. This is evident in the bizarre delusional misidentification syndromes that are associated with RH lesions, particularly in frontal and parietal regions. With RH lesions, the patient can lose a coherent understanding of the body (and by extension the person) within its appropriate context. In Capgras syndrome, someone who is familiar is seen as a stranger or an imposter. For example, an elderly woman was admitted to the hospital accompanied by her home health aide, Maria. The woman was convinced that Maria was not who she said she was. In fact, there were two Marias, one was nice and took care of her—the nice Maria. The other, the bad Maria, was more sinister, in fact an agent of the Honduran government sent to spy on her. Additionally, people can fail to recognize *themselves,* as exemplified by a disorder called mirror agnosia. An elderly man was admitted to the hospital as he was so distressed by his reflection in the mirror or even in a pane of glass, that he became acutely agitated. "Who is that man?" he would cry plaintively. "Why does he keep following me?" Finally, patients with RH lesions can perceive their own body parts as alien, believing their leg belongs to someone else and trying futilely to throw it out of the bed.

Relatedly, facial recognition is largely a RH matter. Faces are very complicated, and it is a difficult and energy intensive process to distinguish and remember the 1,000s of faces we regularly encounter. Thus, we excel at recognizing the gestalt, which is handled in the RH; instead, the LH analyzes faces by parts. Prosopagnosia is a neurological disorder associated with lesions in the right fusiform gyrus, deep within the tempero-occipital cortex. People with this disorder are unable to recognize the gestalt of faces, as famously exemplified in Oliver Sacks' book, *The Man who Mistook his Wife for a Hat* (Sacks, 1985).

McGilchrist notes that, consistent with the RH's sensitivity to holistic processing, flux and continuity over time, it is much more attuned to *living* things. The LH on the other hand is more attuned to *mechanical* function. It can analyze objects in space with greater precision than the RH. In fact, LH damage disrupts tool use far more than RH damage. Thus, the RH appears to be oriented to living, sentient beings, while the LH is a master at understanding the behavior of inanimate objects.

Likewise, the RH processes emotional information far better than the LH, which is limited by its computer-like, mechanical mode. The prosody (nonverbal intonations) of language, emotional facial expressions, and emotional language are all processed preferentially in the RH. Empathy and theory of mind are also reliant on the RH. While one's own suffering is processed in both hemispheres, attunement to others' suffering is predominantly processed in the RH.

Finally, reasoning is processed differently across hemispheres. Effortful, focused and sequential reasoning is mostly processed in the LH, while unpredictable insight and that "aha moment" is more dependent on the RH (p. 65).

Consistent with McGilchrist's conclusions, structural imaging research into BDD has supported the preferential role of the left brain in the kind of detail-oriented, local processing dominant in this disorder (Feusner et al., 2008). In a study investigating neuronal connectivity in patients with BDD, the strongest finding involved heightened white matter connections between the left temporal pole (involved with integrating memory, emotions and object recognition) and the left occipital lobe (visual processing) (Donatello et al., 2013). White matter refers to the brain's axons, the long extensions that connect one neuron's cell body to other neurons' dendrites. Likewise, Happe & Frith postulated a role for heightened left-hemisphere and dampened right hemisphere activity in the cognitive bias towards local, detail-oriented processing over holistic, global information processing characteristic of autism spectrum disorders (Happe & Frith, 2006).

COMMON PSYCHOTHERAPY MODES ON THE ANALYTIC-SYNTHETIC SPECTRUM

Now that we have reviewed the nature of the two different processing modes and their likely neurological substrates, let us consider how this might apply to the different modes of psychotherapy. As noted above, this is important as the different modes have distinct *epistemologies*; they have different standards of what constitutes knowledge. And hence they are likely to dismiss one another as inadequate, when they are simply different. Nonetheless, they both have strengths and limitations and competent therapists will need to employ both modes.

As indicated on Figure 8.1, I have placed cognitive therapy the furthest towards the analytic end of the spectrum, followed by schema therapy and then ACT. As is clear here, I am interpreting the CBT tradition to be heavily indebted to the analytic processing mode. Knowledge is broken down into predetermined parts (e.g., automatic thoughts, specified schemas) and the treatment is guided by clear rules and plans of action. Therapy is manualized and standardized. I have placed psychodynamic therapy in the center as it is far less prescriptive than CBT but also relies on the structure of the therapeutic frame (e.g., the therapeutic hour, therapeutic boundaries, specific theories of what is and is not acceptable in treatment). Humanistic therapies start to move toward the synthetic end of the spectrum with their emphasis on personal growth and unfolding, an emergent process. Mindfulness is seen as even further on the synthetic end of the spectrum. The goal of the process is almost entirely open ended and reached through emergent processes; insight and mental clarity will arise through the simple focus of attention and the emptying of the mind of directed thought. It is as if the process is intended to quiet the analytic mode. Finally, psychedelic therapy is placed on the far end of the synthetic spectrum. The actual psychedelic process is performed with little structure outside of ensuring facilitative set and setting. The process appears to work by breaking down previous mental structures so that new ones can emerge from the wreckage.

What are the strengths and limitations of the two processing modes? Treatments that emphasize the analytic mode are precise; they give clear guidelines and emphasize behavioral change. Change is easy to measure and thus their efficacy can be clearly, if laboriously, tested. They seem to be particularly well suited to disorders at the Pre-Conceptual level, which are not experienced as the core part of self but rather as alien, separate features. In fact, treatment progresses by *objectifying* the behavior, by treating it as an alien entity, as an object to master with manualized treatments. For example, with OCD, it is important for the patient to recognize their symptoms *as* symptoms, as ego-alien, something separate from the self. However, these types of treatment depend on pre-specified concepts of psychopathology. If the patient does not fit into the conditions that the treatment has been designed to treat, the therapist may be at a loss. They may miss the patients as this mode of processing does not adjust well to rapidly changing conditions or unexpected situations. It is not flexible. Moreover, it is not well suited for a holistic understanding of the patient as a person, rather than as an aggregation of symptom clusters or diagnoses. I have noticed in my own clinical supervision of student therapists that those who are trained exclusively in evidence-based modalities have more trouble developing a coherent conceptualization of their patients as people. With these students, it is harder for me to get a sense of who the patient is.

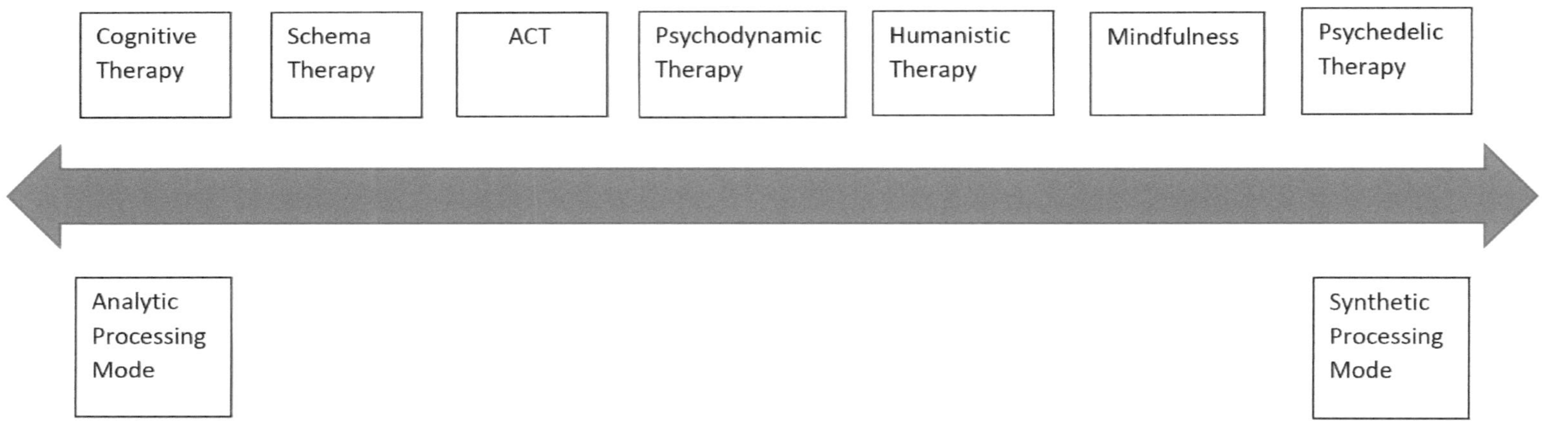

Figure 8.1. Position of different therapies along the spectrum from analytic to synthetic information processing. Image created by Lisa J. Cohen.

In contrast, treatments that emphasize the synthetic mode can be easily customized to the patients' unique presentation and can flexibly adapt to change. Such treatments lend themselves to personalized, comprehensive clinical formulations. For the therapist, a synthetic processing mode promotes the ability to apprehend a holistic gestalt of the patient. It facilitates the therapist's creativity. For the patient, the emphasis on emergence can be *transformative*, giving the person a wholly different experience of themselves in the world. However, this approach is not precise and I will stipulate that it does not work as well with Pre-conceptual pathology, such as obsessive-compulsive disorder, borderline cutting and suicidal gestures, or panic attacks. Instead, its most powerful impact is on the way patients experience themselves and the world around them, the felt sense of self in the world. Thus, it works best with difficulties on the Basic Conceptual level, involving problematic representations of self and others. Additionally, the lack of precision can affect the language used to describe clinical phenomena, which can lead to misunderstandings among practitioners or a dense, impenetrable jargon that serves less to communicate than to delineate insiders from outsiders. This problem has frequently been noted by psychoanalytic writers (c.f. Greenberg & Mitchell, 1985). Finally, although the creative stories generated in the synthetic mode are compelling and can be very trenchant, they are not necessarily *accurate*. After all, it is the synthetic mode that gives us fiction, mythology and even conspiracy theories. But it is the analytic mode, with its careful logic and attention to detail, that tests the accuracy of the synthetic mode's creations.

Interestingly, the practitioners of treatments on the analytic side of the spectrum seem to acknowledge the need for a balanced approach between analytic and synthetic modes. Jeff Young states that schema therapy should be structured but not formulaic, with an iterative approach that continually integrates new information (Young, Klosko & Weishara, 2003, p. 63). Likewise, Judith Beck states that the strict rules of cognitive therapy are mainly used for training purposes. Once the concepts and structures are thoroughly internalized, the therapist can customize the approach to the individual patient, adapting spontaneously and intuitively in the moment (J. S. Beck, 2011, p. 13). The promotion of mindfulness practices in third wave CBT also serves as a corrective to the overly analytic approach. Similarly, the growing popularity of DBT and other CBT approaches speaks to a need to correct for the imprecision of earlier psychodynamic and other synthetic approaches.

Emergence and Personality Change

Now let us consider the role of the synthetic mode in the amelioration of personality pathology and the fostering of healthy personal growth. As noted above, the synthetic mode may play a privileged role in the transformation of interpersonal representations. To consider how this might work, let us go back to our first chapter, which laid out the concepts of Emergent Systems Theory.

As we discussed in Chapter 1, a system is a self-contained entity, defined by the patterns of interactions between its component parts. Different systems interact with one another and form supersystems. In this way, hierarchical structures are created, with multiple levels of subsystems forming the components of higher order systems. We see this at every level of life, from atoms, to molecules, to cells, to tissues, to organisms, to the social group. Importantly, systems are seen as wholes, characterized by emergent qualities that are not explainable by lower levels of the system. The whole is greater than the sum of its parts.

The same process applies to personality structure. As discussed in Chapters 3 and 4, we can conceive of character, the learned component of personality, as a system of interpersonal representations. Across maturation, these representations grow in complexity. Most of the development takes place in childhood but growth generally continues throughout life as most people grow wiser and more mature with greater life experience. Integral to such organizational development are the three inter-related processes of integration, differentiation, and articulation.

In personality pathology, this development is stunted. In fundamental ways, self and others are seen in crude, simplistic ways. Specifically, the representation of self is undifferentiated from that of others, causing, for example, impairment in empathy or overly ego-centric interpretations of others' behavior (he didn't call me back me because he hates me and I am not worth loving). Likewise, the different parts of the self are not integrated over time into a coherent whole, hampering the ability to learn from experience or to take responsibility for prior actions (But that was yesterday. I don't feel that way anymore). Further, representations of others are equally fragmented. During a pleasant interaction, prior bad behavior may be disregarded. Alternatively, in the midst of negative emotions, positive experiences are forgotten. Because of this, people can stay in toxic relationships that they should leave or abandon supportive relationships after a minor rupture. Finally, interpersonal representations are global and unarticulated. People are seen as all good or all bad, often switching from one state to the other. Nuance and complexity are missed, again causing further instability in relationships as well as self-concept (I lost that job so I'm a total loser).

How does this change? I suggest here that the transformation from states of relative simplicity to those of greater complexity (i.e., higher levels of integration, differentiation, and articulation) occurs in an emergent process.

In a somewhat mysterious and unpredictable way, complexity *emerges* out of simplicity. I further propose that use of the synthetic mode is critical in the facilitation of this process. Moreover, this is the case both for the therapist and the patient.

I am not saying that the analytic processing mode is unimportant. For therapists, it is essential for critical thinking. For patients, it helps build an intellectual framework to understand their own psyche. In turn, this serves as a *scaffold* for the emergent processes, like a trellis for a climbing vine. Such an intellectual understanding is also an invaluable aid when trying to control maladaptive responses. People can use self-talk to refute assumptions drawn from maladaptive interpersonal representations (Now, you know she didn't mean it like that. Look at it from her point of view). But ultimately it is the emergent insight that is so powerfully transformative and this arises out of the synthetic processing mode.

What does the synthetic mode look like in therapists? Many authors have described this state of mind before, albeit using different language. Wilfred Bion spoke of entering each session with no memory and no desire. Freud spoke of evenly hovering attention. And the more recent practice of mindfulness encourages moment-to-moment awareness without judgment. In essence, when therapists utilize the synthetic mode, they are practicing mindful psychotherapy.

The cultivation of this state of mind allows us to have the kind of "aha insights" described by the writers Ursula Le Guin and Amy Tan. I often have similar experiences sitting with patients who are clearly struggling with what Jeff Young would call schema activation. They are emotionally activated in a way that appears more related to their internal narrative than to the present situation. If I am not sure what is going on, I listen and wait for the material to talk to me, to tell me what is happening. Almost every time, something reveals itself to me. A narrative unfolds and I have greater understanding of the patient's interpersonal representations, of the patient's inner world. Sometimes it is hard to capture, as evanescent as a dream. Other times it is very clear. I will then offer this interpretation to my patients as a hypothesis. Just as Le Guin describes in her own writing, I have learned to trust this process, to trust that an insight will come to me.

How does the synthetic processing mode work for patients? How can they employ it in their own treatment? Once again, this notion has been previously addressed across different therapeutic modalities. Sigmund Freud instructed his patients to engage in free association. They were asked to say whatever came to mind, without censoring their thoughts or worrying if they made sense. In my own (strongly psychodynamic) graduate training, we encouraged patients to "just sit with" their emotions to see what insights emerged.

In schema therapy, a very different modality, patients engage in imagery exercises to help elucidate early maladaptive schemas, as direct verbal questioning is often insufficient. Despite his CBT background, Jeff Young realized that logical thought is often inadequate to the task of schema identification. Finally, psychedelic treatment relies upon open-ended introspection during a hallucinogenic trip to promote greater self-knowledge, although conscious discussion of the experience after the trip ends is deemed necessary to consolidate the lessons learned.

Now we can ask: What does change look like? What do our patients feel like when their views of self and other are more integrated, differentiated and articulated? In general, patients appear more mature, more grounded, and less reactive. They are wiser, more thoughtful, and have greater empathy for others. They are better able to take others' perspectives without sacrificing their own. They can handle conflict adaptively without rupturing relationships or acting in ways incompatible with their values. Moreover, their sense of self is more solid, more secure, allowing them to handle shame and guilt more easily while still maintaining a stable sense of self. Finally, they are better able to assert themselves without invalidating others' positions or conflicting needs. Ultimately, when character truly shifts, the patient feels like a different person in front of you.

To illustrate, let us contrast the reactions of two different women to their boyfriend's emotional distancing several months into a new relationship. Edith cries out "What's wrong with him? Why doesn't he love me anymore? I don't believe this. What did I do? I know I'm the one for him." Janelle is also upset but can take more perspective. "I understand where he's coming from and I get that he is nervous to commit after a bitter divorce, but I need someone who is more available. If we can't work through this, I don't think it's going to work for me."

What role does emotion play in this process? Remember that interpersonal representations are not strictly cognitive structures. They are maps of the person's entire experience of key events, centrally involving the affective tone of the event. Therefore, a reworking of emotional experience is pivotal to the development of more mature interpersonal representations. Emotion needs to be incorporated into the work; it needs to be part of the emergent process. As psychoanalytic writers have long noted (See Chapter 3), intellectualized insight does not bring about felt change. Jeff Young's schema therapy also recognizes this issue, emphasizing the need to engage emotional experience in schema change.

Nonetheless, with severely traumatized or neglected patients, premature engagement with emotion can be grossly destabilizing (Linehan, 2015; Young, Klosko & Weishaar, 2003). It can precipitate an affect storm that is poorly contained by conceptual abilities and hence results in dangerous and symptomatic behavior such as self-harm, aggression, or substance abuse (Linehan, 2015). More than once I have been told by patients that they have felt overwhelmed and dysregulated after a session, even if the patient seemed to be able to handle the material during the session. In these cases, skills to enhance self-regulation must be focused upon first. Treatments such as DBT, CBT for various problematic behaviors, or relaxation techniques are useful for this purpose. Alternatively, emotionally distressing content can be addressed very gradually or in discussion of less emotionally fraught situations. In some cases, when the trauma is too severe or the patient is too ill, the overall goal of treatment must be redirected, either to regulating Pre-conceptual functioning (e.g., impulse control, affect regulation) or to functioning in the world within the parameters of their limitations, i.e., to an intervention at the Life Structure level.

Length of Treatment

Now, we can ask about the time frame for this kind of change. In general, change is slow and gradual; these shifts in interpersonal representations are often subtle. Thus, it is helpful for the therapist to attune to such subtle shifts, both to mark progress but also to identify areas in need of further growth. But how long should treatment last? Across the entire span of psychotherapies, the length of treatment is highly variable. Although many manualized treatments designed for specific disorders like depression or anxiety last 8 to 20 weeks (Steinert et al., 2017), there is consensus that the treatment of personality disorders generally takes much longer. These treatments can be measured in years rather than months (Gabbard, 2000). In general, it appears that the necessary length of treatment will vary according to the type, length, and complexity of the problem (American Psychological Association, 2017). Short-term, recent onset problems in the context of otherwise high functioning generally need less time to resolve. This might include adjustment disorders, new onset panic attacks, or a recent or mild depression. Complex clinical pictures that include multiple comorbid disorders—as is typical with the more severe personality disorders—can take considerably more time. According to a review by Gabbard (2000), patients with borderline personality disorder may not show notable improvement until at least the second year of treatment.

Nonetheless, there are, on occasion, quick and dramatic shifts in people's understanding of self and other, almost a kind of quantum change. Such changes are not well studied but fit in with broader studies of complex systems, in which sudden shifts in organizational complexity can suddenly occur after the system reaches some kind of critical point (Gell-Mann, 1995). These are very rewarding moments for therapists but do not necessarily signal the completion of the treatment. Nonetheless, it is moments such as these that make the treatment of personality disordered patients so compelling.

In the next chapter, we will consider the role of factors relevant to therapy that operate on the Socio-cultural level. Although we have emphasized the privileged role of interpersonal representations in the origin and perpetuation of personality pathology, it is also crucial to consider the role of the larger social context, not only to the individual patient's clinical picture, but also to the provision of the psychotherapy.

Chapter Nine

The Socio-Cultural Level

In this chapter we are going to discuss the socio-cultural level of the emergent systems hierarchy. To continue the building metaphor, we are going to take a helicopter ride over the city where the building is located. We will see our building within its larger context. Earlier in this book, I have used the term social level; for example, when discussing diagnosis in Chapter 5 and treatments in Chapter 6. But here I wish to be a little more specific and target the socio-cultural level. What does this mean? By socio-cultural level I am referring to larger social systems, outside of any immediate interpersonal group. Here we are considering the larger society, rather than a small social group, such as a family.[1]

Why is this important and why might it merit an entire chapter on its own? Because cultural influences have an enormous impact on personality development and on the expression, assessment, and treatment of emotional distress. Although psychotherapy does not expressly aim to intervene on the socio-cultural level—we do our work on the level of individuals and small groups[2]—we cannot perform our work effectively without being mindful of the larger social and cultural forces shaping our patients' clinical presentation. Likewise, both the American Psychological Association and the DSM-5 emphasize the necessity of taking culture into account in the provision of mental health care. In fact, the issue is so important and complex that entire academic disciplines are devoted to it. Certainly, we cannot do the topic full justice in one chapter, but we can touch upon some key points that are pertinent to psychotherapy in general and the treatment of personality disorders in particular.

Moreover, it is very easy to misdiagnose behavior when we overlook cultural factors. Primarily, there is risk of *pathologizing* behavior that is normative for the patient's culture but not for the clinician's. As a minor example of this, I once interpreted a young man's choice to dye his hair platinum blond as an attempt to return to his childhood (he was a towhead as a child) before I learned that this hair style had become quite fashionable. Perhaps he had been identifying with his childhood self, but he was also following a fashion trend. In another example, White American clinicians with highly individualist values may over-pathologize the familial interdependence of patients from other cultures, where, for example, it is expected that adult children live with their parents until marriage. On the other hand, we can also *normalize* pathological behavior when we are unclear about its cultural context. For example, a patient from an ultra-orthodox Jewish community was admitted to the hospital for excessive praying. His psychiatrist, who was raised in a Communist country with an avowed atheist stance, was afraid to pathologize culturally normative behavior. It was only after his rabbi and other community members confirmed that his praying far exceeded cultural norms and was interfering with basic self-care that the patient received a diagnosis of schizophrenia and obtained appropriate treatment. Religious or not, the patient was psychotic. Finally, a critical part of the treatment of personality pathology is the elucidation of the patient's narrative, the script or schema of who they are in the world. But, as we just saw, we cannot fully understand our patients' narratives unless we understand the larger socio-cultural context in which those narratives have developed.

CULTURE AND EMERGENT SYSTEMS THEORY

How might we understand the influence of culture within the framework of emergent systems theory? In effect, culture exerts *top-down* influence on all the levels of the human system we have addressed so far. It influences the *Life Structure* level by shaping people's work life, families, moral beliefs, and values. Consider the everyday life of someone living in a huge, modern city vs. a small village in the Australian outback. Or of a devout nun vs. a strict atheist. Culture influences the *Verbal Conceptual level* by literally determining what language people speak, as well as by impacting their education and the conscious ways they think about their experience. It shapes how they reason and problem solve. Culture shapes the *Basic Conceptual Level* by influencing parenting styles and hence the unconscious and deeply embedded representations of self in relation to others that result. How we think about ourselves, who we are in the world, and what it means to relate to other people is powerfully affected by the larger social forces that shape our early environment. Culture also impacts self-concept by shaping one's role and value in the larger society. Are we well integrated into our social world, respected and valued? Or are we marginalized and dismissed? Further, culture impacts the *Pre-conceptual* level through the conditioning effects of lived experiences, especially in childhood. Children in high crime or war-torn regions are exposed to chronic levels of stress that condition their emotional responses to remain on high alert. Culture even impacts the *Unlearned Core* through epigenetic changes in gene expression related to socially induced stress (McGowan et al., 2009).

In order to truly understand our patients, therefore, to properly assess their difficulties and to meet them where they live, we must be mindful of the myriad ways that culture can influence every part of their clinical presentation.

The Social Group and Culture

Now, before we go further, let us make a distinction between the social group and culture. I will define the social group as a group of people who share one or more traits and interact with one another (Cohen, 2016). As noted above, we are interested here in larger social groups, not small interpersonal groups. Although the group is interactive, members do not all know each other. A social group can be seen as an emergent system and as such it is defined by certain principles. 1) The system is created by characteristic patterns of interactions among the group members. 2) The group is greater than the sum of its parts; there are characteristics of the whole that cannot be reduced to the behavior of its component parts (i.e., individual people). 3) Subgroups within the group form subsystems. 4) The group interacts with other groups to form supersystems.

Within social groups, the characteristic patterns of interactions can be conceptualized as culture.[3] *We will define culture as a system of norms, values, beliefs, and rules that binds a social group together, lasts over time, and gives the group a common identity* (American Psychiatric Association [APA], 2013; Triandis, 1993). As above, the culture of a group can last far beyond the membership of any particular person. In fact, many cultures persist for centuries or even millennia. Sometimes cultures change very quickly—consider how dramatically Western culture has changed with recent advances in technology—but, in principle, culture is not dependent on the presence of any individual and frequently lasts beyond the lifetimes of its members.

CULTURAL COMPETENCE

Because of the impact of socio-cultural factors on individuals' clinical presentation and the course of therapy, the notion of cultural competence has become an important component of professional development in the mental health fields. Both the American Psychological and Psychiatric Associations incorporate cultural competence into their practice guidelines. Lo & Fung (2003) distinguish between general and specific cultural competence. The former refers to a familiarity with and sensitivity to the general issues that vary across cultures. With specific cultural competence, the clinician becomes familiar with the norms of a particular culture, so as not to misunderstand, misdiagnose or stigmatize culturally different behavior. Meltzer and colleagues introduced the concept of structural competence to focus on the structural barriers to adequate health and health care among minority and low-income populations (Metzel & Hansen, 2014). These can include reduced access to transportation, nutritious food, health care services, and clean air, among many other factors.

The American Psychological Association has incorporated these issues into their code of ethics. When such knowledge is relevant to their work, psychologists are required to be familiar with factors associated with age, gender, gender identity, race, ethnicity, culture, national origin, religion, sexual orientation, disability, language, and/or socioeconomic status or to seek appropriate consultation, supervision, or referrals (American Psychological Association, 2017). In the field of psychiatry, DSM-5 includes a section on cultural formulations, which proposes assessment of the following four categories: 1. Cultural identity of the individual, 2. Cultural conceptualization of distress, 3. Psychosocial stressors and cultural features of vulnerability and resilience, and 4. Cultural features of the relationship between the individual and the clinician (APA, 2013). Note that this formulation addresses positive cultural features as well, those which support health and resilience. These might include religious figures or institutions, community groups or organizations, rituals or rites that mark important life passages, and culturally normative modes of managing stress and personal challenges.

Importantly, it is crucial to recognize (and common sense) that it is not possible to know everything about the cultures and subcultures to which our patients belong. Metzl & Hansen (2014) recommend cultivating "structural humility." By maintaining humility about our limited knowledge, we can better avoid making harmful and arrogant assumptions.

Indeed, there are numerous landmines to consider when addressing cultural factors in psychotherapy. The foremost of which is stereotypes. All cultural descriptors involve generalized statements about a large group of people and generalizations about any social group easily devolve into stereotypes. Once stereotypes are in place, they can have considerable power on both conscious and unconscious thought. Now, to cut us all some slack, it is impossible *not* to evaluate people in terms of generalizations. It is the way the human brain works; we create schemas of the people in the world with whom we interact.

We do this to provide maps to guide our responses to the world. Without such schemas, our world is a mass of buzzing confusion and every step we make must be considered anew. Nonetheless, when these schemas become oversimplified and unmodifiable in the face of new information, we are dealing with stereotypes. A wealth of research shows that stereotypes of other groups develop easily and quickly devolve towards the negative (Brown, 2000; Cohen, 2016; Lin, Kwan, Cheung & Fiske, 2005). Across cultures, we tend to view our own group in a positive light and other groups more negatively (Brewer & Campbell, 1976). Even when stereotypes are ostensibly positive, as the stereotypes of Asian Americans as the "model minority," hardworking and studious, there is a dehumanizing and objectifying effect. The vast complexity of the individual is reduced to a crude and simplistic trope (Cheng, 2021; Lin et al., 2005; Reny & Barreto, 2020).

Secondly, even when one's understanding of cultural norms is accurate and informed, we cannot know how each individual will engage with his or her culture. Not everyone adheres to general cultural norms to the same extent and there are always mitigating factors. Thus, there needs to be a balance in psychotherapy between consideration of the individual and that of culture. In response to this challenge, Lo & Fung suggest that clinicians use cultural knowledge to *generate hypotheses* to then be tested collaboratively with the patient (Lo & Fung, 2003). For example, a therapist might ask, "Is it possible that you and your parents have different cultural expectations about how parents and children should relate to each other? After all you were raised in the United States and your parents were raised in a very different culture. Could that explain some of your disagreements?" Likewise, DSM-5 promotes a "person-centered approach," in order to minimize stereotyped assumptions. Clinicians can ask the patient and family what *their* perception of their situation is. They might ask, "How do your family and the people in your community understand your problems?"

SPECIFIC CULTURAL FEATURES

In light of these caveats, let us consider some of the cultural features that present themselves in treatment. What kinds of cultural norms should we be paying attention to? One distinction that has frequently been made is the difference between collectivism and individualism (Cohen, 2016; Lo & Fung, 2003; Triandis, 1993). In collectivist cultures, as found across Asia and parts of Africa, the individual is seen as embedded within the family or communal group. Identity is largely derived from the group to which one belongs and one's goals, wishes and decisions are oriented towards group harmony rather than individual satisfaction. For example, young adults may assume that they will marry someone of whom their parents approve regardless of their wish to make an independent choice. They may also assume that a good part of the money they make will be sent home to their family, rather than funding independent initiatives. Western cultures, such as those in Europe and North America, emphasize individual responsibility, independence and goal orientation. It is expected that adults will make decisions based on their individual goals rather than their parents' preferences.

Likewise, attitudes towards authority can vary across cultures. Western cultures, such as those of Europe and North America, particularly in the Northern regions of both continents, tend to have a flatter view of hierarchies than do Asian and African cultures or those of the southern regions of Europe and the Americas (Hayes, 2009; Triandis, 1993). It is expected that authority figures will be treated more casually and people will act less deferentially in the former than the latter group of cultures. This can affect parent-child relationships, as parents are the first authority figures that children will meet. This can also play out in therapy as some patients may treat the therapist as an authority figure while others may treat the therapist more like a peer (Lo & Fung, 2003). When people view authority differently than other people in their life, this can lead to conflict and misunderstanding. Further, attitudes towards authority have changed considerably in the last half century, with Western cultures, in particular, showing less deference towards authority than they did as recently as the 1950s.

Norms regarding expression of emotion also vary across cultures. Northern Europeans and their North American descendants are known to be quite contained with regard to emotional expression while Southern Europeans and the cultures of Latin America tend to be far more expressive (Pennebaker, Rime, & Blankenship, 1996; Triandis, 1993). Clearly, this can impact the conduct of psychotherapy, which relies so much upon emotional exploration. Related issues that can differ across cultures include the degree of separation vs. connection between children and parents, the expected amount of closeness vs. distance in intimate relationships, and involvement of the extended family in the nuclear family.

Gender roles also vary tremendously across cultures and have changed considerably in only the past few decades (Kim, Lau & Chang, 2006; Sugihara & Warner, 2002; Mirande, 2018). Traditional gender roles place women in the domestic sphere, responsible for childcare and management of the household, while men operate in the public sphere, responsible for financial support and protection of the family. The degree to which this template is followed generally correlates with a power differential, such that women are dependent upon men for financial survival and tend to be deferent to them in major decisions. Since the middle of the 20th century, however, women now comprise a much larger share of the workforce in most developed countries. Yet there is still considerable variation both between and within cultures, and different expectations of gender roles can underlie many problems in couples (Caetano, Ramisetty-Mikler, Vaeth, & Harris, 2007; Sugihara & Warner, 2002). Likewise, both partners in heterosexual marriages may unwittingly try to hold onto the benefits of the old arrangement while discarding the disadvantages. For example, the husband may enjoy the extra income brought in by his wife but not want to shoulder any additional housework and childcare. Similarly, the wife may enjoy the extra freedom of a more liberal role but resist taking on financial responsibilities. I have often seen this in my own practice. Of course, with the greater acceptance of non-traditional gender roles and family constellations, such as those involving homosexual or transgender individuals and partnerships, we see even more variation in cultural mores and norms, even within the same society.

Likewise, attitudes towards sexuality can vary tremendously across cultures and subcultures. In many traditional cultures, sexuality is tightly controlled and acceptable sexual behavior is highly circumscribed. For example, Catholic teachings state that sex should only occur within heterosexual marriages for the purposes of reproduction. Extra-marital, premarital, homosexual and masturbatory sexual activity is therefore considered sinful. Moreover, across cultures, it is frequently female more than male sexuality that is tightly controlled. Examples of this include clitorectomies in certain African countries, which serve to greatly reduce women's sexual pleasure, and harems, which were quite common across Muslim countries in Asia in prior centuries. In ultra-orthodox Judaism, married women are still expected to shave and then cover their heads so as to not attract attention from men other than their husband. Consider the cultural conflicts engendered, therefore, by the relatively recent liberalization of sexual mores in many Western and economically developed countries, as exemplified by the legalization of homosexual marriage, birth control, and abortion, the explicit sexual depictions in popular media, and the development of alternative sexual subcultures, such as those promoting polyamory and sex parties. Given our complex, cosmopolitan and constantly changing world, many of our patients will grapple with conflicting sexual mores, as they negotiate their competing identifications with different cultures and different generations.

Additionally, patient's sense of self can also be affected by cultural norms. Lo & Fung (2003) distinguish between interdependent vs. independent self-concepts. These dovetail with the distinction between collectivist and individualist societies. In an interdependent sense of self, the person defines him or herself through a web of relationships; personal goals, values and self-esteem are embedded in these relationships. In contrast, people with independent self-concepts set their goals, values and identity on their own individual desires and accomplishments, separate from those of other people in their life (Triandis, 1993). Cultures and subcultures also vary in terms of the individual's sense of agency and perceived ability to effect change. As early as the 1830s, the French writer Alexis de Toqueville remarked upon the American sense of agency, similar to what was later labeled the "can-do spirit," much touted in political campaigns (de Toqueville, 1835/2000). This is in contrast to a kind of fatalism that is found in many other cultures, especially in those members of the culture who fall lower on the social hierarchy.

Hierarchies and Power Relations

Likewise, the structure of social hierarchies and power relations represent an incredibly important element of culture, powerfully influencing individuals' daily life, their interactions with others and their sense of self. In this context we are referring to the norms within the culture that determine allocation of status, resources, and power. In India, for example, there is an ancient and hereditary caste system that explicitly determines one's place on the social hierarchy, although the power of caste is diminishing with modernity. In the Western world, socio-economic status is the great divider, as determined by wealth, education, and occupation. Race and ethnic background also impact one's rung on the social ladder in the United States and many other cultures.

Social status has a tremendous impact on all aspects of mental and physical health as will be discussed below. In fact, research has shown that experiences of racism, poverty, and related stress even impact cellular aging (Chae et al., 2020). Norms determining social hierarchy can be internal (i.e., within the social group or intra-group) or external (i.e., between different social groups or inter-group).[4]

The concept of minority stress is relevant here. It was originally developed to explain the psychological challenges of homosexuals and other sexual minorities, who struggle with a greater level of mental health and substance abuse problems compared to the general population (King et al., 2008; Meyer, 2003). Minority stress is conceptualized as the combined deleterious effects of objectively stressful events and conditions related to social prejudice, expectations of such adverse experiences, and the internalization of negative societal attitudes towards one's minority status (Meyer, 2003). Clearly, this concept can be generalized to many other minority groups or to any social group that falls lower on the social hierarchy.

To summarize, a variety of socio-cultural features come into play when engaging in psychotherapy. These include the norms, values, identity, and subgroups of the cultures and social groups to which our patients belong as well as intra- and inter-group hierarchies of status, resources and power. Keep in mind that we all belong to multiple, intersecting social groups, resulting in a complex interplay of cultural influences in every individual.

RELEVANT SOCIAL GROUPS

Now let us consider a range of social groups that are relevant to psychotherapy and some pertinent cultural features associated with these groups. Here we will review groups characterized according to ethnicity, socio-economic status, race, gender, religion, political ideology, and historical cohort. As above, as therapists we must balance attention to our patients as individuals and to their context within one or more social groups.

Ethnicity

We can define ethnicity as pertaining to a social group with a shared language, history, norms and/or values (see APA, 2013) and which either currently or in the past has belonged to a common political entity. To some extent, ethnicities also reflect genetic population groups who descend from a common tribe, e.g., the Celts or Slavs, although this is frequently diluted by centuries of migration and intermarrying. Colloquially, when we use the term culture, we are typically referring to the norms of an ethnic group. We have already mentioned cultural features of different ethnic groups that can impact therapy, such as the distinction between collectivist vs. individualistic cultures. The role of language is also important as the language that we learn in childhood has an impact on our ways of thinking about ourselves and the world around us. If our language has no name for a specific concept, including emotions, we will be hampered in our ability to think about it. For example, many societies do not have a word that translates into our word for depression. And the way they understand such a condition also varies widely (Kleinman & Good, 1985/2010). Additionally, many of our patients will be bilingual. Such patients may find that therapy in their first language has more direct access to deeper feelings (Kokaliari, Catanzarite, & Berzoff, 2013). Indeed, research suggests neuroanatomical differences between monolingual vs. bilingual speakers (Green & Abutalebi, 2016). Many bilingual people also have emotional ties to the different languages they speak. For example, the well-known Indian-American writer Jhumpa Lahiri recently started to write exclusively in Italian, her third language and one she only learned as an adult. She explained that she did this as she found it freed her from the emotional constriction that she associated with writing in either Hindi or English, her first and second languages respectively (Nunez, 2021).

Immigration is another important aspect of ethnicity and a common phenomenon in the United States and many other countries. Immigrants must negotiate their relationships to two cultures, their culture of origin and the host culture. Frequently, there is felt conflict between the two cultures, resulting in considerable adjustment difficulties (Caetano et al., 2007; Lo & Fung, 2003). A Chinese-American patient once conveyed this conflict to me symbolically by saying, "Sometimes I want to eat rice with chopsticks but other times, I only want to eat hamburgers." A large literature exists on the psychological challenges of immigration and there is consensus that people adjust best when there is a balance between maintaining ties to the original culture and acculturating to the new culture (Lo & Fung, 2003; Berry & Sam, 1996). Sometimes, cultural issues may impede the progress of therapy, as when there is considerable stigma towards mental health care in the culture of origin.

It is also important for therapists to become familiar with and look to the strengths and resources of the patient's culture (APA, 2003; Hayes, 2009; Lo & Fung, 2003). Community and religious institutions, such as the Black church or the orthodox Jewish community, can provide considerable social, emotional, and practical support for our patients. Sometimes, a word from a pastor, rabbi, or traditional healer can offer support for mental health treatment, and thereby reduce stigma.

Socio-Economic Status (SES)

SES can be defined as the relative amount of power, wealth, income, and status one has in the general society. Education is both a marker of SES and a means to move up the social ladder. The United States has long held to a myth of a classless society, in which everyone who wants to work has full access to upward mobility. Given the increasing income and wealth disparities between the upper and lower echelons of society, the fallacy of this myth is increasingly exposed. In fact, SES has extraordinary impact on all health indicators, including physical health, exposure to violence, substance abuse problems, mental health problems and the outcome of mental health treatment, and even life expectancy (Chetty et al., 2016; Cunradi, Caetano, & Schafer, 2002; Sugihara & Warner, 2002; SAMHSA, 2018; Yoshikara, Aber, & Beardslee, 2012).

Keep in mind though that the notion of SES is relative, not absolute. It is how one's resources, wealth, status, and power compare to others that is most psychologically impactful. Happiness studies shows that people in low-income countries can report higher levels of happiness than people in high income countries (Cohen, 2016). While there may be absolute differences in concrete physical resources, such as food, protection against the elements and access to technology and health care, if the culture is cohesive and functional, individuals can still thrive.

Within the United States and other complex societies, low SES confers considerable risk, including more physical and mental health problems, substance abuse, chronic stress, experience of crime both as victims and perpetrators, unemployment, inadequate education, domestic violence, and child maltreatment. There is more contact with the criminal justice system and worse outcome (Hopps & Liu, 2006; Metzl & Hansen, 2014; Sharam & Hulse, 2014; Sugihara & Warner, 2002; SAMHSA, 2018; Western, 2019; Yoshikara et al., 2012). These problems can be mitigated by strong extended families, good social programs, including those supported by the government, and by community institutions such as churches and non-profit organizations (Kasturirangan, Krishnan & Riger, 2004; Metzl & Hansen, 2014; North, Holahan, Moos, & Cronkite, 2008). Most of all, these problems can be mitigated by reducing inequality across socio-economic status, an issue implicitly touched upon in Metzl and colleagues' work on structural competence (Metzl & Hansen, 2014; Yoshikara et al., 2012).

There is psychological danger to high SES as well, however, supporting the notion that social inequities affect all involved. A literature exists on the pressure to achieve in upper-middle class and upper-class youth, who feel that their identity and self-worth are entirely dependent on a very high level of accomplishment (Hirsch, 2019; Luthar, 2003). It is as if they are afraid of losing their elite status, of falling off their high rung on the social ladder. Relatedly, there is also a concept called "failure to launch" (Kins & Beyers, 2010), describing the phenomenon in which affluent young people opt to avoid engaging in work or other age-appropriate tasks to avoid the risk of failure. They may take on the sick role to do this and their parents' continued financial support removes the most immediate disincentive to such behavior (Kins & Beyers, 2010). Along with this over-valuing of professional status, there is a loss of felt community as social relations become tainted with excess competitiveness (Luthar, 2003).

Further, among the very affluent, there is evidence of a disproportionate amount of attachment difficulties and alienation between parents and children (Luthar, 2003). When childcare can be outsourced to paid workers, it is easy to slough off the tiring, stressful, and sometimes tedious but otherwise crucial elements of childcare. The resulting impairment in secure attachments can then get transferred to the next generation.

Race

Race offers a complicated and fraught topic in society today, particularly but not exclusively in the United States. While racial conflicts in the U.S. date back centuries, the issues have become much more front and center since the police killing of George Floyd in 2020. The definition of race is not simple. In fact, whether race exists at all is a controversial and complex question. In general, we can define a racial group as a group of people who share biological features and physical traits and descend from the population of a given continent (European, African, Asian, and Native American). The United States census lists the following racial categories: White, Black or African American, American Indian and Alaskan Native, Asian, Native Hawaiian and other Pacific Islander (U.S. Census Bureau, 2020a).

In prior centuries, race was used as a nonspecific term that referred to any social group, although typically an ethnic group, such as "the Hebrew race." Only after the enslavement of Africans and their descendants became an economic pillar of both European and American wealth was the term used more specifically to distinguish between the descendants of Africans and Europeans. Likewise, some of the earliest "scientific" theories of race came from aristocratic scholars in the 18th century whose families had ties to the trans-Atlantic slave trade (Gates & Curran, 2021). As Isabel Wilkerson notes in her book *Caste* (2020), White people were not White before coming to the US; they were French, German, Polish and Italian (and even more molar, as in Neapolitan rather than Italian). Further, Black people were not Black before coming to the US. Wilkerson cites a Nigerian writer who informed her that even now there are no Black people in Africa—only Sosa, Yoruba, Hutu, etc.

At present, race is understood to be a social construct and not a valid biological classification. The philosopher of race, Naomi Zack, distinguishes between population genetics and race as a biological category (Zack, 2002). Population genetics is the study of genetic commonalities of various groups of people who have shared a relatively circumscribed gene pool. Here we may find a predominance of specific genes for skin color, hair color, and hair texture but also for other phenotypic traits, such as height, immune factors, and various enzymes. Nonetheless, while population genetics is recognized as scientifically valid, race as a delineated biological construct is not. There are several reasons for this. Let us first consider what is necessary to create a valid biological category. For one, the people within the category should have more genetic material in common with each other than they do with people not in the category. Secondly, there should be a boundary around the category. It should be clear who does and does not belong to the category based on biological (i.e., genetic) criteria.

Now, despite some shared genetic inheritance in the populations defined by race, there is also considerable genetic heterogeneity. Within group differences can be very great (Potts & Sloan, 2010). Moreover, the between group differences can be very slight, far less than would be expected based on the social construct of race. Additionally, it is impossible to draw boundaries between racial groups. If you travel around the world, you will see that the physical features of different peoples vary gradually across geographical distances (Potts & Sloan, 2010). The people of Northern China look quite different from those of Indonesia, and certainly from those of India, and there is no exact geographical boundary where the changes are abrupt. And yet they are all considered Asians. Even within one country there can be marked physical variation. The people of Egypt range from light-skinned Semitic-looking people to darker skinned people, who look more similar to their sub-Saharan neighbors. And yet they are all Africans. Additionally, people from very different parts of the world can share traits typically associated with race. Indigenous people from Australia as well as New Guinea have dark skin and curly hair, tightly curled hair in the case of New Guineans. Although their ancestors left Africa maybe 70,000 years ago, long before the ancestors of modern Europeans, they look remarkably like Africans today (Bachman, 2021). Further, people mix and intermarry and have done so across human history and prehistory. African Americans today may have on average about 25 percent European genes, though much of that mixing was likely not consensual (Bryc et al., 2015).

Secondly, population genetics refers to the group, the population. It does not describe the individual. If 60 percent of the population carries a certain genetic variant, it does not mean that any given individual will have that genetic variant. Finally, the differences that are used to characterize different racial groups reflect specific and superficial physical traits, which serve to help individuals adapt to different climates. For example, dark skin, produced by the pigment melanin, protects against overexposure to ultraviolet rays in equatorial areas. In contrast, the loss of melanin and resultant light skin found in Northern climates helps the skin absorb Vitamin D, which is necessary in latitudes with less sun exposure. Crucially, there is no evidence of any relationship between these superficial traits and the phenomenally complex gene/environment interactions that make up our psychology.

While the notion of race is conceptually murky, the concept of racism is much less so. While race may not exist, racism certainly does. This is a critically important socio-cultural phenomenon that has far-reaching downstream effects on lower levels of psycho-social functioning. And as such, it is a dynamic that all psychotherapists need to be aware of. Let us define racism as 1) the assumption that group membership in one or another racial category is reflective of essential features about that person, including the individuals' character, personality, intelligence, and psychological and physical capabilities, and 2) the valuing or devaluing of that person because of his or her racial category. It has been proposed that race in the U.S. functions like a caste system, which refers to a hierarchical social system into which people are born and from which they cannot depart. Change is not possible. In her book on caste, Wilkerson proposes a hierarchy within the U.S. that places White people on the top, Black people on the bottom and other racial groups, such as Latino, Asian, and Native American, in the middle (Wilkerson, 2020).

Certainly, in American history, anti-Black racism has been blunt and phenomenally destructive, from justification of slavery, to tacit governmental support for lynching and other types of racial murder, to segregation, to Jim Crow laws, to the redlining of real estate even into the late 20th century. At present, explicit racism is less common and most explicitly racial laws have been deemed illegal. Nonetheless, profound racial disparities persist, despite many decades of civil rights progress. These disparities were particularly evident in the disproportionate illness and death rate among African Americans during the COVID epidemic (Bray et al., 2021; Yancy, 2020). Other disparities are also glaring, regarding health status, access to healthcare, educational attainment, occupational attainment, income and wealth, housing segregation, rates of homelessness, police killings, contact with and outcome within the criminal justice system (Aronson, Whitehead & Baber, 2003; Bishop, Hopkins, Obiofuma, & Owusu, 2020; DeGue, Fowler, & Calkins, 2016; Fusaro, Levy, & Shaefer, 2018; Hopps & Liu, 2006; Kahlenberg, 2021; Metzl & Hansen, 2014; U.S. Census Bureau, 2020b; SAMHSA, 2018). While these disparities are most dramatic when comparing Black and White Americans, they are also found among other racial minorities within the United States, such as Latino and Native American peoples (Bishop et al., 2020; Fusaro et al., 2018; Hopps & Liu, 20006; U.S. Census Bureau, 2020b; SAMHSA, 2018).

The notion of systemic racism has been proposed to account for this, which suggests that the structure of the entire societal system functions to perpetuate these racial inequities (Feagin & Bennefield, 2014). For example, when public schools are supported by local property taxes, poor localities cannot afford adequate education for their children, dooming them to substandard occupational opportunities. Wealthier families will then flee to more affluent localities to ensure quality education, and in so doing drive up the price of housing in those areas, effectively precluding poorer families from moving in. A related factor is the common practice of zoning affluent areas for single family dwellings only, precluding less expensive multi-family dwellings, which would be affordable for lower income families and therefore allow their children a better education (Kahlenberg, 2021). As such, lower income people are concentrated in specific areas, increasing the socio-pathology associated with poverty and racism, such as increased crime, substance abuse, family dissolution, etc. (Hopps & Lu, 2006; SAMHSA, 2018; Yoshikara et al., 2012). It is important to note here, that although the discussion so far has centered on racism within the U.S., it is not exclusive to the United States, and is found in many areas with racial heterogeneity. For example, similar problems have been evident among indigenous and other ethnic minorities in Australia (Sharam & Hulse, 2014).

So what are the effects of systemic racism? As above, there are dramatic effects in terms of racial disparities, but there are also more direct effects found at all levels of human psychology. There is even evidence that explicit experiences of racial discrimination are directly related to cellular aging (Chae et al., 2020). The concept of minority stress is highly relevant here; the direct experience of stigmatizing interactions, the anticipation of such experiences and the internalizing of negative societal attitudes all contribute to increased mental health difficulties (King et al., 2008; Meyer, 2003). Further, greater exposure to instability and trauma associated with racial disparities leads to a broad range of mental health difficulties. Finally, receiving messages both explicit and implicit about one's inferiority makes it hard to develop the self-confidence necessary to set high aspirations and work towards them.

While it is important for therapists to be aware of these broader social issues regarding race, it's also important to not over-pathologize. A good proportion of the Black population of the U.S. are in the middle class and the median income in 2019 was $46,073 (U.S. Census Bureau, 2020b). The median income for Hispanic families (all races) was $56,113. Although the median income for non-Hispanic Whites was notably higher at $67,027, the median income for all groups fell in the middle class. Moreover, there are many strengths to these different cultures and subcultures. Consider for example the numerous musical, intellectual, artistic, athletic, literary, dance, and political contributions of Black culture over the past century. These cultural innovations have had worldwide impact, far beyond the borders of the United States. Further, as mentioned above, every individual experience is unique, and it is useful to keep in mind the notions of structural and cultural humility when approaching the topic of race in therapy.

A note here about racial stereotypes regarding Asian Americans. Within the United States, Asian immigrants and their descendants have done particularly well. In 2019, their median income was significantly higher than White Americans at $98,174 (US Census Bureau, 2020b). With this has come a stereotype of Asian Americans as the model minority, studious and smart, hardworking, and driven (Lin et al., 2005; Reny & Barreto, 2020). While this involves positive attributes, it is also reductionist, and like all stereotypes is essentially objectifying. Further there is a persistent perception of Asian Americans as foreign and not truly American (Cheng, 2021; Lin et al., 2005). With the COVID pandemic, Asian hate crimes have spiked, and anti-Asian bias has received new attention (Cheng, 2021; Reny & Barreto, 2020). Hence racial stereotypes are prevalent throughout our ethnically diverse society and carry considerable downstream weight on many levels of psychological functioning.

Given that most psychotherapists are White and many clients are not, it is worthwhile to consider the impact of racial differences on the therapeutic relationship. As Lo & Fung (2003) describe, therapists should attune to the patients' level of trust, openness and comfort within the therapeutic relationship and their perception of the inherent power imbalance. Additionally, while ethnic and racial differences in the patient-therapist match can reduce trust and mutual understanding, in some cases it can make the patient feel more secure and open, particularly in cultures and subcultures with considerable stigma against psychotherapy (Lo & Fung, 2003). Lo & Fung further suggest that the way that cultural issues should be addressed depends on the stage of the treatment, how well patient and therapist know each other and how much information has been obtained. Indeed, in my own experience, I have found that it can backfire to address cultural differences between patient and therapist too early in the treatment. If there is need for culturally relevant factual information, I will ask about practices in the patient's community or family as recommended in DSM's cultural formulation section. Otherwise, I follow the patient's lead in addressing cultural/racial differences within the therapeutic dyad. I often find that patients only feel comfortable addressing such issues after a fair amount of trust has been established. Nonetheless, as indicated in the DSM's cultural formulation section, it is always important to consider the cultural implications of the therapeutic relationship.

Additionally, therapists must also attune to their own racial and ethnic biases. We are all products of our time and of our culture and some degree of conscious or unconscious bias is inescapable. Indeed, research into micro-aggressions show that therapists can unwittingly make comments that reinforce devaluing cultural stereotypes rather than transcend them (Sue et al., 2007). These authors define racial micro-aggressions as "brief and commonplace daily verbal, behavioral, and environmental indignities, whether intentional or unintentional, that communicate hostile, derogatory, or negative racial slights and insults to the target person or group" (p. 273). They propose a taxonomy of micro-aggressions, including Alien in their own land (treating Asian or Latinx Americans as foreigners), Myth of meritocracy (denying that race plays a role in life's successes), Pathologizing cultural values (assuming the values/norms of the dominant culture are superior), Color blindness (denying the influence of racial differences between therapist and patient), and Denial of individual racism (denying one's own racism). Sue and colleagues suggest that the only way to counter such tendencies is to foster open communication about race and racism within society. On an individual level, therapists must commit to overcoming their own defensiveness to accept that racism is inescapable and that denial only drives it underground, to leak out perniciously in reflexive, unacknowledged micro-aggressions. Nonetheless, this is no reason for therapists to panic. Rather therapists must cultivate a mindful attention to their own socio-cultural countertransference, much as they would to any other kind of countertransference.

Gender

Gender marks an important social group that we must attend to in therapy. But in today's terminology, gender is not identical to biological sex. Gender refers to the psychosocial characteristics attributed to one's biological sex, including one's gender identity (Walker & Cook, 1998). The role of nature vs. nurture in psychological characteristics associated with sex and gender has always been difficult to determine. Historically, such differences were considered essential, that is somehow innate. But since the mid-20th century and the growth of feminism, there has been much more emphasis on the environmental influences on sex roles and the associated psychological features. More recent research has shown that biology does matter, however, and that despite a considerable amount of variation within each sex, there are on average differences between the sexes. Clearly there are physical differences. Men on average are taller, stronger, and have a greater muscle to fat ratio. Additionally, research indicates that men have better spatial skills and are more aggressive while women are more attuned to fine emotional distinctions (Satherthwaite et al., 2015) and possibly have better verbal skills (Hyde, 1990). There are numerous studies showing sex differences in brain structure and function (Ruigrok et al., 2014; Satherthwaite et al., 2015). Sexuality also varies across the sexes, with men more easily aroused by visual stimuli and maintaining high and steady sex drive while women's sexual desire is much more context-dependent and more fluid in terms of the desired object (Baumeister, 2000). Such differences have been attributed to sex hormones such as testosterone and estrogen (Forbes & Dahl, 2010). They have also been interpreted to reflect the different evolutionary strategies that human males and females have utilized to maximize genetic fitness (Allport, 1997).

Nonetheless, environment and socialization have an enormous impact and gender roles have varied tremendously across cultures and across historical periods. Conflicts between members of a couple often involve different expectations of gender roles, which are frequently unconscious. Elucidating common differences between men and women and the varying social expectations of gender roles can help normalize patients' struggles and allow for a more impartial and less judgmental response from either partner.

More recently, in the past decade or two, the very nature of binary gender identity has come in question. Likewise, transgender identity has become far more socially acceptable and technological advances have allowed for greater biological fluidity between the sexes. For example, when I started performing psychological research several decades ago, I recorded only two sexual categories, male and female. In contrast, I recently consulted on a trainee's project in which subjects were asked to self-identify among 6 gender categories: male, female, nonbinary (born male), nonbinary (born female), trans male, and trans female. This is a sea change in cultural attitudes about gender and will likely be reflected in generational differences in how patients talk about and consider their own gender.

Additionally, as noted above, gender roles will differ across the cultures of many social groups, influenced by ethnicity, religion, generational cohort, and political affiliation. Negotiating these differences can be a challenge for many patients, particularly for those who hold different cultural values from their communities or families. Moreover, the perceived failure to live up to certain gender roles and norms can often be a source of distress and shame for patients and may underlie certain adjustment difficulties. For example, as I have often observed in clinical practice, women who remain single into middle age sometimes feel significant shame at their perceived failure to marry, even if they consciously reject traditional gender roles. Likewise, when men suffer a loss of income and hence their ability to contribute to marital or familial support, they may also feel a tremendous sense of shame regardless of their conscious attitudes toward traditional gender roles.

Religion

Religion might be defined as a culturally normative set of beliefs about moral values and a transcendent reality. Religion is believed to be a cultural universal and there are as many religions as there are cultures. Nonetheless, most of the largest religions vary on a spectrum from orthodoxy to secularism. This means the degree to which religious tenets circumscribe one's daily life will vary. The specific religion people ascribe to and their degree of orthodoxy vs. secularism will deeply impact their values, morals, life goals, community identity, coping strategies, and approaches to many features of daily life. Attending to patients' religious beliefs can thereby shed considerable light on how they make sense of their world as well as sources of strength and/or conflict. Religion can be a tremendous source of comfort, strength, and purpose and there is research showing that people who are religious report higher levels of happiness than secular people (Steger & Frazier, 2005). But religion can also be a significant source of conflict if one's personal values or desires conflict with religious tenets. A common example of this is found with homosexual individuals whose sexual preferences may be deemed unacceptable by their religious doctrine.

Political Ideology

In recent years, political ideology has become an increasingly divisive issue within the United States. The rupture is between political conservatism and liberalism or progressivism, associated with the Republican and Democratic parties, respectively. While tensions between these two groups are nothing new, these differences are currently at an extreme point, such that as of 2021, a large portion of self-identified Republicans believe that the 2020 election, in which the Democratic candidate won, was fraudulent (Kahn, 2021). While the specific positions of conservatives and liberals have varied across the years, the general stance of conservatives is to preserve (i.e., "conserve") the social order whereas liberals/progressives wish to change society towards a more just and equitable ideal (Muller, 1997). Jonathan Haidt suggests that moral values vary across political affiliation. He presents a theory of five moral "instincts," which are genetically based tendencies that serve to maintain cohesion within the social group. These include Harm/Care, In-Group/Loyalty, Authority/Respect, Purity/Sanctity, and Fairness/Reciprocity. In a survey of people of various political affiliations, he found that in general, conservatives emphasized in-group loyalty, respect for authority, and Purity/Sanctity whereas liberals emphasized Harm/Care and Fairness/Reciprocity (Graham, Haidt & Nosek, 2009). Additionally, political affiliation is associated with group identity and as the polarization between different political groups intensifies, the in-group cohesion of each group also intensifies along with the pressure to conform. Nonconformist opinions become socially dangerous, and transgressors are often ostracized, particularly via social media, a phenomenon known colloquially as "cancel culture." Thus, our current political impasse can be understood both in terms of differing moral priorities as well as heightened group dynamics. As many of our patients have strong feelings about politics, it is helpful to keep such issues in mind, but also to make sure to differentiate one's own political stance from the therapeutic role.

Occupation

One's work life plays a huge role in most people's daily life and personal identity and stresses at work are frequently the reason people seek out therapy. Many occupations have their own distinct culture, particularly those with strong and cohesive group identities, such as police officers and fire fighters. For example, psychotherapists value emotional expressiveness and self-disclosure, whereas many other occupational cultures value emotional stoicism, such as those of soldiers, physicians, and investment bankers. Occupational culture can have as much of an influence on people's identity as their membership in other social groups, such as their ethnicity or religion. Additionally, some occupations have more status and authority than others, both within the workplace and within the larger society, which can have far reaching effects on patients' wellbeing (Sharam & Hulse, 2014). This can also impact our patients' aspirations and personal identity, for example in patients who have failed to obtain the elite occupational status upon which they had set their sights. The more therapists learn about the distinct cultures of different occupations, the more they can understand their patients' experience within that culture and hopefully help them negotiate it.

Historical Cohort

Finally, it is worth considering the significant historical events that have impacted our patients' personal narratives. There can also be cross generational effects, particularly of mass trauma. For example, the impact of the Holocaust, the Great Depression, the Armenian genocide, and World War II is still felt, even if most of the people who experienced these mass traumas directly are no longer alive. Their children and grandchildren are still shaped by the impact on their own parents (c.f. Sorscher & Cohen, 1997). Somewhat more recently, the Vietnam war, the social upheavals of the 1960s, and the feminist movement of the 1970s have shaped the life experiences of the Baby Boomer generation and indirectly those of their children, while the economic, military, and social crises of recent years will shape the life structure and social perceptions of people in years to come. And we will have to see how the COVID pandemic, the Black Lives Matter movement, climate change, and the current political polarization will shape the world view of young people growing up now. Certainly, the hegemony of social media has changed the socio-emotional landscape for the millennial generation and younger.

Intersectionality

So far, we have looked at each type of social group in isolation, but we all belong to multiple, overlapping social groups of gender, ethnicity, socio-economic class, and race. "Intersectionality" is a term bandied about in academia that refers to the overlapping and interacting effects of one's simultaneous membership in multiple social groups. It originated in legal scholarship addressing the specific nature of discrimination experienced by Black women (Crenshaw, 1989). In social science research, we speak of "moderating effects." In other words, the psychological effect of belonging to one social group is modified by membership in other social groups. For example, it is different to be Black and poor than to be Black and upper-middle class. It is different to be a woman in a secular Jewish family than in an orthodox Jewish family. This adds multiple layers of complexity when seeking to understand any given patient and thus reinforces the need for "cultural humility" when assessing the relevant socio-cultural influences on that patient.

Case Examples

Now let us consider a few case examples. The first, Sammy, was introduced in Chapter 5 in our discussion of differential diagnosis. The other two, Jeremy and Cheyenne, are new to this chapter.

> Sammy:
>
> Sammy was a 46-year-old man from a wealthy secular Jewish family, who struggled with an undiagnosed learning disability, compromising his focus, attention and reading comprehension. Growing up in an affluent environment with ambitious and successful peers, Sammy felt tremendous pressure to achieve. Given his learning disability, however, such goals were more difficult for him and generally unrealistic. His family helped him out, obtaining a job through family connections. Less than optimal behavior at his work was often overlooked due to his employer's desire to avoid offending his family. This combination of unrealistic expectations and protection from failure stymied the growth of mature coping skills and the ability to manage the inevitable frustrations and failures in life. When his wife started to advance in her career, therefore, he reacted impulsively, leaving his family for another woman and to join a self-help cult. By the time the affair ended and he grew disillusioned with the cult, he had little to return to. His marriage was over and his children were furious with him as were his parents and siblings. At this point, he fell into a serious depressive episode.

In Sammy's case, his religious and ethnic background may be less salient than his family's socio-economic status. His relative privilege both heightened the expectations for his level of accomplishment and shielded him from the consequences of irresponsible behavior. That combination poorly prepared him for the inevitable times when other people would surpass him in one arena or another. No one can win every competition and psychological maturity requires an acceptance of that. Most people learn this in youth. In Sammy's case his family's wealth delayed his psychological maturation into middle age, such that when reality finally hit him, he had much more to lose.

Jeremy:
Jeremy was a 29-year-old Chinese American man, who moved to the U.S. with his parents at the age of eleven. His younger sister was born soon after his family immigrated and hence has only lived in the United States. Jeremy came to therapy because of feelings of stress regarding his relationship with his parents. He was unable to save money because all his money went to his parents, who, while deeply in debt, continued to make unwise business investments. His parents refused to share information about their finances with their son, leaving him with no input into their outlays. Jeremy owned a computer software company and business had slowed during a recession. When under stress, he alternated between the wish to sell his business and move overseas to escape his predicament and the feeling that he needed to submit to his parents' demands without protest. Jeremy was also upset with his younger sister whom he described as sullen and disrespectful to both him and their parents. Therapy focused on delineating different cultural views of obligations towards parents in American and Chinese culture. Could he find a way to set limits on his parents' demands without running away? Is there a middle ground between total cut-off and total submission? Collateral therapy with the sister revealed that she is dating a man of another race and felt the need to hide her sexual relationship from her family. She also sees no middle ground between total cut off and total submission. The collateral session with her focused on their varying cultural expectations of the sibling relationship; in America, such relationships are more peer-like and less hierarchical, whereas in China, they are more dutiful and hierarchical. When he feels he is being helpful, she sees his behavior as controlling and judgmental.

Thus with Jeremy, we see the centrality of issues related to ethnicity and immigration, when different family members vary in their acculturation to the host culture.

Cheyenne:
Cheyenne was a 23-year-old Black woman who sought therapy due to concerns that she had trouble opening up to men in intimate relationships. She felt that she was too closed in and self-protective. She had had some disappointing romantic relationships but did not think that those experiences were sufficient to explain her emotional inhibition. Otherwise, she functioned well and had no difficulty with academic or occupational tasks. Cheyenne was the only child of

a wealthy family. Both parents had worked in banking and her father had advanced to upper management in his bank, a major international corporation. At the top of his field, he had spent decades as one of if not *the* only Black person in the room. Hence, while he loved his career, he often felt isolated in his work environment. Both parents came from modest backgrounds and their marked change in socio-economic status created strain with their own families. They sensed a feeling of envy and resentment from family members, which led to further isolation. In this context, Cheyenne and her parents had formed a tight triad, loving but insular. This had posed no problems for Cheyenne growing up but as a young adult, she recognized that it had compromised her ability to fully trust an outsider within an intimate relationship.

In Cheyenne's case, we see the intersection of race and class and also the necessity of checking any preconceptions that might be held about racial divisions of wealth. Cheyenne did not struggle with the intersection of race and poverty, but rather with race and wealth.

In conclusion, this chapter explored the top-down influence of the socio-cultural level of the emergent system hierarchy. We discussed the broad range of factors operating at this level of analysis and the pervasive and sometimes pernicious impact they can have. Of course, no psychotherapist can catch all cultural influences impacting our patients and many clinical issues fall below the level of culture in the overall system hierarchy. Nonetheless, it is always necessary to consider the possible cultural influences at play.

NOTES

1. This distinction is similar in the nested ecological model (Dasgupta, 2002). In this model, the macro-system refers to the larger societal forces and history, while the exo-system refers to more local communities and organizations.

2. Of course, there are psychologists and mental health professionals who seek to intervene on a societal level. Nonetheless, such activity is different from psychotherapy per se. Rather these professionals engage in social policy, community activism, or other similar endeavors outside the express domain of psychology.

3. Sometimes, however, cultural patterns derive less from within-group than between-group interactions. For example, Chinese Confucian ideals represent intra-group cultural norms, whereas antisemitic stereotypes reflect inter-group cultural norms. The second type of cultural norm often derives from a power imbalance between the groups. It is *imposed* on the first group from the second. Nonetheless, it is still a cultural feature that can influence the group members' lives and psychological functioning.

4. Whether the hierarchies are internal or external depends on one's point of view. If the focus is upon the larger group, say the U.S. as a whole, then racial/ethnic disparities reflect internal hierarchies. When looking at a smaller group, such as Black or native Americans, disparities with white Americans reflect inter-group or external hierarchies.

Conclusion

The purpose of this book was to introduce an integrative model for the many different types of psychotherapy, with an emphasis on personality pathology. Returning to the metaphor of the blind men and the elephant, my goal was to describe the entire elephant, to present it as a unified whole and not just an aggregation of parts—of trunk and tail and legs.

Emergent Systems Theory is a comprehensive model of the mind/brain that integrates clinical psychology with neuroevolutionary science. It proposes a hierarchical model of all human systems. Within the human mind/brain, each system level reflects our species' evolutionary history. Specifically, this model proposes 5 general levels of the mind/brain, each of which dates back to a different point in our evolutionary history and has its own distinct psychological functions and, consequently, distinct forms of psychopathology. Hence many types of psychotherapy differ from one another because they address separate levels of the mind/brain. They are each appropriate for the level(s) they target but no one treatment is a panacea. No one treatment targets all 5 levels (or the additional levels outside of the mind/brain proper, such as the life structure or social levels). Still, we need to repeat a caveat here. The brain functions as a unified system so the separation of levels is far from absolute and there is constant interaction between levels. Nonetheless, I believe there is a meaningful distinction between levels and that such a distinction carries tremendous clinical significance.

We also addressed the distinction between analytic and synthetic modes of information processing and how different types of therapy fall along a spectrum from one mode to the other. Choice of therapy not only involves the identification of the correct level of the mind/brain for intervention, but also a sense of the predominant need for top-down (analytic) or bottom-up (synthetic) therapeutic modes with which to intervene.

It is still very new for clinical psychology and psychotherapists to think about their work in terms of neuropsychology, especially related to the deeper regions of the brain. As Panksepp and colleagues have stated, our prejudices have been toward the higher, cortical levels as these are bigger and easier to study and tie into the most distinctly human functions of conceptual thinking. But, from the vantage point of Emergent Systems Theory, the lower levels of the mind/brain are fundamental to our psychological functioning and provide the targets for many types of psychotherapy, including those highly relevant to personality pathology.

Of course, further research exploring the neuropsychological basis of personality pathology is needed, especially with regard to interpersonal representations. The seminal work of Jaak Panksepp has added a tremendous amount to the neurological study of emotion, a field that was far too long in coming. Future research could aim to expand his work into the higher conceptual domains, to look at how interpersonal relationships are represented in cortical regions. As we better understand the neurobiological substrates of these formative socio-emotional structures, we will enhance our understanding of the psychological processes involved, which can then translate into clinical advances. When we can take apart the car, we are better able to diagnose and then fix its problems.

Further research can also test the associations between the specific levels of the mind/brain and the psychological functions associated with them. Even though this model was based on extant research, the hypotheses presented here have never been tested empirically. Imaging studies would be the most obvious technique, but it is difficult to tease apart the focal findings in imaging research as so many regions of the brain are activated by any one task. As shown by Iain McGilchrist, clinical studies of brain damaged patients can be enormously revealing and might supplement imaging research.

How might Emergent Systems Theory be tested clinically? One way to test the model would be to develop an assessment tool to identity the primary and secondary types of pathology in each patient's presentation and link them to level-specific treatments. We could then customize the patient's treatment according to this assessment. Perhaps the end result may not look so different from what is done in many practices today, especially those of clinicians with an integrative orientation. Nonetheless, the model presented here could serve to systemize this approach, to give it structure and theoretical clarity. It would provide a coherent rationale for treatment selection.

Listed below are four general research questions that might guide future research:

1. Using a priori hypotheses (i.e., research questions posed in advance of data collection rather than afterwards) rather than a review of past literature, can we specifically differentiate the psychological functions attributed to each mind/brain level by the methods of neuroscience (e.g., brain imaging, animal models, neurosurgical techniques, studies of brain damaged patients)?
2. Using a priori hypotheses rather than a review of past literature, does psychopathology attributed to the Unlearned Core have a stronger genetic etiology than that attributed to the higher levels, specifically that of the Basic and Verbal Conceptual level? Genetic correlational studies a la Fox et al. (2015) may be of particular use here.
3. Can assessment and therapy based on Emergent Systems Theory show clinical efficacy? Do patients treated with such an approach show greater clinical improvement than in treatment as usual? Might the treatment effect be stronger with student clinicians than with more seasoned ones?
4. Is Emergent Systems Theory useful as a teaching tool? Will student therapists report greater clarity, confidence, and reduced stress providing psychotherapy after learning this integrative framework than after learning different therapeutic modalities in isolation?

Indeed, it was my experience teaching psychotherapy that motivated me to write this book. Recognizing how students can feel lost in the multiplicity of therapeutic approaches available today, I aimed to present an integrative model that could provide structure and conceptual clarity in the provision of psychotherapy, as well as a coherent rationale for treatment selection. Hopefully, future research can further validate, expand upon, and refine these ideas.

References

Abraham, A., Beudt, S., Ott, D.V.M., & von Cramon, D.Y. (2012). Creative cognition and the brain: Dissociations between frontal, parietal–temporal and basal ganglia groups. *Brain Research, 1482*, 55–70.

Ainsworth, M. (1978). *Patterns of attachment: A psychological study of the Strange Situation*. Hillsdale, N.J.: Erlbaum.

Allen, T.A., & Fortin, N.J. (2013). The evolution of episodic memory. *PNAS, 110* (suppl. 2), 10379-10386. DOI/10.1073/pnas.1301199110.

Allman, J. (1999). *Evolving brains*. New York: Scientific Library.

Allman, J. M., Hakeem, A., Erwin, J. M., Nimchinsky, E., & Hof, P. (2001) The anterior cingulate cortex: The evolution of an interface between emotion and cognition. *Annals of the New York Academy of Sciences, 935*, 107–117.

Allport, S. (1997). *A natural history of parenting: A naturalist looks at parenting in the animal world and ours*. New York: Three Rivers Press.

American Psychiatric Association. (2013). *Diagnostic and statistical manual of mental disorders, 5th Edition: DSM-5*. Washington, D.C.: American Psychiatric Press.

American Psychological Association (2017). Ethical Principles of Psychologists and Code of Conduct. Retrieved from https://www.apa.org/ethics/code (retrieved June 15, 2021).

American Psychological Association (2017). How long will it take for treatment to work? PTSD Clinical Practice Guidelines. APA Division 12 (Society of Clinical Psychology). Retrieved from www.apa.org/ptsd-guildeline (retrieved Feb. 2, 2021).

Anglin, D.M., Ereshefsky, S., Klaunig, M.J., Bridgwater, M.A., Niendam, T.A., Ellman, L.M., DeVylder, J., . . . van der Ven, E. (2021). From womb to neighborhood: A racial analysis of social determinants of psychosis in the united states. *American journal of psychiatry, 178*, 599-610. doi: 10.1176/ appi.ajp.2020.20071091.

Aron, L. & Lechich, M.L. (2012). Relational psychoanalysis. In G.O. Gabbard, B.E. Litowitz, P. Williams (Eds.). *Textbook of Psychoanalysis* (2nd ed.). Washington, D.C.: American Psychiatric Publishing.

Aronson, R. E., Whitehead, T. L., & Baber, W. L. (2003). Challenges to masculine transformation among urban low-income African American males. *American Journal of Public Health, 93*(5), 732–741. https://doi.org/10.2105/ajph.93.5.732.

Ashkenazi, S., Black, J.M., Abrams, D.A., Hoeft, F., & Menon, V. (2013). Neurobiological underpinnings of math and reading learning disabilities. *Journal of Learning Disabilities, 46*(6), 549–569.

Ask, K. & Granhag, P.A. (2007). Hot cognition in investigative judgments: The differential influence of anger and sadness. *Law and Human Behavior, 31*, 537–551. doi: 10.1007/s10979-006-9075-3.

Ayala, F.J. & Cela-Conde, C.J. (2017). *Processes in human evolution: The journey from early hominins to Neanderthals and modern humans*. Oxford, U.K.: Oxford University Press.

Bachmann, D. (2021). Early migrations. Retrieved from https://commons.wikimedia.org/wiki/File:Early_migrations_mercator.svg.

Bakker, T.C.M. (1994). Genetic correlations and the control of behavior, exemplified by aggressiveness in sticklebacks. *Advances in the Study of Behavior, 23*, 135–171.

Barger, N., Hanso, K.L., Teffer, K., Schenker-Ahmed, N.M., & Semendeferi, K. (2014). Evidence for evolutionary specialization in human limbic structures. *Frontiers in Human Neuroscience, 8*, 277. doi: 10.3389/fnhum.2014.00277.

Barlow, D.H., Craske, M.G., Cerney, J.A., & Kiosko, J.S. (1989). Behavioral treatment of panic disorder. *Behavior Therapy, 20*, 261–282.

Baron-Cohen, S., Wheelwright, S., Robinson, J., & Woodbury-Smith, M. (2005). The Adult Asperger Assessment: A diagnostic method. *Journal of Autism and Developmental Disorders*, doi: 10.1007/n10803-005-0026-5.

Barratt, F.S., Johnson, M.W., & Griffiths, R.R. (2015). Validation of the revised Mystical Experience Questionnaire in experimental sessions with psilocybin. *Journal of Psychopharmacology, 29*(11), 1182–1190. doi: 10.1177/0269881115609019.

Bastin, C., Harrison, B.J., Davey, C.G., Moll, J., & Whittle, S. (2015). Feelings of shame, embarrassment and guilt and their neural correlates: A systematic review. *Neuroscience and Biobehavioral Reviews, 71*, 455–471.

Bateman, A. & Fonagy, P. (Eds.) (2019). *Handbook of mentalizing in mental health practice* (2nd ed.). Washington, D.C.: American Psychiatric Association Publishing.

Bateman, A., Kongerselv, M., & Hansen, S.B. Group therapy for adults and adolescents. In Bateman, A., & Fonagy, P. (Eds.). (2019). *Handbook of mentalizing in mental health practice* (2nd ed.). (pp. 117–134). Washington, D.C.: American Psychiatric Press.

Bateman, A., Unruh, B., & Fonagy, P. (2019). Individual therapy techniques. In Bateman, A., & Fonagy, P. (Eds.). (2019). *Handbook of mentalizing in mental health practice* (2nd ed.). (pp. 103–116). Washington, D.C.: American Psychiatric Press.

Baumeister, R. F. (2000). Gender differences in erotic plasticity: The female sex drive as socially flexible and responsive. *Psychological Bulletin, 126*(3), 347–374.

Beauchamp, T. & Childress, J.F. (2001). *Principal of biomedical ethics* (5th ed.). New York: Oxford University Press.

Beck, A. T. (2019). A 60-year evolution of cognitive theory and therapy. *Perspectives on Psychological Science, 14*(1), 16–20. doi:10.1177/1745691618804187.

Beck, A.T., Emery, G., & Greenberg, R.L. (2005). *Anxiety disorders and phobias: A cognitive perspective*. New York: Basic Books.

Beck, A.T., & Haigh, E. A. P. (2014). Advances in cognitive theory and therapy: The generic cognitive model. *Annual Review of Clinical Psychology, 10*, 1–24. doi:10.1146/annurev-clinpsy-032813-153734.

Beck, J. S. (2011). *Cognitive behavior therapy: Basics and beyond.* (2nd ed.). New York: Guilford Press.

Beebe, B. & Lachmann, F. [with Markese, S., Buck, K., Chen, H., Cohen, P., Bahrick, L., Andrews, H. & Feldstein, S.]. (2014). *The origins of attachment: Infant research and adult treatment.* New York: Routledge Press.

Berr, J. W. & Sam, D. (1996). Acculturation and adaptation. In Berry, J.W., Segall, M.H., & Kagitcibasi, C. (Eds.). *Handbook of cross-cultural psychology: Social behavior and applications* (Vol. 3, pp. 291–325). Boston: Allyn and Bacon.

Binder, M., Hirokawa, N., & Windhorst, U. (Eds.) (2009). *Encyclopedia of Neuroscience*. New York: Springer.

Bingman, V.P., Salas, C., & Rodriguez, F. (2009). Evolution of the hippocampus. In Binder, M.D., Hirokawa, N., & Windhorst, U. (Eds.). *Encyclopedia of Neuroscience.* Berlin, Germany: Springer.

Bishop, E.T., Hopkins, B., Obiofuma, C., & Owusu, F. (2020, September). *Racial disparities in the Massachusetts criminal system: A report by The Criminal Justice Policy Program, Harvard Law School.* Submitted to Chief Justice Ralph D. Gants, Supreme Judicial Court of Massachusetts. Cambridge, MA: Harvard Law School.

Blacker, K. (2016). Debunking the left-brain/right-brain myth. *Science of Learning Institute*, John Hopkins University. Retrieved from http://scienceoflearning.jhu.edu/science-to-practice/resources/debunking-the-myth-about-left-brain-right-brain-learning-styles.

Blatt, S. J., Brenneis, C. B., Schimek, J. G., & Glick, M. (1976). The normal development and the psychopathological impairment of the concept of the object on Rorschach. *Journal of Abnormal Psychology, 85*, 364–373.

Bloch-Elkouby, S., Knopf, L., Gold, J., & Muran, J. C. (2016, December 15). Assimilative psychodynamic psychotherapy: A critical case study reconsideration. *Journal of Psychotherapy Integration, 27*(2), 254–264. doi.org/10.1037/int0000062.

Bonduriansky, R. (2011). Of mice and men: how things got tricky when we split from Mickey. *The Conversation*. Retrieved from https://theconversation.com/of-mice-and-men-how-things-got-tricky-when-we-split-from-mickey-3924.

Bourne, E.J. (2010). *The Anxiety & Phobia Workbook* (5th ed.). Oakland, CA: New Harbinger Publications.

Bowlby, J. (1969). *Attachment and loss, Vol. 1: Attachment*. New York: Basic Books.

———. (1973). *Attachment and loss, Vol. 2: Separation: Anxiety and anger*. New York: Basic Books.

———. (1980). *Attachment and loss, Vol. 3: Loss: Sadness, and depression*. New York: Basic Books.

Bownds, M.D. (1999). *Biology of the mind: Origins and structures of mind, brain and consciousness.* Bethesda, MD: Fitzgerald Science Press.

Bray, M. J. C., Daneshvari, N.O., Radhakrishnan, I., Cubbage, J., Eagle, M., Southall, P., & Nestadt, P. S. (2021). Racial Differences in Statewide Suicide Mortality Trends in Maryland During the Coronavirus Disease 2019 (COVID-19) Pandemic. *JAMA Psychiatry, 78*(4). doi:10.1001/jamapsychiatry.2020.3946.

Brewer, M. B. & Campbell, D.T. (1976). *Ethnocentricism and intergroup attitudes: East African evidence*. New York: Sage Publications.

Brisch, R., Saniotis, A., Wolf, R., Bielau, H., Bernstein, H. G., Steiner, J., . . . Gos, T. (2014). The role of dopamine in schizophrenia from a neurobiological and evolutionary perspective: Old fashioned, but still in vogue. *Frontiers in psychiatry*, *5*, 47. doi:10.3389/fpsyt.2014.00047.

Britton, R. (2012). Klein and Bion. In G.O. Gabbard, B.E. Litowitz, & P. Williams (Eds.). *Textbook of psychoanalysis* (2nd ed.). Washington, D.C.: American Psychiatric Publishing.

Brown, R. (2000). *Group processes*. Oxford, U.K.: Blackwell Publishing.

Brownell, P. (2010). *Gestalt therapy: A guide to contemporary practice*. New York: Springer Publishing Company.

Bryc, K., Durand, E. Y., Macpherson, J. M., Reich, D., & Mountain, J. L. (2015). The genetic ancestry of African Americans, Latinos, and European Americans across the United States. *American journal of human genetics*, *96*(1), 37–53. doi:10.1016/j.ajhg.2014.11.010.

Burns, D. (2000). *Feeling good: The new mood therapy*. New York: Quill/Harper Collins.

Caetano, R., Ramisetty-Mikler, S., Vaeth, P., & Harris, T. (2007). Acculturation stress, drinking, and intimate partner violence among Hispanic couples in the U.S. *Journal of Interpersonal Violence*, *22*(11), 1431–1447.

Caligor, E., & Clarkin, J. F. (2010). An object relations model of personality and personality Pathology. In J.F. Clarkin, P. Fonagy, & G.O. Gabbard (Eds.). *Psychodynamic psychotherapy for personality disorders: A clinical handbook* (pp. 3–35). Washington, D.C.: American Psychiatric Publishing, Inc.

Carhart-Harris, R. L. (2019). How do psychedelics work? *Current Opinion Psychiatry, 32*, 16–21. doi:10.1097/YCO.0000000000000467.

Carhart-Harris, R. L., Leech, R., Hellyer, P. J., Shanahan, M., Feilding, A., Tagliazucchi, E., Chialvo, D. R. & Nutt, D. (2014). The entropic brain: A theory of conscious states informed by neuroimaging research with psychedelic drugs. *Frontiers in Human Neuroscience, 8* (20). doi: 10.3389/fnhum.2014.00020.

Chae, D.H., Martz, C.D., Yip, T., Fuller-Rowell, T. E., Matthews, K.A., Spears, E.C., Wang, Y., . . . Epel, E.S. (2020). Racial discrimination and telomere shortening among African Americans: The Coronary Artery Risk Development in Young Adults (CARDIA) Study. *Health Psychology, 39*(3), 209–219. doi:10.1037/hea0000832.

Cheng, A. A. (2021). What this wave of anti-Asian violence reveals about America. *New York Times*, Feb. 21st. Retrieved from https://www.nytimes.com/2021/02/21/opinion/anti-asian-violence.html.

Chetty, R., Stepner, M., Abraham, S., Lin, S., Scuderi, B., Turner, N., Bergeron, A., & Cutler, D. (2016). The association between income and life expectancy

in the United States, 2001–2014. *JAMA, 315*(16), 1750–1766. doi:10.1001/jama.2016.4226.
Churchland, P. S. (2002). *Brain-wise: Studies in neurophilosophy*. Cambridge, MA: The MIT Press.
Clark, D. A., & Beck, A. T. (1999). *Scientific foundations of cognitive theory and therapy of depression*. New York: Wiley.
Clarkin, J. F., Cain, N., Lenzenwenger, M. F., & Levy, K. N. (2018). Transference Focused Psychotherapy for the personality disorders. In W. Livesley & R. Larstone (Eds.), *Handbook of personality disorders* (pp. 571–585). New York: Guilford Press.
Cloninger, C. R., Svrakic, D.M., & Przybeck, T. R. (1993). A psychobiological model of temperament and character. *Archives of General Psychiatry, 50*, 975–990.
Cohen, L. J. (2015). Sex addiction: The fire down below. In M.S. Ascher & P. Levounis (Eds.). *The Behavioral Addictions*. Washington, D.C.: American Psychiatric Publishing.
Cohen, L. J. (2016). *The handy psychology answer book* (2nd ed.). Canton, MI: Visible Ink Press.
Cohen, L. J., Ardalan, F., Tanis, T., Halmi, W., Galynker, I., von Wyl, A., & Hengartner, M.P. (2016b). Attachment anxiety and avoidance as mediators of the association between childhood maltreatment and adult personality dysfunction. *Attachment & Human Development, 19*(1), 1–18. doi: 10.1080/14616734.2016.1253639/.
Cohen, L. J., Ardalan, F., Yaseen, Z. S., & Galynker, I. I. (2017). Suicide Crisis Syndrome mediates the relationship between long-term risk factors and lifetime suicidal phenomena. *Suicide and Life-Threatening Behavior, 48*(5), 613–623. doi: 10.1111/sltb.12387.
Cohen, L. J., Foster, M., Nesci, C., Tanis, T., Halmi, W., & Galynker, I. I. (2013). How do different types of childhood maltreatment relate to adult personality pathology? *Journal of Nervous and Mental Disease, 201*, 234–243. doi: 10.1097/NMD.0b013e3182848ac4.
Cohen, L. J., Tanis, T., Ardalan, F., & Galynker, I.I. (2016c). Maladaptive interpersonal schemas as sensitive and specific markers of borderline personality disorder among psychiatric inpatients. *Journal of Psychiatric Research, 242*, 395–403. doi: 10.1016/j.psychres.2016.06.007.
Cole, M., Yeung, N., Freiwald, W., & Botvinick, M. (2009). Cingulate cortex: Diverging data from humans and monkeys. *Trends in Neurosciences, 32*(11), 566–574. doi: 10.1016/j.tins.2009.07.001.
Coveney, P. & Highfield, R. (1995). *Frontiers of complexity: The search for order in a chaotic world*. New York: Fawcett Columbine.
Crenshaw, K. (1989). Demarginalizing the intersection of race and sex: A black feminist critique of antidiscrimination doctrine, feminist theory and antiracist politics. *University of Chicago Legal Forum, 1989*(1), 139–167. Retrieved from http://chicagounbound.uchicago.edu/uclf/vol1989/iss1/8.
Cunradi, C., Caetano, R., & Schafer, J. (2002). Socioeconomic predictors of intimate partner violence among White, Black, and Hispanic couples in the United States. *Journal of Family Violence, 17*(4), 377–389.

Cuthbert, B.N. & Insel, T.R. (2013). Toward the future of psychiatric diagnosis: The seven pillars of RDoC. *BMC Medicine, 11*(1), 1–8.

Damasio, A. (2003). *Looking for Spinoza: Joy, sorrow, and the feeling brain.* Orlando, FL: Harcourt Brace.

———. (1999). *The feeling of what happens: Body and emotion in the making of consciousness.* New York: Harcourt, Inc.

D'Angelo, E. (2020). *The handy Western philosophy answer book.* Canton, MI: Visible Ink Press.

Dasgupta, S. D. (2002). A framework for understanding women's use of nonlethal violence in intimate heterosexual relationships. *Violence Against Women, 8*(11), 1364–1389.

Davis, A. K., Barrett, F. S., & Griffiths, R. R. (2019). Psychological flexibility mediates the relations between acute psychedelic effects and subjective decreases in depression and anxiety. *Journal of Contextual Behavioral Science, 15,* 39–45. doi: 10.1016/j.jcbs.

Davis, K. L. & Panksepp, K. L. (2018). *The emotional foundations of personality: A neurobiological and evolutionary approach.* New York: W. W. Norton & Co.

DeGue, S., Fowler, K. A., & Calkins, C. (2016). Deaths due to use of lethal force by law enforcement: Findings from the National Violent Death Reporting System, 17 U.S. States, 2009–2012. *American Journal of Preventive Medicine, 51*(5 Suppl 3), S173–S187. doi: 10.1016/j.amepre.2016.08.027.

Dennett, D. (1991). *Consciousness Explained.* New York: Little, Brown and Co.

de Toqueville, A. (1835/2000). *Democracy in America.* (Mansfield, H.C. & Winthrop, D. translators). Chicago, IL: University of Chicago Press.

Di, X. & Biswal, B. B. (2014). Modulatory interactions between the default mode network and task positive networks in resting-state. *PeerJ, 2,* e367. doi: 10.7717/peerj.367.

Donatello, A., Leow, A., Brown, J. A., Zhan, L., GadElkarim, J., Hovav, S. & Feusner, J. D. (2013). Abnormal brain network organization in body dysmorphic disorder. *Neuropsychopharmacology, 38,* 1130–1139.

Doss, M. K., May, D. G., Johnson, M.W., Clifton, J. M., Hedrick, S. L., Prisinzano, T. E., Grifths, R. R., & Barrett, F. S. (2020). The acute effects of the atypical dissociative hallucinogen Salvinorin A on functional connectivity in the human brain. *Nature Research: Scientific Reports, 10*(1), 1–12. doi: 10.1038/s41598-020-73216-8.

Dunbar, R. I. M. & Shultz S. (2007). Understanding primate brain evolution. *Philosophical Transactions of the Royal Society of London B: Biological Sciences, 362*(1480), 649–658. doi: 10.1098/rstb.2006.2001.

Dyson, F. (2004, May 13). The world on a string. *The New York Review.* Retrieved from https://www.nybooks.com/articles/2004/05/13/the-world-on-a-string/.

Edwards, A. C., Ohlsson, H., Mósciciki, E., Crump, C., Sudquisk, J., Lichtenstein, P., Kendler, K., & Sundquist, K. (2021). On the genetic and environmental relationship between suicide attempt and death by suicide. *American Journal of Psychiatry, 178*(11), 1060–1069.

Eisenberg, D. P., London, E. D., Matochik, J. A., Derbyshire, S. W. G., Cohen, L. J., Steinfeld, M., Prosser, J., & Galynker, I. I. (2005). Education-associated cortical glucose metabolism during sustained attention. *Neuroreport, 16*(13), 1473–1476.

Eisenberg, N., Sadovsky, A., & Spinrad T. L. (2005). Associations of emotion-related regulation with language skills, emotional knowledge, and academic outcomes. *New Directions in Child and Adolescent Development, 109*, 109–118.

Ellamil, M., Dobson, C., Beeman, M., & Christoff, K. (2012). Evaluative and generative modes of thought during the creative process. *NeuroImage, 59*, 1783–1794.

Elston, G. N. (2007). Specialization of the neocortical pyramidal cell during primate evolution. *Evolution of Nervous Systems, 4*, 191–242. doi.org/10.1016/B0-12-370878-8/00164-6.

Fast, I. (1985). *Event Theory: A Piaget-Freud integration*. Hillsdale, NJ: Erlbaum Associates.

Fast, I., Marsden, K. G., Cohen, L., Heard, H., & Kruse, S. (1996). Self as subject: A formulation and an assessment strategy. *Psychiatry, 59*, 34–47. doi:10.1080/00332747.1996.11024749.

Feagin, J., & Bennefield, Z. (2014). Systemic racism and U.S. health care. *Social Science & Medicine, 103*, 7–14.

Feinberg, T. E. & Mallatt, J. M. (2016). *The ancient origins of consciousness: How the brain created experience*. Cambridge, MA: MIT Press.

Feusner, J. D., Yaryura-Tobias, J., & Saxena, S. (2008). The pathophysiology of body dysmorphic disorder. *Body Image, 5* (1), 3–12. doi: 10.1016/j.bodyim.2007.11.002.

Foa, E. B., & Rothbaum, B. O. (1998). *Treatment manuals for practitioners. Treating the trauma of rape: Cognitive-behavioral therapy for PTSD.* New York: Guilford Press.

Foa, E. B., Yadin, E., & Lichner, T. K. (2012). *Exposure and response (ritual) prevention for obsessive compulsive disorder: Therapist guide (treatments that work)* (2nd ed.). New York: Oxford University Press.

Fonagy, P. (2015). The effectiveness of psychodynamic psychotherapies: An update. *World Psychiatry, 14*, 137–150.

Fonagy, P. & Bateman, A. (2019). Introduction. In Bateman, A., Fonagy, P. (Eds.). *Handbook of mentalizing in mental health practice* (2nd ed., pp. 3–20). Washington, D.C.: American Psychiatric Press.

Forbes, E. E., & Dahl, R. E. (2010). Pubertal development and behavior: Hormonal activation of social and motivational tendencies. *Brain and Cognition, 72,* 66–72. doi: 10.1016/j.bandc.2009.10.007.

Fox, A. S. & Kalin, N. H. (2014). A translational neuroscience approach to understanding the development of social anxiety disorder and its pathophysiology. *American Journal of Psychiatry, 171*(11), 1162–1173. doi: 10.1176/appi.ajp.2014.14040449.

Fox, A. S., Oler, J. A., Shackman, A. J., Shelton, S. E., Raveendran, M., McKay, D. R., Converse, A. K., . . . Kalin, N. H. (2015). Intergenerational neural mediators of early-life anxious temperament. *Proceedings of the National Academy of Sciences of the United States (PNAS), 112*(29), 9118–9122. doi.10.1073/pnas.1508593112.

Freud, A. (1966). *The ego and the mechanisms of defense* (revised edition). Madison, CT: International Universities Press.

Fujii, T., & Suzuki, M. (2009). Episodic memory. In M. D. Binder, N. Hirokawa, & U. Windhorst (Eds.). *Encyclopedia of neuroscience*. Berlin, Germany: Springer.

Fulginiti, A., Rhoades, H., Mamey, M. R., Klemmer, C., Srivastava, A., Weskamp, G., & Goldbach, J. T. (2020). Sexual minority stress, mental health symptoms, and suicidality among LGBTQ youth accessing crisis services. *Journal of Youth and Adolescence, 50*(5), 893–905. doi.org/10.1007/s10964-020-01354-3.

Fusaro, V. A., Levy, H. G., Shaefer, H. L. (2018). Racial and ethnic disparities in the lifetime prevalence of homelessness in the United States. *Demography, 55*(6), 2119–2128. doi:10.1007/s13524-018-0717-0.

Gabbard, G. O. (2000). Psychotherapy of personality disorders. *Journal of Psychotherapy Practice and Research, 9*(1), 1–6.

Gansler, D. A., Moore, D. W., Susmaras, T. M., Jerram, M.W., Sousa, J., & Heilman, K. M. (2011). Cortical morphology of visual creativity. *Neuropsychologia, 49*, 2527–2532.

Gates, H. L. & Curran, A. S. (2021). Inventing the science of race. *The New York Review of Books, 68*(20), 52–57.

Gell-Mann, M. (1995). Complex adaptive systems. In H. J. Morowitz & J. L. Singer (Eds.). *The mind, the brain, and complex adaptive systems*. Proceedings Vol. XXII, Santa Fe Institute Studies in the Science of Complexity (pp. 11–23). Boulder, CO: Westview Press.

Gold, J. (2013). Psychotherapy integration and integrative psychotherapies. In G. Stricker, T. A. Widiger, & I. B. Weiner (Eds.,), *Handbook of psychology: Clinical psychology* (pp. 345–366). Hoboken, NJ: John Wiley & Sons, Inc.

Göstas, M. W., Wiberg, B., Engström, I., & Kjellin, L. (2012). Self-reported anxious- and avoidant-related attachment correlated to interpersonal problems by patients starting psychotherapy. *E-Journal of Applied Psychology, 8*(1), 9–17.

Gottlieb, R. M. (2012). Classical psychoanalysis: Past and present. In G.O. Gabbard, B. E. Litowitz, P. Williams (Eds.). *Textbook of Psychoanalysis, 2nd Edition* (pp. 155–169). Washington, D.C.: American Psychiatric Publishing.

Gould, S. J. (1977). *Ontogeny and Phylogeny*. Cambridge, MA: Belknap Press of Harvard University Press.

———. (1995). *Dinosaur in a Haystack: Reflections in Natural History*. New York: Harmony Books.

Graham, J., Haidt, J. & Nosek, B. A. (2009). Liberals and conservatives rely on different sets of moral foundations. *Journal of Personality and Social Psychology, 96* (5), 1029–46.

Green, D. W., Abutalebi, J. (2016). Language control and the neuroanatomy of bilingualism: In praise of variety. *Language, Cognition and Neuroscience, 31*(3), 340–344. doi:10.1080/23273798.2015.1084428.

Greenberg, J. R. & Mitchell, S. A. (1985). *Object relations in psychoanalytic theory*. Cambridge, MA: Harvard University Press.

Gruber, T., Clay, Z., & Zuberbühler, K. (2010). A comparison of bonobo and chimpanzee tool use: Evidence for a female bias in the Pan lineage. *Animal Behaviour, 80*(6), 1023–1033. doi: 10.1016/j.anbehav.2010.09.005.

Guerin, P. J., Jr. (Ed.) (1976). *Family Therapy: Theory and Practice*. New York: Gardner Press.

Gurin, L., & Bloom, S. (2017). Delusions and the right hemisphere: A review of the case for the right hemisphere as a mediator of reality-based belief. *Journal of Neuropsychiatry and Clinical Neuroscience, 29*, 225–235. doi: 10.1176/appi.neuropsych.16060118.

Hamilton, J. P., Furman, D. J., Chang, C., Thomason, M. E., Dennis, E., & Gotlib, I. H. (2011). Default-mode and task-positive network activity in major depressive disorder: implications for adaptive and maladaptive rumination. *Biological psychiatry, 70*(4), 327–333. doi:1 0.1016/j.biopsych.2011.02.003.

Happé, H., & Frith, U. (2006). The Weak coherence account: Detail-focused cognitive style in autism spectrum disorders. *Journal of Autism and Developmental Disorders, 36*(1), 5–25. doi: 10.1007/s10803-005-0039-0.

Harnad, S. (1995). Why and how we are not zombies. *Journal of Consciousness Studies, 1*, 164–167.

Harris, A. (2012). Transference, countertransference, and the real relationship. In G. O. Gabbard, B. E. Litowitz, P. Williams (Eds.). *Textbook of Psychoanalysis* (2nd ed., pp. 255–268). Washington, D.C.: American Psychiatric Publishing.

Hatchard, T., Mioduszewski, O., Zambrana, A., O'Farrell, E., Caluyong, M., Poulin, P. A., & Smith, A. M. (2017). Neural changes associated with mindfulness-based stress reduction (MBSR): Current knowledge, limitations, and future directions. *Psychology & Neuroscience, 10*(1), 41–56. https://doi.org/10.1037/pne0000073.

Hayes, P. A. (2009). Integrating evidence-based practice, cognitive–behavior therapy, and multicultural therapy: Ten steps for culturally competent practice. *Professional Psychology: Research and Practice, 40*(4), 354–360.

Hayes, S. C., Follette, V.M., Linehan, M.M. (2004). *Mindfulness and acceptance: Expanding the cognitive-behavioral tradition*. New York: The Guilford Press.

Hayes, S. C. with Smith S. (2015). *Get out of your mind and into your life: The new Acceptance and Commitment Therapy*. Oakland, CA: New Harbinger Publications.

Heaven, D. (2014, July 23). Worm neuron hack to probe the mysteries of our brains. *NewScientist*, 2979. Retrieved from https://www.newscientist.com/article/mg22329792-300-worm-neuron-hack-to-probe-the-mysteries-of-our-brains/.

Hengartner, M. P., Von Wyl, A., Tanis, T., Halmi, W., Galynker, I., & Cohen, L. J. (2015). Severity of personality disorders and domains of general personality dysfunction related to attachment: General personality dysfunction related to attachment. *Personality and Mental Health, 9*(3). doi: 10.1002/pmh.1297.

Hirsch, C. (2019). Attachment to the social construct of success and the myth of the "good college": Effects of toxic stress on affluent adolescents. (*Doctoral Dissertation)*. Retrieved from *Scholarly Commons, 125*. https://repository.upenn.edu/edissertations_sp2/125.

Honos-Webb, L. (2008). *The gift of adult ADD: How to transform your challenges and build on your strengths*. Oakland, CA: New Harbinger Publications.

Hopps, J. A., & Liu, W. M. (2006). Working for social justice from within the health care system: The role of social class in psychology. In R. L. Toporek, L. H. Gerstein, N. A. Fouad, G. Roysircar, & T. Israel (Eds.), *Handbook for social justice in counseling psychology: Leadership, vision, and action* (pp. 318–337). Thousand Oaks, CA: Sage Publications, Inc. https://doi.org/10.4135/9781412976220.n23.

Horgan, J. (2017, July 5). Tripping on peyote in Navajo Nation: A journalist exploring psychedelics' therapeutic potential participates in a ceremony of the Native American Church. *Scientific American*. Retrieved from https://blogs.scientificamerican.com/cross-check/tripping-on-peyote-in-navajo-nation/.

Hunt, M. (2007). T*he story of psychology* (2nd ed.). New York: Anchor Books.

Huntingford, F. A. (1976). The relationship between anti-predator behavior and aggression among conspecifics in the three-spined stickleback, *gastrosteus aculeatus. Animal Behavior, 24,* 245–260.

Hurvich, M. (1989). Traumatic moment, basic dangers, and annihilation anxiety. *Psychoanalytic Psychology*, *6*, 309–323.

Hyde, J.S. (1990). Meta-analysis and the psychology of gender differences. *Signs, 16*, 55–73.

Iatrou, A., Kenis, G., Rutten, B. P., Lunnon, K., & van den Hove, D. L. (2017). Epigenetic dysregulation of brainstem nuclei in the pathogenesis of Alzheimer's disease: Looking in the correct place at the right time?. *Cellular and molecular life sciences: CMLS*, *74*(3), 509–523. https://doi.org/10.1007/s00018-016-2361-4.

Imperial College London. (2008, May 15). What's the difference between a human and a fruit fly?. *ScienceDaily*. Retrieved from www.sciencedaily.com/releases/2008/05/080512172904.htm.

Jarvis, B. (2021, November 7). The global dream lab. *The New York Times Magazine*. pp. 22–45. Retrieved from https://www.nytimes.com/2021/11/03/magazine/pandemic-dreams.html.

Johnson, M. W., Hendricks, P. S., Barrett, F. S., Griffiths, R. R. (2019). An integrative review of epidemiology, therapeutics, mystical experience, and brain network function. *Pharmacological Therapy, 197*, 83–102. doi: 10.1016/j.pharmthera.2018.11.010.

Joska, J. A. & Stein, D. J. (2008). Mood disorders. In R. E. Hales, S. C. Yudofsky, & G. O. Gabbard (Eds.). *The American Psychiatric Publishing textbook of psychiatry* (5th ed., pp. 457–503). Arlington, VA: American Psychiatric Publishing, Inc.

Kaas, J. H. (2012). The evolution of neocortex in primates. *Progress in Brain Research, 195*, 91–102. doi:10.1016/B978-0-444-53860-4.00005-2.

Kabat-Zinn, J. (2011). Some reflections on the origins of MBSR, skillful means, and the trouble with maps. *Contemporary Buddhism, 12*, 281–306. doi:10.1080/14639947.2011.564844.

———. (2013). *Full catastrophe living (revised edition): Using the wisdom of your body and mind to face stress, pain and illness*. New York: Bantam Books.

Kahlenberg, R. (2021, April 19). The 'new redlining' is deciding who lives in your neighborhood. The New York Times Opinion Section, *The New York Times*.

Kahn, C. (2021, May 24). 53% of Republicans view Trump as true U.S. president Reuters/Ipsos. *Reuters*. Retrieved from https://www.reuters.com/world/us/53-republicans-view-trump-true-us-president-reutersipsos-2021-05-24/.

Kahr Nilsson, A. K., Jorgensen, C. R., Nielsen Staarup, K., Licht, R. W. (2010). Severity of affective temperament and maladaptive sef-schemas differentiate borderline patients, bipolar patients and controls. *Comprehensive Psychiatry, 51*, 486–491. doi: 10.1016/j.comppsych.2010.02.006.

Karen, R. (1998). *Becoming Attached: First relationships and how they shape our capacity to love*. New York: Oxford University Press.

Kasturirangan, A., Krishnan, S., & Riger, S. (2004). The impact of culture and minority status on women's experience of domestic violence. *Trauma, Violence, & Abuse*, *5*(4), 318–332.

Kendler, K. S., Aggen, S. H., Czajkowski, N., Røysamb, E., Tambs, K., Torgersen, S., & Reichborn-Kjennerud, T. (2008). The structure of genetic and environmental risk factors for DSM-IV personality disorders: A multivariate twin study. *Archives of General Psychiatry, 65*(12), 1438–1446. doi.org/10.1001/archpsyc.65.12.1438.

Kim, I. J., Lau, A. S., & Chang, D. F. (2006). Family violence among Asian Americans. In F. T. Leong, A. G. Inman, A. Ebreo, L. Yang, L. M. Kinoshita, & M. Fu (Eds.), *Handbook of Asian American psychology* (2nd ed., pp. 363−378). Thousand Oaks, CA: Sage.

King, D. B., Viney, W., & Woody, W. D. (2009). *A history of psychology: Ideas and context*. New York: Pearson Education, Inc.

King, M., Semlyen, J., Tai, S. S., Killaspy, H., Osborn, D., Popelyuk, D., & Nazareth, I. (2008). A systematic review of mental disorder, suicide, and deliberate self-harm in lesbian, gay and bisexual people. *BMC Psychiatry*, *8*(1), 70.

Kins, E., & Beyers, W. (2010). Failure to launch, failure to achieve criteria for adulthood? *Journal of Adolescent Research, 25*(5), 743–777. doi: 10.1177/0743558410371126.

Kleinman, A. & Good, B. (1985/2010). Introduction to culture and depression. R. A. LeVine (Ed). *Psychological anthropology: A reader on self in culture* (pp. 112–116). Hoboken, NJ: Wiley-Blackwell.

Kluetsch, R. C., Schmahl, C., Niedtfeld, I., Densmore, M., Calhoun, V. D., Daniels, J., . . . Lanius, R. A. (2012). Alterations in default mode network connectivity during pain processing in borderline personality disorder. *Archives General Psychiatry, 69* (10), 993–1002. doi: 10.1001/archgenpsychiatry.2012.476.

Kokaliari, E., Catanzarite, G., & Berzoff, J. (2013) It is called a mother tongue for a reason: A qualitative study of therapists' perspectives on bilingual psychotherapy—Treatment implications. *Smith College Studies in Social Work, 83*(1), 97–118. doi: 10.1080/00377317.2013.747396.

Kristan, W. (2016). Early evolution of neurons. *Current Biology, 26*, R937–R980.

Lamm, C. & Majdandzic, J. (2015). The role of shared neural activations, mirror neurons, and morality in empathy: A critical comment. *Neuroscience Research, 90*, 15–24. doi.org/10.1016/j.neures.2014.10.008.

Lederman, L. with Teresi, D. (1993). *The God particle: If the universe is the answer, what is the question?* New York: Dell Publishing.

LeDoux, J. (2003). The emotional brain, fear, and the amygdala. *Cellular & Molecular Neurobiology, 23*(4–5), 727–38.

Le Guin, U. K. (2004). *The wave in the mind: Talks and essays on the writer, the reader, and the imagination*. Boulder, CO: Shambala Publications, Inc.

Letheby, C. (2020). Psychedelics show religion isn't the only route to spirituality. *Psyche.* Retrieved from https://psyche.co/ideas/psychedelics-show-religion-isnt-the-only-route-to-spirituality.

Levenson, D. (1979). *Seasons of a man's life.* New York: Ballantine Books.

———. (1997). *Seasons of a woman's life*. New York: Ballantine Books.

Lewis, M. (1997). The self in self-conscious emotions. In J. G. Snodgrass, R. L. Thompson (Eds.) *The Self Across Psychology: Self-Recognition, Self-Awareness, and the Self Concept*. Annals of The New York Academy of Sciences, 818, New York, NY.

Lewis, T., Larson, M., Korcuska, J. (2017). Strengthening the planning process of motivational interviewing using goal attainment scaling. *Journal of Mental Health Counseling, 39*(3), 195–210.

Limandri, B. (2018). Psychopharmacology for borderline personality disorder. *Journal of Psychosocial Nursing, 56*(4), 8–11.

Lin, M., Kwan, V., Cheung, A., & Fiske, S. (2005). Stereotype content model explains prejudice for an envied outgroup: Scale of Anti-Asian American Stereotypes. *Personality & Social Psychology Bulletin, 31*, 34–47. doi:10.1177/0146167204271320.

Linehan, M.M. (1993). *Skills training manual for treating borderline personality disorder*. New York: Guilford.

———. (2015). *DBT skills training manual, (2nd ed.)*. New York: The Guilford Press.

———. (2020). *Building a life worth living: A memoir.* New York: Random House.

Linehan, M. M., Comtois, K. A., Murray, A. M., Brown, M. Z., Gallop, R. J., Heard, H. L., Lindenboim, N. (2006). Two-year randomized controlled trial and follow-up of dialectical behavior therapy vs therapy by experts for suicidal behaviors and borderline personality disorder. *Archives of General Psychiatry, 63*, 757–766.

Linnman, C., Moulton, E. A., Barmettler, G., Becerra, L. & Borsook, D. (2012). Neuroimaging of the periaqueductal gray: State of the field. *Neuroimage, 60*(1), 505–522. doi: 10.1016/j.neuroimage.2011.11.095.

Lo, H-T. & Fung, K. P. (2003). Culturally competent psychotherapy. *Canadian Journal of Psychiatry, 48*, 161–170.

Louis, J. P., Wood, A. M., Lockwood, G., Ho, M.-H. R., & Ferguson, E. (2018). Positive clinical psychology and Schema Therapy (ST): The development of the Young Positive Schema Questionnaire (YPSQ) to complement the Young Schema Questionnaire 3 Short Form (YSQ-S3). *Psychological Assessment, 30*(9), 1199–1213. doi.org/10.1037/pas0000567.

Luthar, S. S. (2003). The culture of affluence: Psychological costs of material wealth. *Child Development, 74*(6), 1581–1593.

MacLean, P. D. (1974). *Triune conception of the brain and behavior* (The Clarence M. Hincks Memorial lectures). Toronto, ON: University of Toronto Press.

MacLean, P. D. (1982). On the origin and progressive evolution of the triune brain. In E. Armstrong and D. Falk (Eds.) *Primate brain evolution: Methods and concepts* (pp. 291–316). New York: Plenum.

Main, M., Cassidy, J., & Kaplan, N. (1985). Security of attachment in childhood, adolescence, and adulthood: A move to the level of representation. In I. Bretheron & E. Waters (Eds.) *Growing points in attachment: Monograph for the Society for Research in Child Development, 50*(1 & 2), 66–104. Chicago: University of Chicago Press.

Marques, D. R., Gomes, A. A., Clemente, V., Moutinho dos Santos, J., Duarte, I.C., Caetano, G., Castelo-Branco, M. (2018). Self-referential dysfunction and default-mode hyperactivation in psychophysiological insomnia patients: A case-control fMRI Study. *Journal of Psychophysiology, 32*(3), 140–155. doi: 10.1027/0269-8803/a000194.

Martín-Blanco, A., Ancochea, A., Soler, J., Elices, M., Carmona, C. & Pasqual, J.C. (2017). Changes over the last 15 years in the psychopharmacological management of persons with borderline personality disorder. *Acta Psychiatrica Scandinavica, 136*(3), 323–331. https://doi.org/10.1111/acps.12767.

Maslow, A.H. (1971). *The farther reaches of human nature*. New York: The Viking Press.

———. (1968). *Toward a psychology of being.* Princeton, N.J.: D. Van Nostrand Company, Inc.

Matthews, D., Deary, I. J., & Whiteman, M. C. (2003). *Personalty traits* (2nd ed.). New York: Cambridge University Press.

Mayseless, N., Eran, A., Shamay-Tsoory, S. G. (2015). Generating original ideas: The neural underpinning of originality. *Neuroimage, 116*, 232–239. doi.org/10.1016/j.neuroimage.2015.05.030.

McGilchrist, I. (2009). *The master and his emissary: The divided brain and the making of the Western world.* New Haven, CT: Yale University Press.

McGowan, P., Sasaki, A., D'Alessio, A., Dymov, S., Labonte, B., Szyf, M., . . . Meaney, M.J. (2009). Epigenetic regulation of the glucocorticoid receptor in human brain associates with childhood abuse. *Nat Neurosci, 12*, 342–348. doi.org/10.1038/nn.2270.

McGuffin, P., Rijsdijk, F., Andrew, M., Sham, P., Katz, R., & Cardno, A. (2003). The heritability of bipolar affective disorder and the genetic relationship to unipolar depression. *Archives of general psychiatry*, *60*(5), 497–502.

Metzl, J. M. & Hansen, H. (2014). Structural competency: Theorizing a new medical engagement with stigma and inequality. *Social Science & Medicine, 103*, 126–133.

Meyer, I. H. (2003). Prejudice, social stress, and mental health in lesbian, gay, and bisexual populations: Conceptual issues and research evidence. *Psychological Bulletin, 129*, 674–697.

Miles, H. L. (1986). How can I tell a lie? Apes, language and the problem of deception. In R. W. Mitchell, & N. S. Thompson (Eds.). *Deception: Perspectives on human and nonhuman deceit* (pp. 245–266). Albany, NY: State University of New York Press.

Miller, A. (2012). *Instructor's manual for Aaron Beck on cognitive therapy with Aaron T. Beck, M.D.* Mill Valley, CA: Psychotherapy.net, L. L. C.

Miller, W.R. (2009). A conversation with William R. Miller. *Addiction, 104*, 883–893. doi:10.1111/j.1360-0443.2009.02544.x.

Miller, W. R. & Rollnick, S. (1991). *Motivational interviewing: Preparing people to change addictive behavior*. New York: Guilford Press.

Miller, W. R., Zweben, A., DiClemente, C. C., & Rychtarik, R. G. (1992). Motivational enhancement therapy manual: A clinical research guide for clinicians treating individuals with alcohol abuse and dependence. Project MATCH monograph series, vol. 2. National Institute on Alcohol Abuse and Alcoholism.

Mirandé, A. (2018). *Hombres y machos: Masculinity and Latino culture*. New York: Routledge.

Muller, J. Z. (Ed.). (1997). *Conservatism: An anthology of social and political thought from David Hume to the present*. Princeton, NJ: Princeton University Press.

Muran, J. C., Safran, J. D., Gorman, B. S., Samstag, L. W., Eubanks-Carter, C., & Winston, A. (2009). The relationship of early alliance ruptures and their resolution to process and outcome in three time-limited psychotherapies for personality disorders. *Psychotherapy (Chic), 46*(2), 233–248. doi:10.1037/a0016085.

Morowitz, H. J. & Singer, J. L. (Eds) (1994). The mind, the brain and complex adaptive systems. *Studies in the science of complexity*, Proceedings Vol. XXII, Santa Fe Institute. Boulder, CO: Westview Press.

Muran, J. C., Safran, J. D., Eubanks, C. F., & Gorman, B. S. (2018). The effect of an alliance-focused training on cognitive-behavioral therapy for personality disorders. *Journal of Consulting & Clinical Psychology, 86*, 384–397.

National Institute of Mental Health (NIMH). Research Domain Criteria (RDoC). Retrieved from https://www.nimh.nih.gov/research/research-funded-by-nimh/rdoc/about-rdoc.

Newberg, A. B., & Iversen, J. (2003). The neural basis of the complex mental task of meditation: Neurotransmitter and neurochemical considerations. *Medical Hypotheses, 61*(2), 282–291. doi:10.1016/S0306-9877(03)00175-0.

Nguyen, T. (2010). Total number of synapses in the adult human neocortex. *Undergraduate Journal of Mathematical Modeling: One + Two*, 3(1). doi: http://dx.doi.org/10.5038/2326-3652.3.1.26.

North, R., Holahan, C. J., Moos, R. H., & Cronkite, R. C. (2008). Family support, family income, and happiness: A 10-year perspective. *Journal of Family Psychology, 22*(3), 475–483. doi: 10.1037/0893-3200.22.3.475.

Northoff, G., Heinzel, A., De Greck, M., Bermpohl, F., Dobrowolny, H., & Panksepp, J. (2006). Self-referential processing in our brain—A meta-analysis of imaging studies on the self. *NeuroImage, 31*, 440–457.

Nunez, S. (2021, May 27). Lost, at sea, at odds. *The New York Review*. Retrieved from https://www.nybooks.com/articles/2021/05/27/jhumpa-lahiri-lost-at-sea-at-odds/.

Oldham, J. M. (2005). Guideline watch: Practice guideline for the treatment of patients with borderline personality disorder. *Focus, 3*(3), 396–400.

Pabba, M. (2013). Evolutionary development of the amygdaloid complex. *Frontiers in Neuroanatomy, 7*, 27. doi: 10.3389/fnana.2013.00027.

Panksepp, J. (1998). *Affective neuroscience: The foundations of human and animal emotions*. New York: Oxford University Press.

Panksepp, J. & Biven, L. (2012). *The Archaeology of mind: Neuroevolutionary origins of human emotions*. New York: W.W. Norton & Co.

Patterson, F.G. (1981). Ape language. *Science, 211*(4477), 86–87. doi: 10.1126/science.211.4477.86-a.

Patterson, F., Linden, E. (1981). *The education of Koko*. New York: Holt, Rinehart, and Winston.

Pennebaker, J. W., Rimé, B., & Blankenship, V. E. (1996). Stereotypes of emotional expressiveness of Northerners and Southerners: A cross-cultural test of Montesquieu's hypotheses. *Journal of Personality and Social Psychology, 70*(2), 372–380. doi.org/10.1037/0022-3514.70.2.372.

Perls, F., Goodman, P., & Hefferline, F. (1951). *Gestalt therapy: Excitement and growth in the human personality.* New York: Dell.

Piaget, J. (1954). *The construction of reality in the child.* New York: Ballantine Books.

Pillai, R., Zhang, M., Yang, J., Boldrini, M., Mann, J., Oquendo, M., . . . DeLorenzo, C. (2018). Will imaging individual raphe nuclei in males with major depressive disorder enhance diagnostic sensitivity and specificity? *Depression and Anxiety, 35*(5), 411–420. doi:10.1002/da.22721.

Pollan, M. (2018). *How to change your mind: What the new science of psychedlice teaches us about consciousness, dying, addiction, depression, and transcendence*. New York: Penguin Press.

Potts, R. & Sloan, C. (2010). *What does it mean to be human*? Washington, D.C.: National Geographic.

Power, R.A. & Pluess, M. (2015). Heritability estimates of the Big Five personality traits based on common genetic variants. *Translational Psychiatry, 5*, e604. doi:10.1038/tp.2015.96.

Rapoport, S. I., Basselin, M., Kim, H. W., Rao, J. S. (2009). Bipolar disorder and mechanisms of action of mood stabilizers. *Brain Research Reviews, 61*(2), 185–209. doi.org/10.1016/j.brainresrev.2009.06.003.

Rees, D. & Rose, S. (2004). *The new brain sciences: Perils and prospects*. Cambridge, U.K.: Cambridge University Press.

Reny, T. T. & Barreto, M. A. (2020): Xenophobia in the time of pandemic: Othering, anti-Asian attitudes, and COVID-19. *Politics, Groups, and Identities.* doi: 10.1080/21565503.2020.1769693.

Rolls, E. T. (2004). The functions of the orbitofrontal cortex. *Brain and Cognition, 55*, 11–29. doi:10.1016/S0278-2626(03)00277-X.

Ruggero, C. J., Zimmerman, M., Chelminski, I., & Young, D., 2010. Borderline personality disorder and the misdiagnosis of bipolar disorder. *Journal of Psychiatric Res*earch, *44*(6), 405–408.

Ruigrok, A. N. V., Salimi-Khorshidi, G., Lai, M., Baron-Cohen, S., Lombardo, M. V., Tait, R. J., & Suckling, J. (2014). A meta-analysis of sex differences in human brain structure. *Neuroscience & Biobehavioral Reviews, 39*, 34–50. https://doi.org/10.1016/j.neubiorev.2013.12.004.

Sabelli, H. C., & Carlson-Sabelli, L. (1989). Biological priority and psychological supremacy: A new integrative paradigm derived from process theory. *American Journal of Psychiatry, 146*, 1541–1551.

Sacks, O. (1985). *The Man who Mistook his Wife for a Hat and Other Clinical Tales*. New York: Summit Books.

Safran, J. D. & Muran, J. C. (2003). *Negotiating the therapeutic alliance: A relational treatment guide*. New York: Guilford Press.

Satel, S. & Lilienfeld, S. (2013). *Brainwashed: The seductive appeal of mindless neuroscience*. New York: Basic Books.

Satterlie, R. A. (2011). Do jellyfish have central nervous systems? *The Journal of Experimental Biology, 214*, 1215–1223.

Satterthwaite, T. D., Wolf, D. H., Roalf, D. R., Ruparel, K., Erus, G. Vandekar, S., Gennatas, E. D., Gur, R. C. (2015). Linked sex differences in cognition and functional connectivity in youth. *Cerebral Cortex*, *25*(9), 2383–2394. doi.org/10.1093/cercor/bhu036.

Schafer, M. & Schiller, D. (2018). Navigating social space. *Neuron, 100*(2), 476–489. doi.org/10.1016/j.neuron.2018.10.006.

Schofield, D. P., McGrew, W. C., Takahashi, A., & Hirata, S. (2018). Cumulative culture in nonhumans: Overlooked findings from Japanese monkeys? *Primates, 59*, 113. doi.org/10.1007/s10329-017-0642-7.

Schore, A. N. (2003). *Affect Dysregulation and Disorders of the Self.* New York: Norton.

———. (1994). *Affect Regulation and Disorders of the Self.* New York: Norton.

Searle, J. R. (1992). *The rediscovery of the mind.* Cambridge, MA: MIT Press.

Shapiro, D. (1965/1999). *Neurotic Styles*. New York: Basic Books.

Sharam, A. & Hulse, K. (2014). Understanding the nexus between poverty and homelessness: Relational poverty analysis of families experiencing homelessness in Australia. *Housing, Theory and Society, 31*(3), 294–309. doi: 10.1080/14036096.2014.882405.

Skinner, B. F. (1948). *Walden Two.* Indianapolis: Hackett Publishing Company.

Sorscher, N. & Cohen, L. (1997). Trauma in children of Holocaust survivors: Transgenerational effects. *American Journal of Orthopsychiatry, 67*(3), 493–500.

Steger, M. F. & Frazier, P. (2005). Meaning in life: One link in the chain from religiousness to well-being. *Journal of Counseling Psychology, 52*(4), 574–582.

Stein, D. (2021). *Problems in living: Perspectives from philosophy, psychiatry and cognitive-affective science*. London, U.K.: Academic Press.

Stein, D. J., Black, D. W., & Pienaar, W. (2000). Sexual disorders not otherwise specified: Compulsive, addictive or impulsive? *CNS Spectrums: International Journal of Neuropsychiatric Medicine, 5*(1), 60–64.

Steinert, C., Munder, M., Rabung, S., Hoyer, J., & Leichsenring, F. (2017). Psychodynamic therapy: As efficacious as other empirically supported treatments? A meta-analysis testing equivalence of outcomes. *American Journal of Psychiatry, 174*(10), 943–953.

Stern, D. N. (1977). *The first relationship: Infant and mother*. Cambridge, MA: Harvard University Press.

———. (1985). *The interpersonal world of the infant*. New York: Basic Books.

Stricker, G. (2010). A second look at psychotherapy integration. *Journal of Psychotherapy Integration, 20*(4), 397–405. doi.10.1037/a0022037.

Stroup, T. S., Lawrence, R. E., Abbas, A. I., Miller, B. R., Perkins, D. O., & Lieberman, J. A. (2014). Schizophrenia Spectrum and other psychotic disorders. In R. E. Hales, S. C. Yudofsky, & L.W. Roberts (Eds.) *The American Psychiatric Publishing Textbook of Psychiatry* (6th ed., pp. 273–210). Arlington, VA: American Psychiatric Publishing, Inc.

Substance Abuse and Mental Health Services (SAMHSA). Administration Center for Behavioral Health Statistics and Quality (2018, September 7). *Results from the 2017 National Survey on Drug Use and Health: Detailed tables*. Retrieved from https://www.samhsa.gov/data/sites/default/files/cbhsq-reports/NSDUHDetailedTabs2017/NSDUHDetailedTabs2017.pdf.

Sue, D. W., Capodilupo, C. M., Torino, G. C., Bucceri, J. M., Holder, A. M. B., Nadal, K. L., Esquilin, M. (2007). Racial microaggressions in everyday life: Implications for clinical practice. *American Psychologist, 62*(4), 271–286.

Sugihara, Y., & Warner, J. A. (2002). Dominance and domestic abuse among Mexican Americans: Gender differences in the etiology of violence in intimate relationships. *Journal of Family Violence, 17*(4), 315–340. doi.org/10.1023/A:1020318532350.

Sullivan, P. F., Kendler, K. S., & Neale, M. C. (2003). Schizophrenia as a complex trait: Evidence from a meta-analysis of twin studies. *Archives of General Psychiatry, 60*(12), 1187–1192.

Tallis, R. (2014). *Aping mankind: Neuromania, Darwinitis and the misrepresentation of humanity*. Abington-on-Thames, U.K.: Routledge.

Tan, A. (2017). *Where the past begins: Memory and imagination.* New York: HarperCollins.

Tasca, G. A., Szadkowski, L., Illing, V., Trinneer, A., Grenon, R., Demidenko, N., . . . Bissada, H. (2009). Adult attachment, depression, and eating disorder symptoms: The mediating role of affect regulation strategies. *Personality and Individual Differences, 47*(6), 662–667.

Thomas, N., Gurvich, C., & Kulkarni, J. (2019). Borderline personality disorder, trauma, and the hypothalamus-pituitary-adrenal axis. *Neuropsychiatric Disease and Treatment, 15*, 2601–2612. doi.org/10.2147/NDT.S198804.

Triandis, H. (1993). Collectivism and individualism as cultural syndromes. *Cross-cultural Research, 27*(3–4), 155–180. doi.org/10.1177/106939719302700301.

Trut, L. N. (1999). Early canid domestication: The Farm-Fox Experiment: Foxes bred for tamability in a 40-year experiment exhibit remarkable transformations that suggest an interplay between behavioral genetics and development. *American Scientist, 87*(2), 160–169.

United States Census Bureau. (2020a). *About Race*. Retrieved from https://www.census.gov/topics/population/race/about.html. (Last updated 10/6/2020).

United States Census Bureau. Bureau of the Census for the Bureau of Labor Statistics. (2020b). Current population survey: 2020 annual social and economic (ASEC) supplement. Retrieved from https://www2.census.gov/programs-surveys/cps/techdocs/cpsmar20.pdf.

Viamontes, G. I., Beitman, B. D., Viamontes, C. T., & Viamontes, J. A. (2004). Neural circuits for self-awareness: Evolutionary origins and implementation in the human brain. In B. D. Beitman & J. Nair (Eds.) *Self-Awareness Deficits in Psychiatric Patients: Neurobiology, Assessment, and Treatment*. New York: W. W. Norton & Co.

Vinogradov, S., Yalom, I. D. (1989). *A concise guide to group therapy*. Washington, DC: American Psychiatric Press.

Von Bertalanffy, L. (1969/2003). *General systems theory: Foundations, development, applications* (Rev. ed.). New York: George Braziller, Inc.

Werner, H. & Kaplan, B. (1963/1984). *Symbol formation*. Hillsdale, NJ: Erlbaum Assoc.

Wachtel, P. L. (1977). *Psychoanalysis and behavior therapy: Toward an integration*. New York: Basic Books.

Walker, P. L. & Cook, D. C. (1998). Brief communication: Gender and sex: Vive la difference. *American Journal of Physical Anthropology, 106*, 255–259.

Wampold, B. E., Baldwin, S. A., Holtforth, M. G., Imel, Z. E. (2017). What characterizes effective therapists? In L. G. Castonguay and C. E. Hill (Eds.) *How and Why Are Some Therapists Better Than Others? Understanding Therapist Effects*. (pp. 37–53). Washington, DC: American Psychological Association. dx.doi.org/10.1037/0000034-003.

Weissman, M. M., Markowitz, J. C., & Klerman, G. K. (2000). *Comprehensive guide to interpersonal psychotherapy*. New York: Basic Books.

Western, B. (2019). Poverty, criminal justice and social justice. *IRP Focus, 35*(3), 3–13.

White, H. A. & Shaw, P. (2011). Creative style and achievement in adults with attention-deficit/hyperactivity disorder. *Personality and Individual Differences, 50*(5), 673–677. doi.org/10.1016/j.paid.2010.12.015.

White, T. L. & DePue, R. A. (1999). Differential association of traits of fear and anxiety with norepinephrine- and dark-induced pupil reactivity. *Journal of Personality and Social Psychology, 77*(4), 863–877.

Wilkerson, I. (2020). *Caste: The origins of our discontent*. New York: Random House.

Williams, P. (2012). Object relations. In G.O. Gabbard, B.E. Litowitz, P. Williams (Eds.). *Textbook of Psychoanalysis* (2nd ed.). Washington, DC: American Psychiatric Publishing.

Willyard, C. (2018). New human gene tally reignites debate. *Nature, 558*, 354–355. doi: 10.1038/d41586-018-05462-w.

Winnicott, D. W. (1971). *Playing and Reality*. London: Tavistock.

Winston, A., Rosenthal, R. N., & Pinsker, H. (2011). *Learning supportive psychotherapy: An illustrated guide* (1st ed.). Washington, DC: American Psychiatric Publishing.

Winston, A., Rosenthal, R. N., & Roberts, L. W. (2019). *Learning supportive psychotherapy: An illustrated guide* (2nd ed.). Washington, DC: American Psychiatric Association Publishing.

Wolf-Man [Pankejeff, S.]. (1971). My recollections of Sigmund Freud. In M. Gardner, (Ed.) *The Wolf-Man and Sigmund Freud* (pp. 135–152). London: Routledge.

Wray, N. R. & Gottesman, I. I. (2012). Using summary data from the Danish National Registers to estimate heritabilities for schizophrenia, bipolar disorder, and major depressive disorder. *Frontiers in Genetics, 3*(118). doi: 10.3389/fgene.2012.00118.

Yancy, C. W. (2020). COVID-19 and African Americans. *JAMA*, *323*(19), 1891–1892. doi:10.1001/jama.2020.6548.

Yoshikawa, H., Aber, J. L., & Beardslee, W. R. (2012). The effects of poverty on the mental, emotional, and behavioral health of children and youth implications for prevention. *American Psychologist, 67*(4), 272–284. doi: 10.1037/a0028015.

Youle, R. J. (2019). Mitochondria—Striking a balance between host and endosymbion. *Science, 365*(6454), eaaw9855. doi: 10.1126/science.aaw9855.

Young, J. E., Klosko, J. S., & Weishaar, M. E. (2003). *Schema therapy: A practitioner's guide*. New York: The Guilford Press.

Zack, N. (2002). *Philosophy of science and race*. New York: Routledge.

Zhang, Y. E., Landback, P., Vibranovski, M. D., & Long, M. (2011). Accelerated recruitment of new brain development genes into the human genome. *PLoS Biol 9*(10): e1001179. doi: 10.1371/journal.pbio.1001179.

Zimmerman, M., Ruggero, C. J., Chelminski, I., & Young, D. (2008). Is bipolar disorder over diagnosed? *Journal of Clinical Psychiatry, 69*(6), 935–940.

Zimmer, C. (2009). *The tangled bank: An introduction to evolution*. Greenwood Village, CO: Roberts & Company.

Zwir, I., Arnedo, J., Del-Val, C., Pulkki-Råback, L., Konte, B., Yang, S. S., . . . Cloninger, C. R. (2020). Uncovering the complex genetics of human character. *Molecular Psychiatry*, *25*, 2295–2312. dx.doi.org/10.1038/s41380-018-0263-6.

Index

Page references for figures are italicized.

About the Author

Lisa J. Cohen serves as Clinical Professor of Psychiatry at the Carl Icahn School of Medicine at Mount Sinai/Mount Sinai Beth Israel, where she is involved with teaching, research, and clinical work. Her research has included studies of obsessive-compulsive disorder, bipolar disorder, suicide, childhood trauma, personality disorders, and minor attraction. She has published over 100 scientific articles and is the author of the *Handy Psychology Answer Book*, *1st* and *2nd editions*.

www.ingramcontent.com/pod-product-compliance
Ingram Content Group UK Ltd.
Pitfield, Milton Keynes, MK11 3LW, UK
UKHW040857081026
15587UKWH00016B/751

9 781793 610102